Y0-DKE-783

ELECTROSURGERY
FOR HPV-RELATED DISEASES
OF THE LOWER GENITAL TRACT

A Practical Handbook
for Diagnosis and Treatment By
Loop Electrosurgical Excision
and Fulguration Procedures

ELECTROSURGERY FOR HPV-RELATED DISEASES OF THE LOWER GENITAL TRACT

A Practical Handbook for Diagnosis and Treatment By Loop Electrosurgical Excision and Fulguration Procedures

Thomas C. Wright, Jr., M.D.
Assistant Professor of Pathology
College of Physicians and Surgeons of Columbia University
New York, New York

Ralph M. Richart, M.D.
Professor of Pathology and Obstetrics and Gynecology,
College of Physicians and Surgeons of Columbia University and
Director, Obstetrical and Gynecological Pathology and Cytology,
Columbia Presbyterian Medical Center
New York, New York

Alex Ferenczy, M.D.
Professor of Pathology and Obstetrics and Gynecology
McGill University and the
Sir Mortimer B. Davis - Jewish General Hospital,
Montreal, Quebec

PUBLISHED BY
Arthur Vision, Incorporated
216 Congers Road
New City, New York, USA
and
BioVision, Incorporated
7816 Bodinier
Anjou, Quebec, Canada

© 1992 by Arthur Vision, Incorporated and BioVision, Incorporated
ISBN 0-9696002-0-8

All rights reserved. No part of the contents of this book may be reproduced or transmitted in any form or by any means, electronic, mechanical, photocopying, recording or otherwise, without prior written permission from the publisher.

COVER ILLUSTRATION
© Teri J. McDermott M.A., 1991.
Reprinted courtesy of Medical Economics Company.

Neither the authors nor publishers accept legal responsibility for errors or omissions, and make no warranty, express or implied, with respect to material contained herein. Although the authors and publisher have attempted to insure that the information in this book is correct, because of the rapidly changing nature of medical practice, in every individual case, the clinician (user) must verify the clinical applicability of a particular procedure, type of equipment, or drug by consulting other literature or package insert or equipment instruction manual.

Printed in Canada

TABLE OF CONTENTS

Acknowledgments … vii

Chapter 1	History of the Development of Electrosurgery	1
Chapter 2	Glossary of Electrosurgical Terms	13
Chapter 3	Principals of Electrosurgery	9
Chapter 4	Equipment for the Loop Excision Procedure and Electrosurgical Safety	45
Chapter 5	Development of Loop Excision Procedures	67
Chapter 6	The Etiology of Epithelial Cancer and Precursor Lesions in the Lower Male and Female Anogenital Tract	93
Chapter 7	Loop Excisional Procedures for Treating Cervical Intraepithelial Neoplasia (CIN)	121
Chapter 8	Electrosurgery of the Cervix: A Step-by-Step Guide	155
Chapter 9	Diagnosis and Management of Vaginal and External Anogenital HPV-Related Diseases	171
Chapter 10	Electrosurgery for Vaginal and External Anogenital Lesions	193
Chapter 11	Electrosurgery of the Vagina and External Anogenital Tract: A Step-by-Step Guide	219
Chapter 12	The Pathology of Specimens Produced Using Loop Electrodes	235
Chapter 13	Clinical Implications of Electrosurgical Excision Procedures	249

ACKNOWLEDGMENTS

We are indebted to Susan Young for the many hours spent typing and designing this book and without whose help this book would not have been possible. We would like to thank the following companies for providing either photographs, figures, illustrations, equipment or financial support for publication: Aspen Labs, Cabot Medical Corporation, Canderm Pharmacal Ltd., CooperSurgical, Inc., Digene Diagnostics, Inc., Euro-Med, Inc., V. Montegrande and Company, Oclassen Pharmaceuticals, Inc., the Purdue Frederick Company, Simpson/Basye, Inc., Utah Medical Products and Wallach Surgical Devices, Inc.

CHAPTER 1

HISTORY OF THE DEVELOPMENT OF ELECTROSURGERY

Modern electrosurgical generators (ESUs) incorporate solid state electronics and microprocessor-controlled circuitry in order to produce complex, blended waveforms. These waveforms allow the surgeon to excise large pieces of tissue from highly vascularized regions of the body with a minimal amount of thermal damage and a minimal amount of bleeding. If clinicians are to use these modern ESUs safely and to their fullest capacity, it is important that they have a firm grasp of the fundamentals of electricity and electrosurgery. In this chapter, the history of the development of electrosurgery and the theory behind how ESUs cut and coagulate tissue will be reviewed. A glossary of electrosurgical terms is provided in Chapter 2.

BEGINNINGS OF ELECTROSURGERY

Thermal Cautery

The application of electricity for treating diseases, both philosophically and practically, developed as an outgrowth of the application of heat as a therapeutic modality.[1] Heat has been used medically since the beginning of recorded time as a method for treating disease. Prehistoric skeletons, unearthed in archaeological digs, have evidence that thermal cautery was used as a way of treating injuries and one of the earliest written records, the Edwin Smith papyrus, describes the use of thermal cautery for treating tumors and ulcers of the breasts. Similarly, in India and the Far East, hot cautery had been used for millenia as a treatment for disease. The Hindu God of surgery, Susruta, said, "Caustic is better than the knife, cautery is better than either".[1] Hippocrates is credited with the saying, "Fire will succeed, where other methods fail". Cautery was commonly used throughout the Greek, Roman and Medieval periods.[1] In the United States, cautery was used through the American Civil War. Heat was applied to tissues by a variety of methods ranging from the simple placing of a red hot poker on a wound, to placing an ignitable substance such as gunpowder or boiling liquids within a wound or abscess cavity. In order to facilitate the cauterization of different tissues and different types of wounds, cautery irons or pokers were built in a variety of ingenious shapes. Cautery was felt to be especially advantageous for sterilizing wounds and stopping hemorrhages.

Development of Electrocautery

The medical use of electric current to produce electrocautery developed as an outgrowth of thermal cauterization methods. A number of prominent scientists of the 18th century, including Benjamin Franklin and Mesmer, were interested in studying the effects of electric energy on tissues.[2] These men, and many others, experimented with taking the output from early model electric generators and applying it directly to body tissues to treat a variety of disorders. Early electrical therapeutics included the continuous application of direct current from batteries to treat systemic disorders such as gout, and the application of sparks produced by static generators for ablating lesions.

Although the concept of using electrocautery therapeutically was advanced first by Pravas and Joseph Recamier (1774 - 1856), who reportedly used electrocautery with "red hot" electrodes to destroy tumors of the neck of the uterus, the first well-documented therapeutic use of electrocautery was by Gustav Crusell, a Finnish surgeon, in 1847.[3] Crusell had a patient with a large, ulcerated tumor of the forehead and face that obscured the eye. The tumor was encircled with a thin platinum wire which was heated until it was red hot by passing direct current through it. The wire was then tightened until the tumor was excised. Upon removal of the tumor, a healthy eye was revealed and the operation was deemed a success. Daguerreotypes were taken of the patient before and after treatment in order to document the procedure. Subsequently, Crusell used galvano-cautery (electrocautery) to treat other tumors and conditions including opening the urethral orifice in patients with urethral strictures.

After Crusell had demonstrated its usefulness, electrocautery began to be used for a variety of operations. Different types of electrosurgical instruments were designed for various uses including specially configured cutting loops for excising tumors. Many of these instruments had handles with on-off switches and uniquely configured wire electrodes that allowed cautery and cutting at sites that could not be reached with conventional knives (Figure 1.1).

HISTORY OF THE DEVELOPMENT OF ELECTROSURGERY

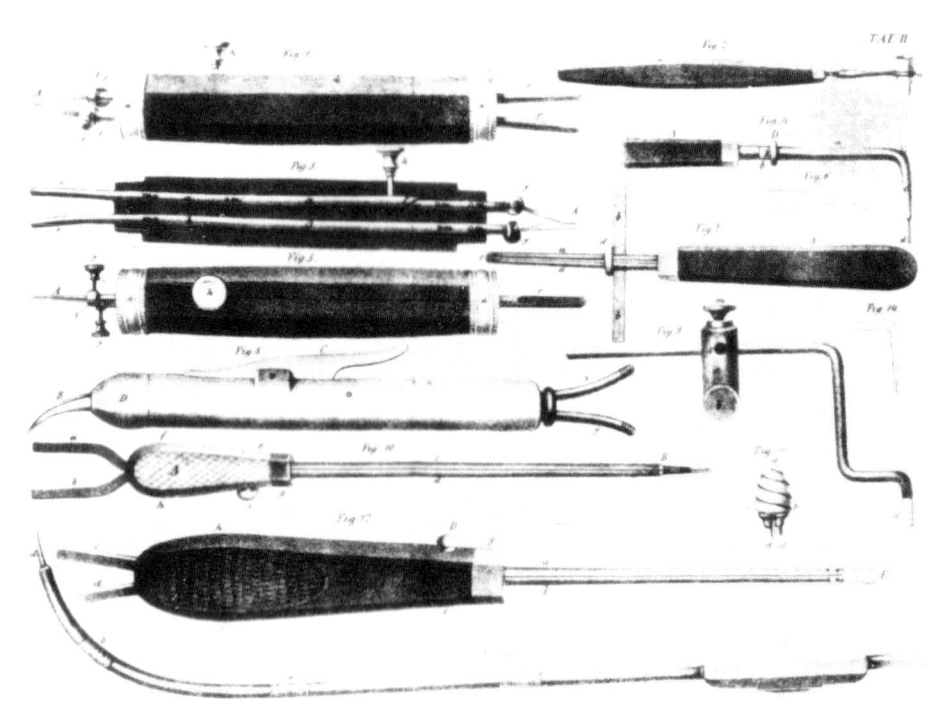

Figure 1.1. Electrocautery instruments used in the 1800s and designed by Middeldorpf. *(From ref. 4.)*

Galvanism and Electrolytic Effects

In the early 1800s, investigators took the output of direct current (D.C.) batteries (galvanic current) and applied it to biological tissues such as skin. It was found that when D.C. was applied to skin for a prolonged period of time, a blister with serous fluid would develop at the negative pole. By the early 1800s, galvanism, as this technique came to be called, was used to induce suppuration in tumors. In 1867, Julius Althous from Britain introduced the concept that chemical effects caused by direct current, as opposed to the heating effects, could cause tissue destruction. In a series of animal experiments on the disruption of tissues with galvanic current, Althous demonstrated that this technique, which he called electrolysis, was a safe and effective method for shrinking and destroying a variety of tissues and tumors including large nevi, skin tumors, ulcers, hemorrhoids and goiters.

After Althous' studies, electrolysis was used widely for treating many types of disorders including some related to the uterus and cervix. One of the most interesting gynecological applications was the use of electrolysis for alleviating the hemorrhage and pain associated with large uterine fibroids. Many prominent clinicians, such as Sir Thomas Spencer Wells of London and Horatio Bigelow of Philadelphia, advocated the insertion of a specially designed platinum needle electrode (positive pole) into the uterine cavity and placing a large negative electrode of moist clay on the abdomen. They would then pass a galvanic current of 60-70 mA for 5-15 minutes through the circuit twice a week. This method appeared to be quite palliative in women with menorrhagia. Ninety percent of patients had a reduction in bleeding and up to 50% experienced relief of their pain.[5] Despite its apparent efficacy and ease of use, many clinicians felt that electrolysis had little advantage over other surgical methods for treating symptomatic uterine fibroids. Similar arguments are being made today (almost 150 years later) by the proponents and opponents of electrosurgical endometrial ablation techniques.

EARLY EXPERIMENTS ON THE PHYSIOLOGIC EFFECTS OF ELECTRICITY
Arsène D'Arsonval

In the late 19th century, the early attempts at electrotherapy became more scientific as inventors/scientists/physicians began carefully documenting the effects of high-frequency alternating currents on biological organisms. The list of these inventors/scientists/physicians is long, but most prominent are Arsène D'Arsonval, Nikola Tesla, Elihu Thomson, and William J. Morton. D'Arsonval is now recognized as the first person to use high-frequency alternating current (as opposed to direct current) therapeutically.[3]

D'Arsonval was a French physiologist and inventor who helped develop the microphone, telephone, and moving coil galvanometer. While observing the effects of electric currents on nerve and muscle preparations, he established a number of key observations that form the basis of much of our current concepts of electrophysiology (Table 1.1).

Table 1.1

D'Arsonval's Key Observations

The physiological effects of current on nerves and muscle is the same regardless of the source if the waveform of the current is the same.

Galvanic current (direct or continuous wave current) has no observable effect on living organisms whereas sinusoidal currents (alternating currents) produce striking results in living organisms.

The response of nerve and muscle to a sinusoidal current is dependent on the frequency of the current.

In studies on the effects of the frequency of an alternating current on sensation and neuromuscular excitability, D'Arsonval found that at very low frequencies (several cycles per second) alternating current did not result in contractions or pain. As the frequency increased, individual muscular contractions occurred at the rate of two per oscillation of current. As the frequency increased to 20-30 cycles per second, the muscular contractions increased and fused so that the muscle tetanized. The intensity of the tetany produced by the alternating current increased further as the frequency approached 2,500 cycles per second and then the intensity began to decrease. At a frequency of over 10,000 cycles per second, no effects were observed.

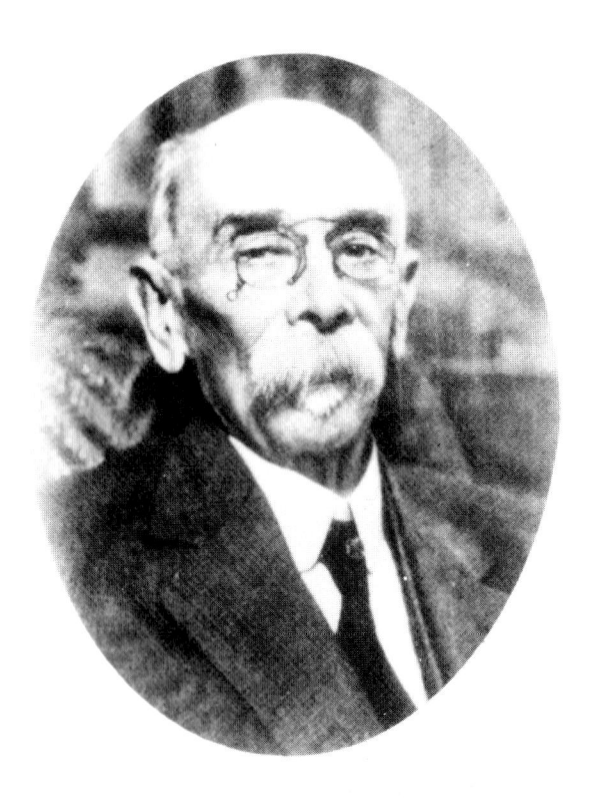

Figure 1.2. Arsène D'Arsonval. *(Used with permission from ref. 3.)*

While D'Arsonval was pursuing these studies in Paris, Nikola Tesla, a Czechoslovakian-born U.S. immigrant, was designing high-frequency alternating current generators with Elihu Thomson. Together they developed the Tesla Generator, capable of producing a very high-frequency alternating current, which D'Arsonval used in his later physiological studies. D'Arsonval often used himself as an experimental subject and observed that when high-frequency alternating currents passed through his body, he felt no sensation except for warmth in his hands where he held the wires. He quickly became famous throughout Europe for personally demonstrating during his lectures that a high-frequency alternating current flowing through his body would make an electric light bulb held in his hands illuminate without causing ill effects.

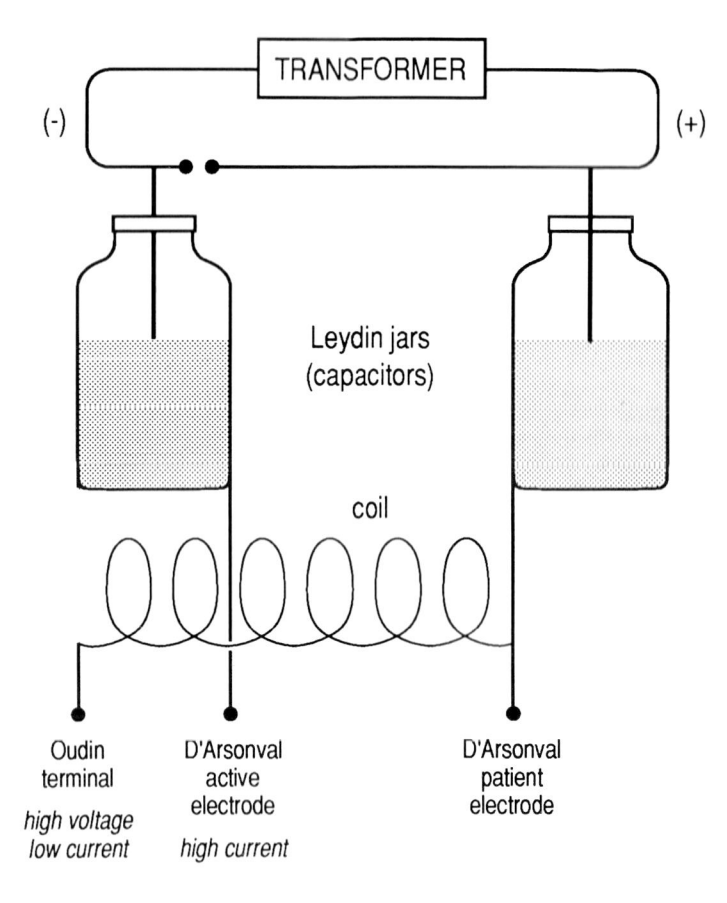

Figure 1.3. Drawing of an "Oudin Resonator" in which a transformer is connected to two Leydin jars (capacitors) that are connected in parallel with the coil. The free end of the open end coil serves as a high voltage, low current whereas the D'Arsonval outputs provide high current outputs. (*Modified from ref. 6.*)

During the course of his studies, D'Arsonval observed that sparks produced by high-frequency alternating generators produced burns when they fell on his hands. In later work with Paul Oudin, D'Arsonval modified the high-frequency generator of Tesla so that it was safer and produced a higher frequency output. This modified generator became known as the "Oudin Resonator" and was widely used, with only slight modifications, in medical applications through the early 1900s. The basic design of this early generator consisted of two Leydin jars (condensers) in series that were connected through a spark gap. As a method of raising the voltage in the circuit, a secondary coil was attached to the primary coil in a way that resulted in a powerful brush discharge in the secondary coil by self induction (Figure 1.3).

Studies Investigating The Therapeutic Effects of High-Frequency Alternating Current

Together, Oudin and D'Arsonval investigated, from 1893 - 1897, the medical effects of the high tension spark discharge obtained from the Oudin Resonator on a variety of dermatological disorders including acne, anal and vulvar pruritis, eczema, and lupus. They also investigated the effects of the current on various gynecological conditions including gonorrhea. These experiments led them to conclude that the sparks from the Oudin generator were anesthetic and could produce relief from neuralgia, sciatica, lumbago, and various muscular conditions. They also demonstrated that it destroyed small skin tumors. Joseph Riviere, an associate of D'Arsonval, performed extensive studies on the treatment of tumors (predominantly skin tumors) using high tension sparks produced by the Oudin-type generators and, in 1907, the term "fulguration" was introduced by Pozzi for the use of high-tension sparks to destroy tissue. Fulguration became widely used for destroying small tumors and, because it made cancer resections much less bloody, it began to be used to pretreat tumors prior to surgical excision.

In addition to his studies with the Oudin generator, D'Arsonval worked on the therapeutic effects of other types of electric current. One of his more interesting electrotherapeutic modalities involved placing patients in full body cages of electric wire through which a high-frequency alternating current was passed. These "large solenoids" produced extremely strong magnetic fields around the patients. Although no sensation was felt by the patients, a light bulb held in their hands would begin to glow as the alternating current was passed around the cage (Figure 1.4). This was referred to by D'Arsonval as "autoinduction". This type of electrical therapy became popular in the early 1900s in Europe as a means of alleviating the symptoms of a variety of systemic diseases but, by the 1920s, "autoinduction" had fallen into disfavor.

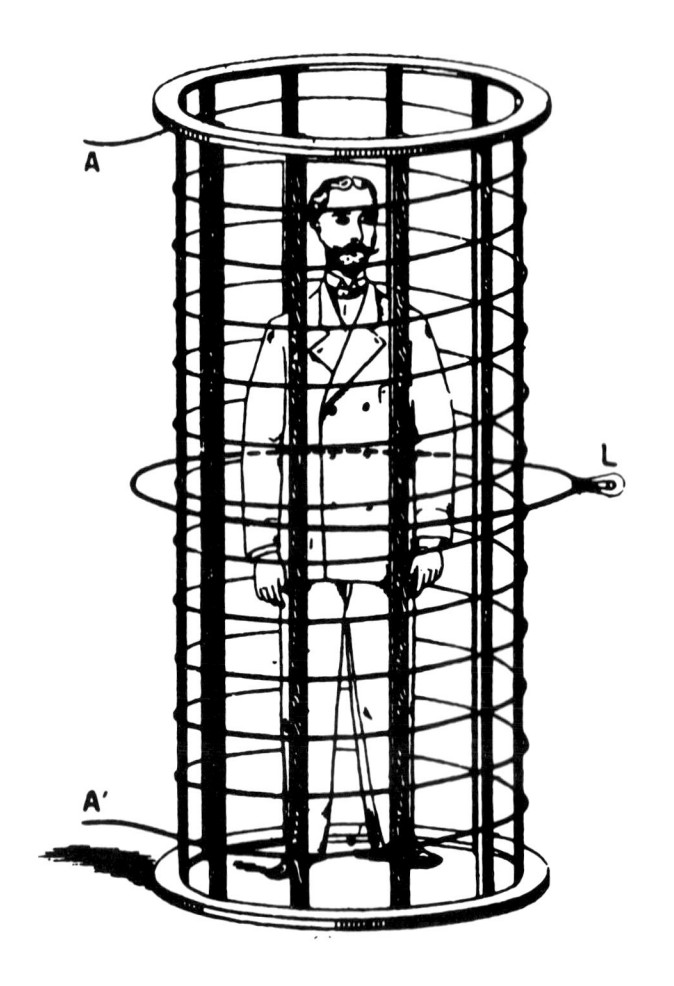

Figure 1.4 Large solenoid into which a patient was placed and subjected to strong magnetic fields. *(From Comptes Rendus, 1893, as shown in ref. 3.)*

Electrosurgical Diathermy

Another therapeutic effect of electric current that was investigated by the French scientists was to take the output from the Oudin resonator and pass it through the body from the feet to the hands. This type of systemic electrotherapy was thought to be beneficial for a variety of systemic disorders including diabetes and obesity and became the most widely used form of electrotherapy throughout the late 1800s and early 1900s. With the development of more powerful generators capable of producing undampened currents, numerous investigators became interested in the therapeutic effects of low-current, high-frequency alternating currents. In Germany and Austria it was first demonstrated that the body temperature of small animals could actually be increased by passing a high-frequency alternating current through them. Carl Frans Nagelschmidt introduced the term "diathermy" to refer to the phenomenon by which heat is generated in a tissue by the oscillation of molecules in response to high-frequency currents. Nagelschmidt also developed diathermy apparatti for the application of this technology in hospitals. These apparatti are still widely used by physiotherapists. In Europe, the term diathermy is frequently used to refer to any use of electrosurgery.

DEVELOPMENT OF MODERN ELECTROSURGICAL PROCEDURES IN THE UNITED STATES

Events in the United States unfolded independently, but synchronously, with those in Europe. Edwin Beer, an American who appears to have done his studies while largely unaware of the work going on in Europe, began using high-frequency alternating currents produced by Oudin resonators together with cystoscopes, to fulgurate bladder tumors around 1910. The use of electrosurgical fulguration for treating bladder tumors was expanded by Hugh Young, who, in 1913, presented a study of over 100 patients treated by cystoscopically-directed fulguration (Figure 1.5).[6]

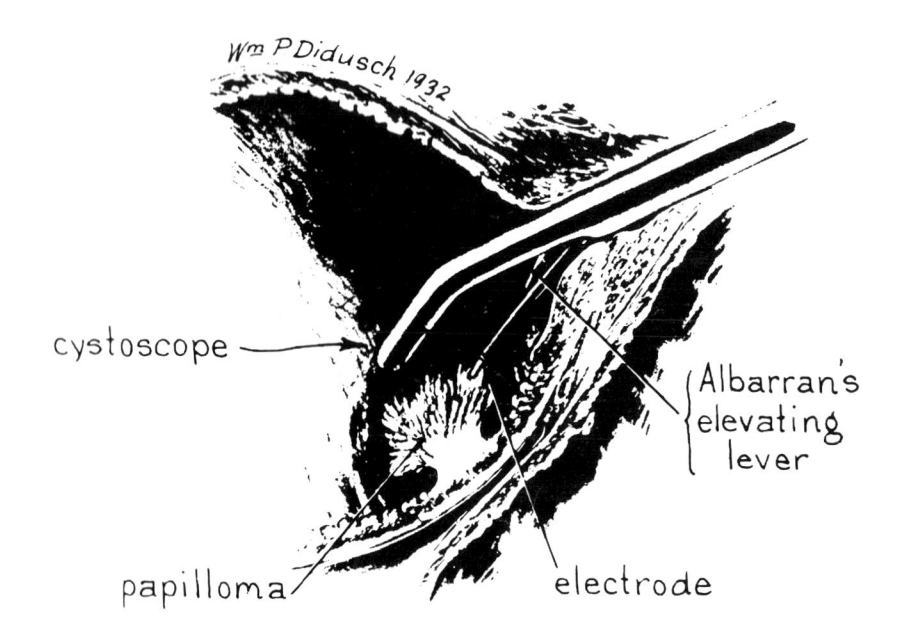

Figure 1.5. Drawing of the use of cystoscope to direct fulguration of bladder papilloma as performed by Beer. *(Used from ref. 6.)*

By the early 1900s, it was recognized that different types of tissue effects could be obtained using electrosurgical current. Riviere (who was a student of D'Arsonval) demonstrated that when high-frequency alternating currents were applied to tissues in the absence of sparking, a process which he called "white coagulation" occurred. Tissue that has undergone "white coagulation" is firm and desiccated but is not charred. This effect is quite different from that of fulguration which develops when sparking is allowed to occur. When strong electric arcs produce charring of a tissue (fulguration) the temperatures in the tissues can reach as high a 600°C, whereas the temperatures that are reached in the absence of sparks (white coagulation) rarely exceed 50°C to 70°C.

In the early 1900s, an American, William Clark, used Oudin Resonators coupled with a powerful Wimhurst static generator to produce very strong, high-frequency alternating currents for electrosurgery. He applied these currents directly to tissues with needle electrodes in order to desiccate them (Table 1.2). Initially, Clark demonstrated that desiccation was very useful for the destruction of cutaneous nevi.[7] Later, he began using this technique for treating epitheliomas, granulation tissue, tatoos, x-ray keratoses, and bladder papillomas. Clark's work helped to popularize the use of electrosurgery in the United States and led to the widespread acceptance and application of the electrosurgical desiccation technique by American surgeons because of advantages over other surgical approaches.

The next major advance in electrosurgery came with the development of the triode vacuum tube in the 1920s. The triode vacuum tube allowed electrosurgical generators to be developed that produced high-frequency, continuous, sinewave currents. These currents, when applied to scalpel-like electrodes, allowed surgeons to cut tissues quickly and easily in the absence of significant charring. Because the spark-gap generators and the triode vacuum tube generators produced widely varying effects on tissues, they were combined together into a single electrosurgical unit (ESU) by Harvey Cushing and William Bovie in the late 1920s.[8] There was a vacuum tube electrosurgical generator that produced a continuous, sinewave, electrosurgical current which was good for cutting on one side of these early model Bovie generators. On the other side of the cabinet, there was a spark-gap Oudin-type Resonator that produced an intermittent spark-gap current excellent for tissue fulguration and hemostasis. The early model Bovie generator was widely adopted throughout

Table 1.2

Advantages of Clark's Electrosurgical Desiccation

It was relatively bloodless due to coagulation of blood vessels. Therefore, no clamps were required to prevent blood loss.

The wound was essentially sterile.

---

the United States and Western Europe and underwent only minor changes until the early 1970s, when modern, solid-state, electrosurgical generators were produced. This was a major advance for electrosurgery since solid-state generators are capable of producing complex, high-frequency blended currents that combine both good electrosurgical cutting with excellent hemostatic effects. In addition, the use of solid-state electronics has allowed the introduction of numerous safety features in the generators. It is these solid state generators that have facilitated the development of the electrosurgical loop excision procedure.

REFERENCES

1. Licht, S. The history of therapeutic heat. In *Therapeutic Heat and Cold,* 2nd ed. Elizabeth Licht Publications, New Haven, CT, 1965.
2. Pearce, J. *Electrosurgery.* Wiley Medical, New York, 1986.
3. Rowbottom, M. and Susskind, C. *Electricity and Medicine: History of Their Interaction.* San Francisco Press, Inc., San Francisco, 1984.
4. Middeldorpf, A.T. *Die Galvanocaustik.* Breslau, Max, 1854.
5. Morgan, C.E. *Electro-physiology and Therapeutics.* New York, 1868.
6. Kelly, H.A. and Ward, G.E. *Electrosurgery.* W.B. Saunders, Philadelphia and London, 1932.
7. Clark, W. L. Oscillatory desiccation in the treatment of accessible malignant growths and minor surgical conditions. *J. Adv. Therapy.* 29:169-183, 1911.
8. Bovie, W. T. and H. Cushing. Electrosurgery as an aid to the removal of intracranial tumors. *Surg. Gyn. Obstet.* 47:751-784, 1928.

CHAPTER 2

GLOSSARY OF ELECTROSURGICAL TERMS

A.C. Leakage Current: A 60 Hz current which is transmitted from the electrosurgical generator to ground. This current can flow through the patient or operator to ground.

Active Electrode: The electrode with the small surface area at which an electrosurgical effect is obtained, i.e., the electrode used for cutting or coagulation.

Alternating Current (A.C.): A current in which electrons flow first in one direction and then in the other direction, i.e., a current in which the polarity alternates.

Ampere (Amp): The unit of measurement of the number of electrons flowing through an electric circuit. One ampere is defined as 6.24×10^{18} electrons flowing past a given point in one second (i.e., one coulomb).

Arc: An electric discharge (flow of current) through gas. Occurs when a high voltage is applied across a gas and the gas molecules become sufficiently ionized for current to flow. When this occurs, light and sound are produced.

Bipolar Technique: The coagulation of tissue using an instrument such as forceps that directs the current between the two ends of the instrument.

Blended Current: A current with a complex electrosurgical waveform that combines electrosurgical cutting effects with coagulation effects.

Capacitance: A measure of the ability of a capacitor to conduct an alternating current or store direct current charge.

Capacitor: Two pieces of conductive material separated by a relatively nonconductive material. Capacitors store direct current and conduct high-frequency alternating current.

ELECTROSURGERY FOR HPV-RELATED DISEASES

Capacitive Coupling: Connection from one circuit to another by capacitance rather than conductance. Capacitive coupling allows current to flow from one circuit to another even though the circuits are separated by an insulator.

Carrier Frequency: The frequency of the principle alternating current waveform produced by an ESU. With continuous sinewaves the carrier frequency is the same as the fundamental frequency. For complex, blended waveforms there may be several cycles of the carrier frequency in each repeated pulse.

Cautery: The destruction of tissue by the application of heat or a caustic substance.

Charge: The relative absence or presence of electrons on a conductor.

Circuit: Pathway that electrons take.

Coagulation: The process of causing bleeding to cease by clotting blood and contracting the ends of blood vessels. Electrosurgically, the type of current that promotes coagulation.

Conductor: Any substance or material through which electrons can flow.

Coulomb: 6.24×10^{18} electrons.

Current: Flow of electrons through a conductor. Current is measured in amperes.

Cutting: The severing of tissue. Electrosurgically, a current that promotes tissue separation with minimal thermal and coagulation effects.

Desiccation: The drying of tissue which results in tissue necrosis. Electrosurgically, a type of coagulation that occurs in the absence of sparks.

Diathermy: The generation of heat diffusely throughout the body secondary to the passage of a high-frequency electric current. In European literature, used synonymously with electrosurgery.

Direct Current (D.C.): Circuit in which electrons flow in only one direction.

GLOSSARY OF ELECTROSURGICAL TERMS

Dispersive Electrode: The electrode with a large surface area at which no observable electrosurgical effects occur. Can be thought of as the electrode that directs current flow from the patient back to the generator. Often referred to as the patient return electrode.

Duty Cycle: The percentage of time that voltage is applied to a circuit having a repetitive waveform compared with the total time of the cycle.

Electrosurgery: The cutting, desiccation and coagulation of tissue using high-frequency alternating current.

Electrode: The terminal of an electric circuit through which electrons pass.

Electrolysis: The necrosis of tissue due to the effects of a direct current. Occurs secondary to chemical cauterization as ions become polarized within cells in response to a strong electrical field.

Energy: The capacity for doing work.

ESU: Abbreviation for an electrosurgical generator.

Fulguration: Destruction of tissue or production of hemostasis (coagulation) by means of sparks from a high-frequency alternating current.

Frequency: Rate of repetition of identical voltage or current patterns. Measured in hertz (Hz) which is cycles per second.

Galvanism: The therapeutic use of a direct current. Named after Luigi Galvani.

Ground: Conductor connected to earth. Grounded conductors have the same potential and no current can flow between them.

Ground Referenced ESU: An ESU in which the dispersive electrode is grounded via the metal chassis of the ESU. With these generators, current can flow from the active electrode to any grounded object.

Hertz (Hz): Measure of frequency. One hertz is one cycle per second.

Impedance: Resistance to flow of an alternating current. Impedance includes not only simple resistance to flow of a direct current but resistance secondary to capacitance and inductance of the circuit.

Inductance: A property of a coil of wire in which energy is stored in a magnetic field around the wire as direct current flows through the wire.

Isolated Output: An ESU in which the voltage carried is not referenced to ground. With this type of ESU, current will not flow from the active electrode through any grounded object. Instead, current will flow only through an object connected to the return electrode terminal of the ESU.

Leakage current: A current that flows through a circuit other than the one desired. For example, current flowing from a patient to ground during electrosurgery.

Monopolar technique: Electrosurgical technique in which current flows from the active electrode through the patient's body to the dispersive electrode.

Ohm: The unit of measurement of electrical resistance. One ohm is the amount of resistance that requires one volt to cause a current of one ampere.

Ohm's Law: The equation defining the relationship between voltage, current and resistance.

Patient Electrode: Another term for dispersive electrode or return electrode.

Power: Energy produced or consumed over time.

Radiofrequency: Alternating current frequencies above the audible frequency range, i.e., higher than 15,000 Hz. The term radiofrequency is usually used to refer to a frequency between 550,000 Hz. and 3,000,000 Hz.

Rectification: A reduction in the frequency of the alternating current. A rectifier changes an alternating current to a direct current.

Return Electrode: Another term for dispersive electrode or patient electrode.

RMS Voltage: Root mean square voltage. Term used to define the "average" voltage of an alternating current.

GLOSSARY OF ELECTROSURGICAL TERMS

Solid State: Circuitry that uses transistors as opposed to vacuum tubes or spark gaps.

Spark: Electric discharge across air (i.e., an arc). Occurs when a high voltage is applied across a gas and the gas molecules become sufficiently ionized for current to flow, producing light and sound.

Spark-gap generator: A generator that produces a discontinuous current when the voltage in the circuit becomes great enough that sparks cross an air gap incorporated into the generator.

Voltage: The force that pushes electrons through a circuit. The electric potential.

Volt: The unit of measurement of voltage.

Watt: The unit of measurement of electrical power. Power in watts is related to heat production since one watt is defined as one joule of energy consumed per second.

CHAPTER 3

PRINCIPLES OF ELECTROSURGERY

In order to understand the theory behind electrosurgery and to use it to its full advantage, it is important to have a basic understanding of electric circuits and electrical principles. This chapter will serve as a primer of electricity to refamiliarize the clinician with electric circuits and electrical principles. A detailed glossary of electrosurgical terms is given in Chapter 2.

BASIC CONCEPTS IN ELECTROSURGERY
Definitions

Table 3.1

	Electrical Definitions
Circuit:	Pathway that electrons take
Current: (amperes)	Number of electrons flowing through a circuit
Voltage: (volts)	Force that drives electrons through a circuit
Power: (watts)	Energy produced or consumed over time
Resistance: (ohms)	Difficulty that a substance presents to electron flow

Electric current is defined as the flow of electrons through a substance or tissue secondary to an electrical potential or an electromotive force (EMF) which is placed across the substance. The term current is used to refer to the number of electrons that are flowing through the substance. The unit of measurement of current is the ampere (A). One ampere of current is defined as 1 coulomb (C) of electrons flowing through the circuit in 1 second. This definition translates into 1 ampere being exactly 6.24×10^{18} electrons moving by a given point in a circuit in 1 second. For electrosurgical purposes this is a relatively large amount of current. Electrosurgical applications usually involve milliamperes of current as opposed to amperes of current. A milliampere (mA) is 1/1,000 of an ampere and is the unit of measurement usually referred to in electrosurgery.

> 1 ampere (A) = 1 coulomb (C) of electrons flowing per second
> 1 coulomb = 6.24 x 10^{18} electrons

The pathway that the electrons take as they flow through a substance or tissue forms the circuit. The amount of current that flows through a circuit involves two factors. One is the electric potential or electromotive force (EMF) across the circuit and the other is the resistance that the circuit provides to the current.

Electromotive force should be thought of as the force that drives the electrons through the circuit. This is the electrical potential difference between the two ends of the circuit and is due to an imbalance in the density or number of electrons at the two ends of the circuit. If there is a large disparity in the number of electrons at the two ends there is a large EMF. EMF is measured in volts. A volt is defined as the EMF which will produce a current of 1 ampere through a conductor with a resistance of 1 ohm. Voltages produced by ESUs typically range from 2,000 to 12,000 volts.

> Volt = EMF that produces 1 ampere of current through 1 ohm resistance

Resistance is the second factor that will determine the amount of current that flows through a circuit. Resistance refers to the difficulty which a substance presents to the flow of electrons through that substance. Resistance is measured in ohms. One ohm is defined as the amount of resistance offered by a column of mercury 106.3 cm long and 1 mm^2 in cross-sectional area. The

> Ohm = Resistance offered by column of mercury 106.3 cm long and 1 mm^2 in cross-sectional area

resistance of a material to direct current is an inherent property of the material and is determined by its chemical make-up since the flow of current through a material is determined by the availability of free electrons for conducting the current. The resistance of a material to an alternating current (as opposed to a direct current) is referred to as impedance. Impedance is determined by the resistance of a material to direct current and to the resistance secondary to the capacitance and inductance of the circuit.

The resistance of biological tissues varies greatly and ranges from a high of 100,000 ohms (essentially nonconductive) found in dry, calloused palmar

PRINCIPLES OF ELECTROSURGERY

skin to approximately 200 ohms (very conductive) for highly vascularized tissue (with a high water and electrolyte content) such as the cervix.[1] The extremely high resistance (nonconductivity) offered by dry calloused skin explains why electricians can occasionally handle lines containing live household current without shocking themselves. Other tissues with high

Table 3.2

Resistance of Biologic Tissues

Tissue	Resistance in Ohms
Calloused skin	100,000
Adipose	2,000
Cervix	200

resistance include bone and adipose tissue. The latter is composed predominantly of nonconductive lipids and has a resistance of approximately 2,000 ohms.

In addition to the inherent properties of the material through which the current is flowing, the resistance of a circuit is also dependent on the length of the circuit, its cross-sectional area and the temperature of the conductor. The larger the circuit and the narrower its cross-sectional area, the greater the resistance of the circuit.

Ohm's Law

Interrelationships between current, EMF (voltage) and resistance are defined by Ohm's Law which states "the current in an electrical circuit is directly proportional to the voltage and inversely proportional to the resistance."

$$\text{Voltage} = \text{current} \times \text{resistance}$$
$$V = I \times R$$

Therefore, as the resistance of a circuit increases, an increased voltage (EMF) is required to obtain the same current flow. Similarly, as the voltage increases, more current will flow through a circuit of a fixed resistance. The

ELECTROSURGERY FOR HPV-RELATED DISEASES

practical importance of this relationship is that as tissue dries out (desiccates), a higher voltage will be required to pass a current through it. The higher voltage will result in significantly more tissue damage and will reduce the quality of an electrosurgically excised specimen for pathological examination.

Electrosurgical generators generally do not allow the operator to adjust the actual voltage produced by the instrument. Instead, they allow the operator to adjust the output power which is more difficult to conceptualize than is voltage. Power is the energy produced or consumed over a period of time.

$$1 \text{ watt} = 1 \text{ joule / sec}$$

Power can be directly related to heat output and is often measured in heat units such as joules, calories or British Thermal Units (BTUs). In many electrical applications, power is measured in watts. One watt is defined as being 1 joule of heat produced per second.

Output power is related to the voltage and current by the following equation:

$$\text{Power (watts)} = \text{EMF (volts)} \times \text{current (amperes)}$$
$$P = V \times I$$

Inserting Ohm's law into this equation allows the power output of an ESU to be defined in terms of the electrical resistance (impedance) of the circuit and either voltage or current.

$$P = V \times I$$
$$P = I^2 \times R$$
$$P = V^2 \times R$$

Electrical power supplied to a tissue results in tissue heating (see below). The amount of power supplied to a tissue increases as a function of the square of the current or of the voltage. Therefore, doubling the current will result in the power applied to a tissue increasing four times.

Basic Circuits

The easiest form of circuit to understand is termed a simple direct current (D.C.) circuit. In this type of circuit, current flows in a single direction and the amount of current is directly related to Ohm's Law (given above). Figure 3.1 presents a prototypical simple D.C. circuit in which a light bulb is connected to a D.C. battery.

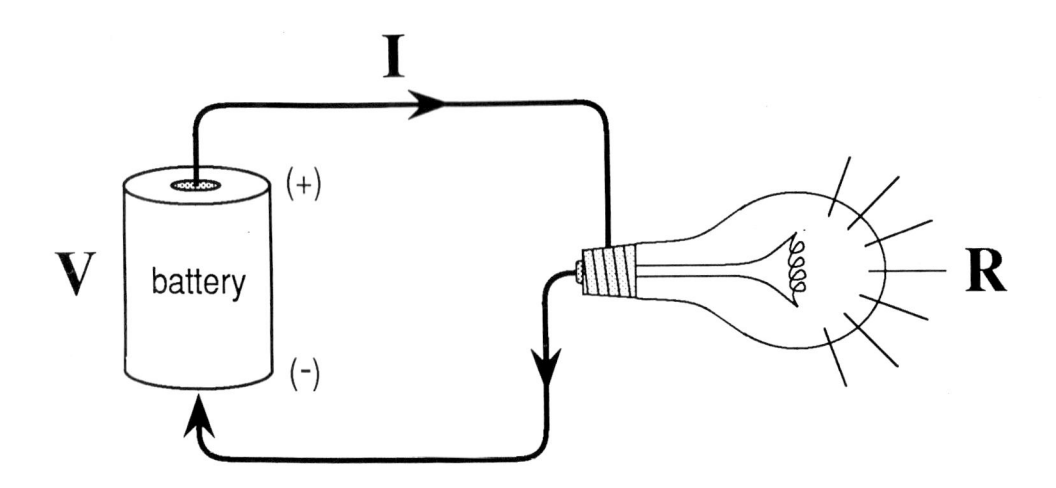

Figure 3.1. Prototypical D.C. circuit in which a D.C. battery is attached to a light bulb.

A D.C. battery has a specific polarity. One side (pole) is negatively charged and the other is positively charged. Electrons are diagrammed as flowing from the positive pole through the circuit to the negative pole. (Real electrons actually flow in the opposite direction from the negative pole, where they are overrepresented, to the positive pole, where they are underrepresented. So much for the precision of electrical engineering!) When the electrons flow through the light bulb, as diagrammed in Figure 3.1, they encounter a resistance due to the small diameter and composition of the filament in the light bulb. As the electrons flow through this high resistance, both heat and light are emitted.

If two light bulbs in series are placed in the circuit with the same battery, only half the current will flow through each light bulb as compared to a circuit with only one light bulb since the resistance is now twice as high. Therefore, each light bulb will produce less heat and light. This is because Ohm's Law states:

$$V = I \times R$$
$$I = V/R$$

Characteristics of Different Types of Current

The simplistic circuit diagram given above is useful for demonstrating the interrelationships between current, voltage and resistance. However, ESUs do not use direct current. Instead, a high-frequency alternating current (A.C.)

ELECTROSURGERY FOR HPV-RELATED DISEASES

is used to produce their tissue effects. In an alternating current the polarity of the current (i.e., direction of electron flow) periodically reverses. The periodicity with which the reversal of polarity occurs is described in terms of cycles per second or hertz. One hertz (Hz) equals 1 cycle per second. Figure 3.2 diagrams common household alternating current operating at 60 Hz.

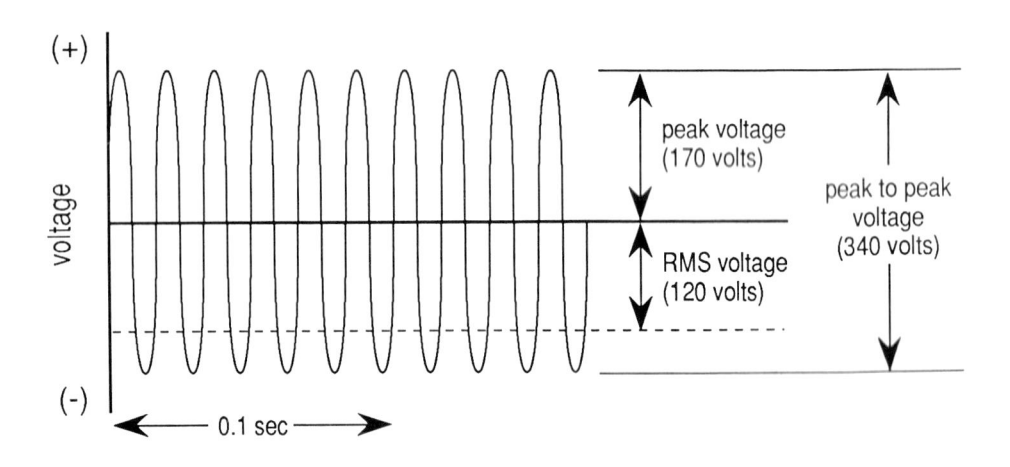

Figure 3.2. An alternating current operating at 60 Hz. The polarity of the current changes sixty times a second.

The important characteristics of an alternating current are voltage, waveform, duty cycle and periodicity.

Table 3.3

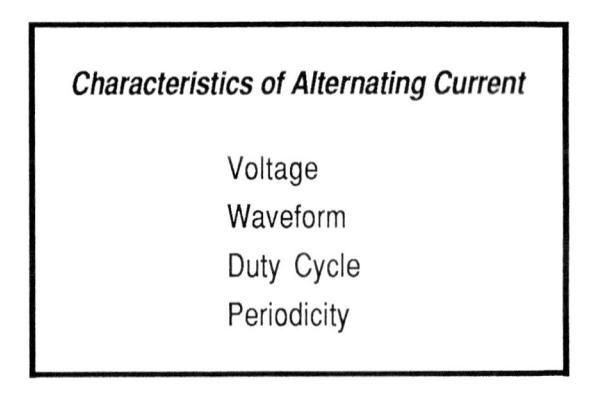

Characteristics of Alternating Current

Voltage
Waveform
Duty Cycle
Periodicity

PRINCIPLES OF ELECTROSURGERY

Unlike the voltage of a direct current, the actual voltage of an alternating current varies throughout the cycle. Depending on the specific effect of the current one is observing, different types of voltage measurements are used for describing the voltage of an alternating current. The two easiest voltage measurements to comprehend are the peak voltage and peak to peak voltage (Figure 3.2). Peak voltage is the highest voltage obtained during a cycle whereas peak to peak voltage describes the voltage change from the lowest negative voltage to the highest positive voltage. These two voltage measurements are important in electrosurgery since the peak voltage and peak to peak voltage will determine how strong an electric spark can be produced. With the common household alternating current shown in Figure 3.2, the peak voltage is 170 volts and the peak to peak voltage is 340 volts.

If a perfectly symmetrical, alternating current waveform is described (i.e., a sinewave current), the average voltage of the current will be 0 since the positive voltage produced in 1 cycle will be negated by the identical negative voltage produced in the same cycle. Therefore, average voltage will have little descriptive power for such a current (i.e., the average voltage of common household alternating current is 0). To get around this problem, the term root mean square voltage (RMS) is used to describe the "average" voltage of an alternating current (Figure 3.2). The RMS voltage of common household current is 120 volts. This is the voltage that is used in all electrical calculations.

The periodicity of alternating currents can vary between less than 1 Hz (cycle per second) to more than 880 million Hz (MHz). The frequency spectra of various types of alternating current is given in Figure 3.3.

Nerve and muscle stimulation by an alternating current (termed faradic effects) occurs maximally at frequencies between 10 and 100 Hz. These faradic effects cause muscular tetany and may result in electrocution which is why common household current presents such an electrical danger. As D'Arsonval originally described in the 1800s (see Chapter 1), at frequencies above 2,500 Hz the faradic effects of an alternating current gradually diminish and at frequencies of above 300,000 Hz (i.e., 300 kHz) they are essentially absent. This is why modern ESUs produce an alternating current with a frequency above 500 kHz.

The term radiofrequency is often used to refer to the very high-frequency alternating currents used for electrosurgery. By definition any alternating current which is beyond the audible range (15,000 Hz) should be referred to as a radiofrequency current. However, since AM radio broadcasts are in the frequency ranges of 550 kHz to 1.6 MHz, the term radiofrequency is commonly used to refer to all alternating currents with frequencies above 550 kHz. FM radio and TV broadcasts use even higher frequency alternating currents (up to 187 MHz). Since modern ESUs generally produce an alternating current with a frequency between 500 kHz and 3 MHz they are often referred to as radiofrequency generators.. One word of caution about the use of the term radiofrequency. It is sometimes stated that ESUs that operate at particularly high frequencies, such as 3.8 MHz, are "radiofrequency generators," whereas those that operate at lower frequencies, such as 550 KHz, are not. As the above discussion indicates, this is clearly incorrect. ESUs produced for operating room use and operated at a frequency above 500 KHz can all be considered "radiofrequency generators".

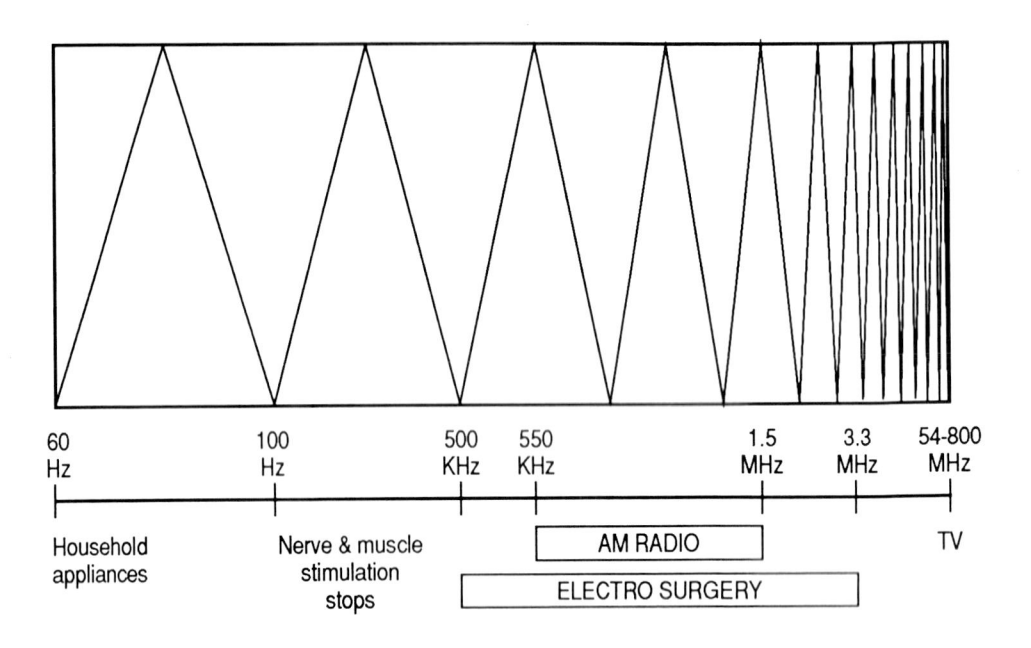

Figure 3.3. Alternating current frequency spectra.

It has been recognized for more than 100 years (see below) that the waveform and duty cycle of a current will influence the effects of that current on tissue. All forms of current can be produced as a continuous or a discontinuous form. With direct current the direction of electron flow is constant but the actual flow of electrons in the circuit can be turned on and off by inserting a switch into the circuit. The repetitive turning on and off of a direct current produces a discontinuous or interrupted current (Figure 3.4). This is sometimes referred to as a pulsed current.

PRINCIPLES OF ELECTROSURGERY

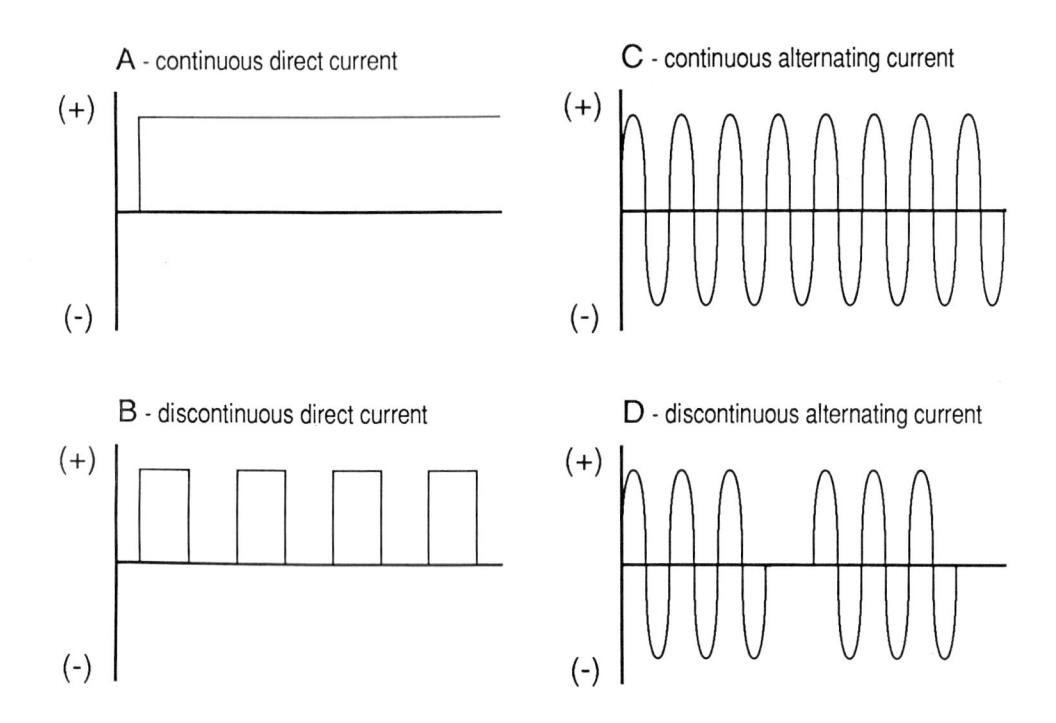

Figure 3.4. Different types of current.

Similarly, alternating current can be produced in either a continuous or discontinuous fashion (Figure 3.4). The term duty cycle is often used to describe a discontinuous alternating current. Duty cycle is defined as the percentage of time that current actually flows (Figure 3.5). In a 100% duty cycle, alternating current flows the entire time the ESU is activated, whereas in a 50% duty cycle, current actually flows just 50% of the time the ESU is activated.

The shape of the pulses of direct current produced when a discontinuous current is used can be varied and play an important role in determining the effects of the current on the tissue. The most important parameter of pulse configuration is the rate of rise of the voltage since this will determine the capacity of the current to depolarize cell membranes and excite nervous and muscular tissue. Figure 3.6 demonstrates the various configurations of D.C. pulses that are used for electrotherapy.

ELECTROSURGERY FOR HPV-RELATED DISEASES

A - 100% duty cycle

B - 75% duty cycle

C - 50% duty cycle

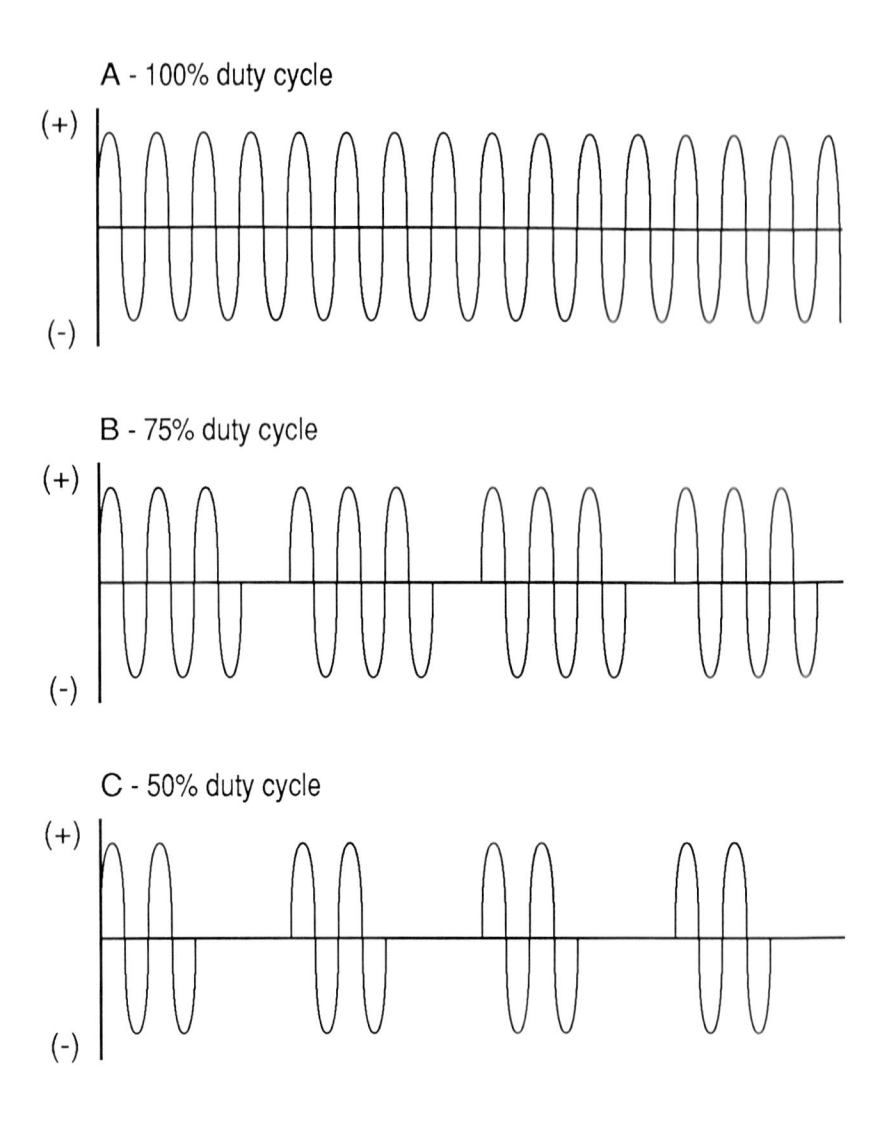

Figure 3.5. Duty cycle of alternating current produced by ESUs. A) 100% duty cycle. B) 75% duty cycle. C) 50% duty cycle.

Solid state ESUs can produce very complex alternating current waveforms for different electrosurgical applications. The two prototypical A.C. electrosurgical waveforms are the spark-gap waveform and the continuous sinewave (Figure 3.7). The spark-gap waveform is both discontinuous and

PRINCIPLES OF ELECTROSURGERY

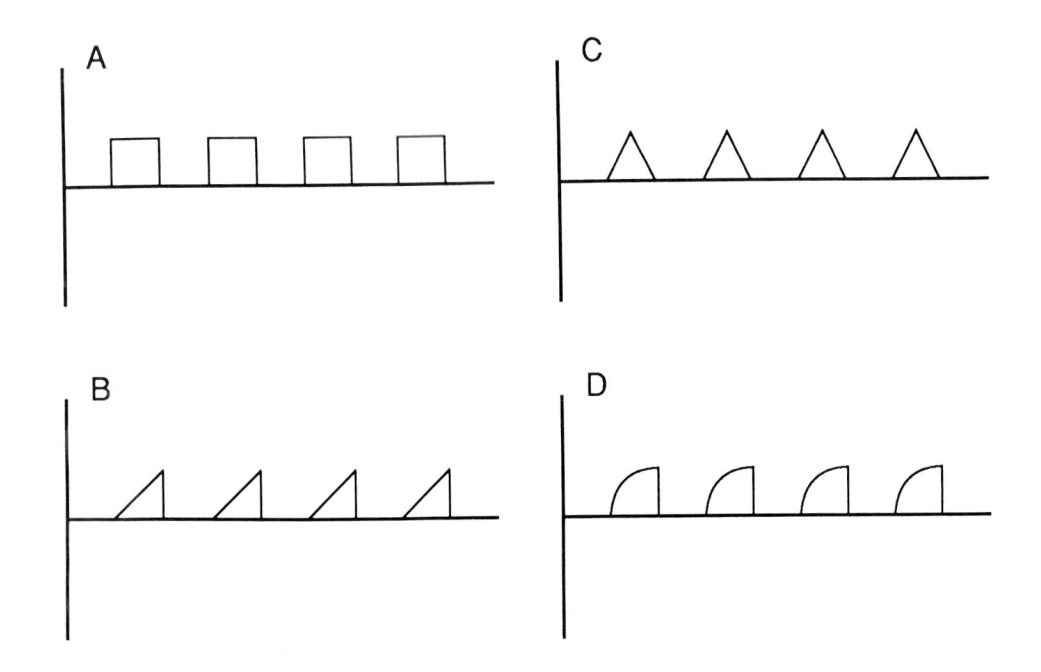

Figure 3.6. Configuration of different types of D.C. pulses used for electrotherapy. A) Interrupted square. B) Sawtooth. C) Triangular. D) Surged pulse.

asymmetric. In other words, current only flows during part of the cycle (i.e., it has a low duty cycle) and the peak voltage varies as current flows. Spark-gap alternating current produces good hemostasis and extensive tissue necrosis but is not suitable for electrosurgical cutting. With continuous sinewave alternating current, the peak voltage is the same throughout the entire cycle. Continuous sinewave alternating current produces little hemostasis but is excellent for electrosurgical cutting.

Concept of Ground

When a metal stake is driven deeply into the ground and attached by a wire to another metal stake driven into the earth there would be very little electrical resistance between the two stakes. If two objects were connected to these stakes, no electric potential would exist between the objects (i.e., they would be at the same voltage) and no current would flow between the objects. These objects would therefore be grounded with respect to each other.

ELECTROSURGERY FOR HPV-RELATED DISEASES

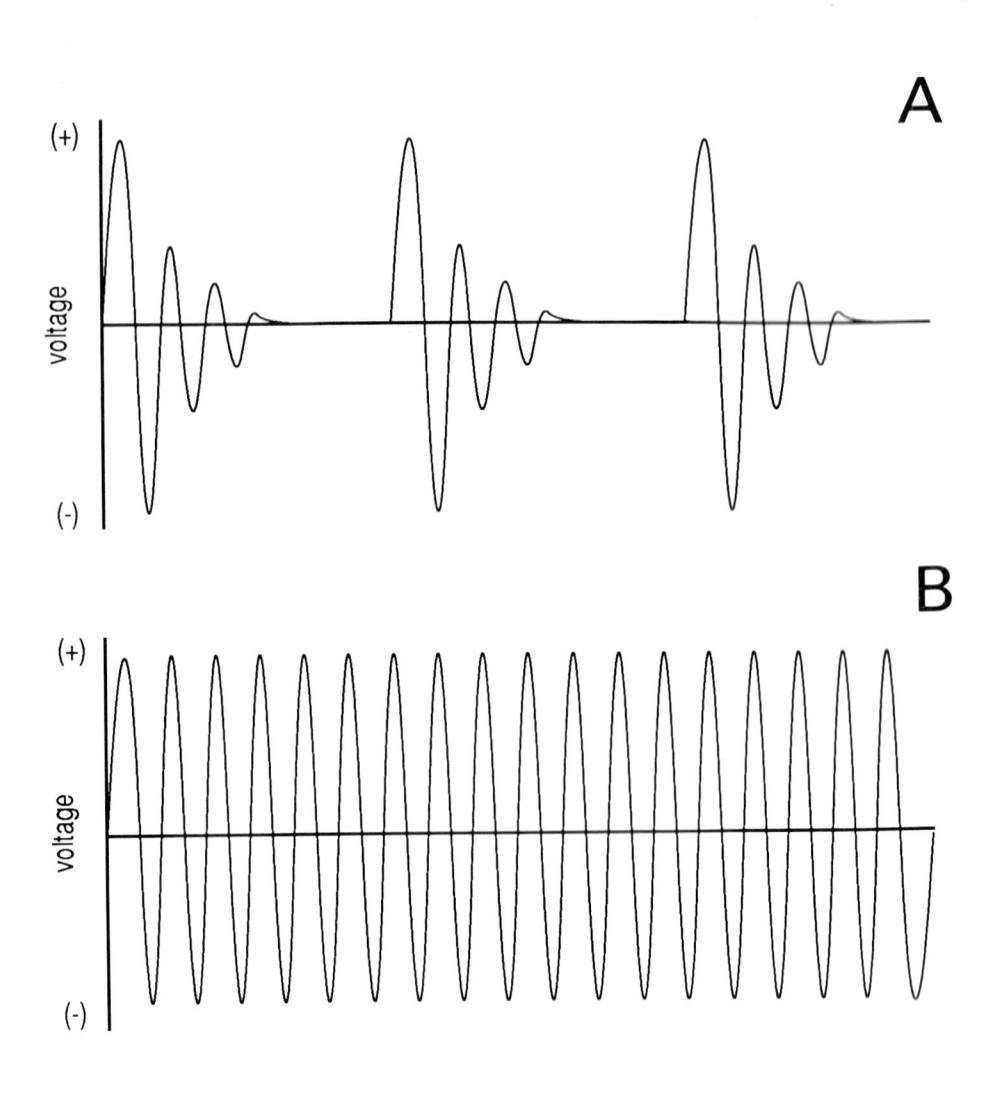

Figure 3.7. A) Spark-gap type alternating current. B) Continuous sinewave alternating current.

Grounding is usually obtained by connecting the appliance or ESU to metal that comes in contact with the earth such as water pipes. ESUs that are ground referenced have the chassis connected to ground via the ground wire in the three pronged electrical plug. Although such units generally operate quite safely, there is always a potential for breaks to occur in the electrical wiring. If this occurs and if a grounded operator or patient touches the ESU there is potential for a serious electrical shock.

Another safer method of wiring an ESU is termed isolated circuitry. In this type of circuitry, the main power is isolated by passing it through an isolation transformer. This eliminates the potential for the patient or operator to

PRINCIPLES OF ELECTROSURGERY

receive a shock should the wiring fail. Only ESUs with isolated circuitry should be utilized for electrosurgery since they are inherently safer. Only generators with isolated circuitry meet the AMSI Standard for Electrosurgical Devices (see Chapter 4, Equipment and Electrosurgical Safety).[2]

ELECTROSURGICAL CONCEPTS

In order to complete an electric circuit, it is necessary that two electrodes be used. Depending on the configuration of the electrodes that complete the electric circuit, electrosurgical techniques can be divided into either monopolar or bipolar techniques (Figure 3.8). In monopolar procedures, one electrode is termed the active electrode and is the electrode at which electrosurgical cutting or coagulation takes place. This electrode is relatively small and can be fabricated in any of a number of shapes including blades, loops, needles or rectangles depending on the particular application. The other electrode is termed the patient return electrode or "neutral" electrode. The return electrode is relatively large compared to the active electrode. In monopolar procedures, electric current flows from the active electrode through the patient's body to the return electrode (Figure 3.8).

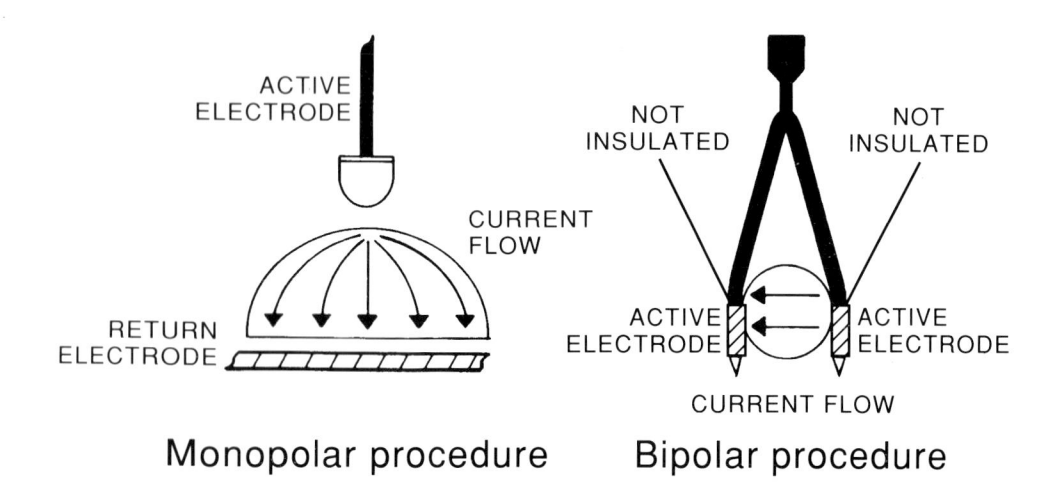

Figure 3.8. Types of electrosurgical procedures.

In bipolar procedures, two active electrodes are used which usually are combined into a surgical instrument, such as a pair of coagulation forceps. The electric current flows from one active electrode to the other active electrode and the current path is limited to the small amount of tissue between the two electrodes (Figure 3.8). In bipolar procedures, current does not flow through the patient's body back to a return electrode.

A key difference between monopolar and bipolar techniques is current density. In monopolar techniques, there is a very high current density at the active electrode and a very low current density at the patient return electrode. This results in good electrosurgical cutting at the active electrode and no electrosurgical effect at the return electrode. In contrast, with bipolar techniques, there is a moderate current density in all of the tissue held between the two poles of the electrode. This results in desiccation of the tissue between the two electrodes but not in electrosurgical cutting or fulguration.

EFFECTS OF RADIOFREQUENCY CURRENT ON BIOLOGICAL TISSUES

When a radiofrequency electric current passes through a tissue three different effects can occur: Thermal effects, faradic effects, and electrolytic effects (Figure 3.9). The relative magnitude of these effects will depend on the waveform, current density and how long the current is flowing.

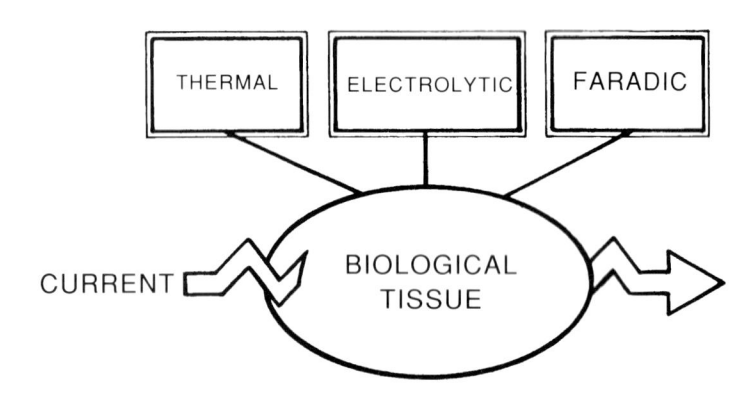

Figure 3.9. Biological effects that occur when an alternating current passes though tissue.

Faradic Effects

Faradic effects are the stimulation of nerve and muscle cells to produce a sensation of pain or a muscle contraction. The faradic effects of an alternating current were originally described by D'Arsonval in the 1800s and are dependent

PRINCIPLES OF ELECTROSURGERY

on the frequency of the alternating current. The optimum frequency of alternating current to produce faradic effects is 100 Hz. Above 300 kHz faradic effects do not occur, since the frequency of the current is too high to allow membrane depolarization to occur. Since modern ESUs operate at frequencies in excess of 300 kHz, faradic effects usually are not observed. However, faradic effects can occasionally occur during electrosurgery due to rectification of the high-frequency alternating current during the procedure.

Rectification is a process whereby some cycles of the high-frequency A.C. are filtered out so that the tissues actually experience a much lower frequency than that which is produced by the ESU. Rectification can be due either to tissues filtering some of the voltage (uncommon) or to the sparking process between the electrode and the tissue acting as a rectifier (more common). As will be described below, under conditions of electrosurgical cutting or fulguration, current passes from the active electrode to the patient in sparks. Sparks are a random and relatively inefficient way of transferring the current. Therefore, even though the generator is producing an A.C. of 500 kHz, if only 1 out of 10 cycles produces a spark, the tissue would experience a current of only 50 kHz which could produce faradic effects. To circumvent this problem, most modern ESUs are equipped with blocking capacitors that prevent low frequency current from flowing in either the active or the patient circuits. If rectification occurs, electrosurgery should be stopped immediately and the plan outlined in Table 3.4 carried out.

Table 3.4

What to do if Faradic Effects are Observed

Stop the procedure.

Check all connections to insure that metal-to-metal sparks are not occurring.

Reposition / replace the patient return electrode.

If faradic effects occur again, have qualified personnel check for 60 cycle leakage currents to ground and to insure that blocking capacitors are intact.

In our personal experience with almost 1,000 patients treated electrosurgically for HPV-related diseases of the lower genital tract, faradic effects were observed in a single case and the effect was eliminated as soon as the patient return electrode was removed and repositioned.

Electrolytic Effects

Electrolytic effects are defined as the tissue effects that occur when ions within a tissue become polarized in the strong electric field (Figure 3.10).

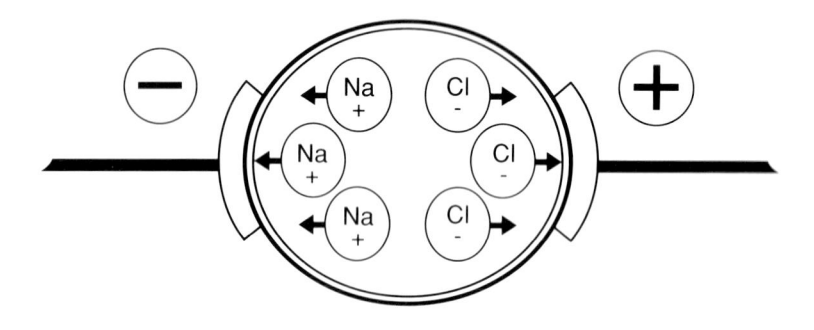

Figure 3.10. Electrolytic effects within a tissue.

When ions become polarized within a tissue due to the presence of an electrical field, chemical cauterization of the tissue can occur. This is the process used to destroy unwanted hairs when electrolysis is performed. The cells in the hair follicle undergo chemical cauterization and die. Electrolytic effects occur principally when direct current is applied to tissues for prolonged periods of time.

Due to the high frequency of the alternating current used for electrosurgery, electrolytic effects are minimal. The polarity of the current changes so rapidly that the ions within the cells do not have sufficient time to move to their respective poles. Instead, the ions move rapidly back and forth trying to align themselves with the electrical field. The kinetic energy that is released results in a temperature rise within the tissue, and it is this temperature rise that produces electrosurgical cutting (Figure 3.11). There is a crucial

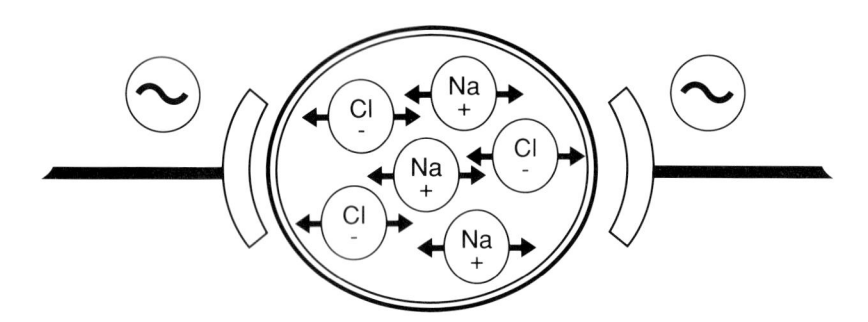

Figure 3.11. Effects of a high-frequency alternating current on ions in biological tissues.

difference between modern electrosurgical cutting and older therapies based on electrocautery. In electrocautery, an electric current is used to heat an electrode and this "red hot" electrode is used to cauterize and cut tissue. In modern electrosurgical applications the electrodes are used to focus the high-frequency alternating current on a particular spot. The focused high-frequency alternating current causes the tissues themselves to become heated. Electrosurgical cutting should not be thought of as taking a "red hot" electrode and excising tissue with it.

Thermal Effects

The thermal equilibrium of a tissue through which an electric current is passing is the balance between the amount of heat imparted to the tissue as a result of the current flow and the amount of heat dissipated from the tissue either through the evaporation of water or through thermal conduction to adjacent tissues (Figure 3.12).

A number of factors influence the rate of heat given off from the tissue. Perhaps the most important factor is the water content of the tissue. Water is an excellent medium for maintaining thermal equilibrium of a tissue due to its constant temperature of vaporization. Another important factor is the vascularity of the tissue, since blood flow helps to dissipate heat away from the tissue.

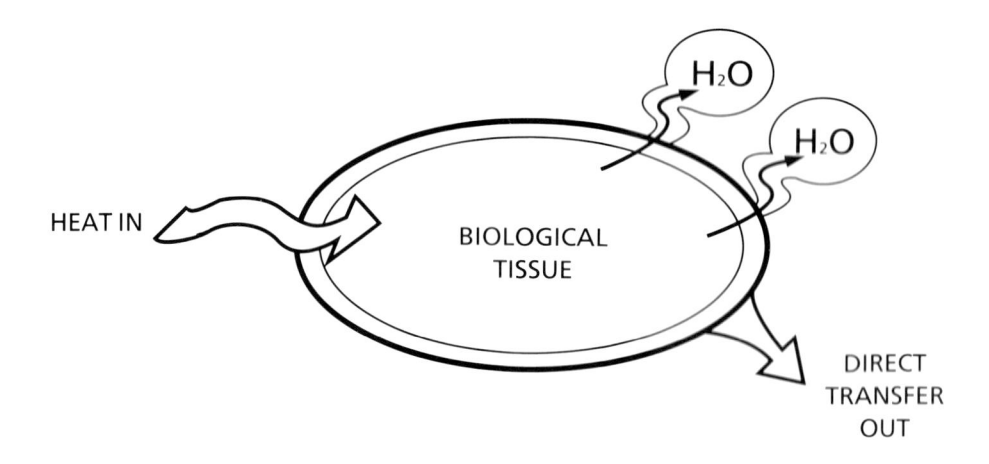

Figure 3.12. Thermal equilibrium of a biological tissue exposed to an electric current.

The effect of a temperature rise on a biological tissue is dependent on the actual temperature obtained and on the time that the temperature is maintained.[3] Table 3.5 lists the time required and the mechanisms thought to be responsible for irreversible cellular injury when metal probes of different temperatures are placed in contact with the shaved skin of a rabbit or dog.[4,5] Even at very low temperatures, such as 40-45°C, cell death will occur provided the elevated temperature is maintained for several hours. This is due to accelerated metabolism within the cell and the production of a lactic acidosis.

When a metal probe of greater than 50°C is placed on a tissue, cell death will begin to occur more rapidly. At these temperatures, the process causing cell death is that of denaturation of critical cellular proteins, such as enzymes, required for oxidative metabolism. At a temperature of 50°C, it takes about 10 minutes for sufficient denaturation to have occurred to result in cell death. However, as the temperature increases, the time it takes for proteins to denature is shortened and at temperatures of over 70°C, irreversible damage occurs in less than 1 second. These effects are similar to those observed when an egg is placed in boiling water and irreversible protein denaturation (coagulation) occurs.

Another process that occurs at temperatures above 70°C is that water evaporates slowly from the cell. When the temperature within a cell is less than 100°C the rate at which water evaporates is relatively slow. The evaporation consumes energy and acts to reduce the temperature within the tissue. Over time, however, even the slow evaporation of water will result in firm, dry, desiccated tissue. Such tissue develops a very high electrical resistance which prevents it from conducting electrical current. Although cell death occurs, there is no physical destruction of the tissue (Figure 3.13).

PRINCIPLES OF ELECTROSURGERY

Table 3.5

Time to Transepidermal Tissue Necrosis

Temp	Mechanism	Time
40-45°C	Accelerated Metabolism	> 2 hrs.
50°C	Protein Denaturation	10 mins.
70°C	Coagulum Desiccation	< 1 sec.
100°C	Vaporization	millisec.

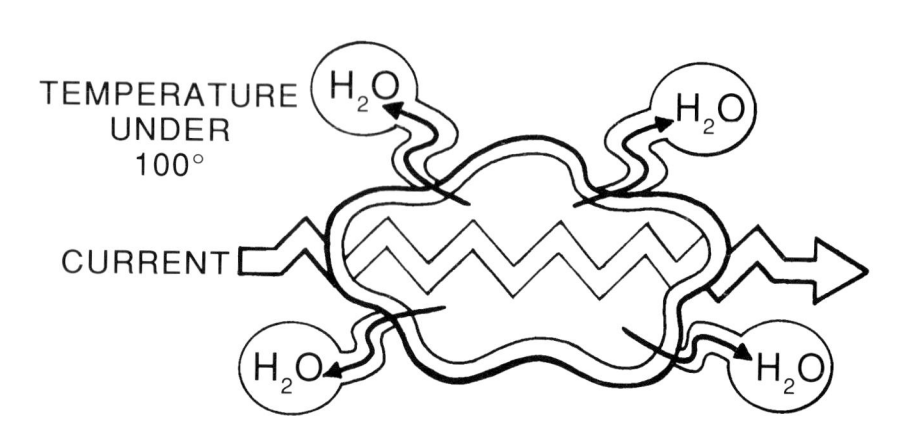

Figure 3.13. Tissue damage through desiccation at temperatures of less than 100°C.

At temperatures of 100°C or more, both intracellular and extracellular water rapidly vaporizes into steam. Since the volume of water vapor is 6 times the volume of liquid water, only a small proportion of intracellular water can vaporize before the intracellular volume expands to the point at which the cell membranes rupture and the cell dies. This process of vaporization and cell rupture occurs less than a millisecond after the temperature reaches 100°C and is essential to electrosurgical cutting. In fact, during electrosurgery, the temperature within the tissue often exceeds 600°C. With this type of superheating, explosive vaporization can occur. This leads to rapid expansion of the intracellular volume and to the production of highly disruptive pressure and acoustic forces that tear the tissues apart and play a role in electrosurgical cutting (Figure 3.14).[6]

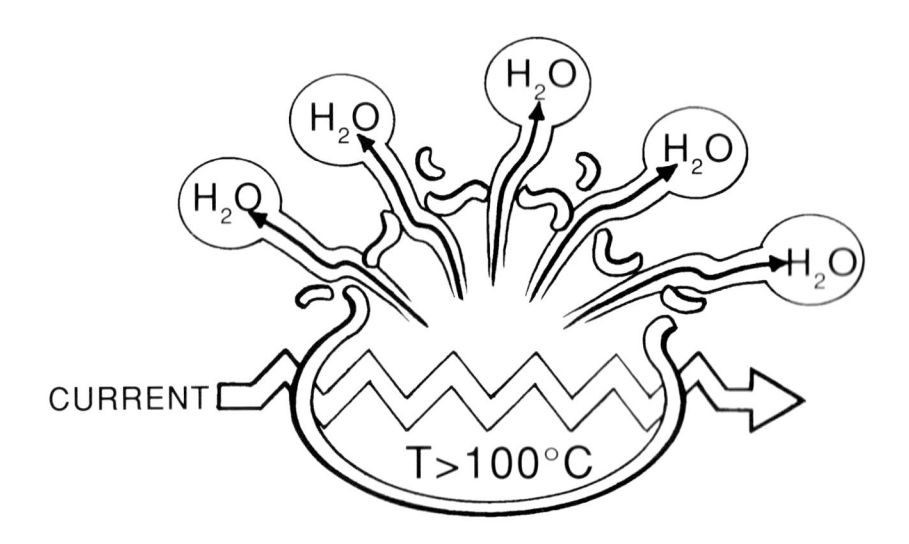

Figure 3.14. Tissue damage through rapid vaporization of intracellular water at temperatures of above 100°C.

In summary, for any given tissue, two divergent thermal effects can occur and the effect of a given temperature will depend on both the rate and the extent of the temperature rise. When temperature rises slowly, intracellular and extracellular water evaporates at a sufficient rate to maintain the temperature under 100°C. As this occurs, the tissue desiccates and the proteins within the tissue become thermally coagulated. This results in hemostasis and cell death, but does not cause actual physical destruction of the tissue. In contrast, when tissue is rapidly heated at high temperatures, evaporation and heat transfer cannot maintain thermal equilibrium within the tissue, the intracellular temperature rises to over 100°C and the rapid vaporization of intracellular water causes a marked volume change. Pressure within the cell increases to the point at which cellular membranes are ruptured and the tissue destruction required for good electrosurgical cutting occurs.

FACTORS INFLUENCING THE THERMAL EFFECTS OF HIGH-FREQUENCY ALTERNATING CURRENT

The thermal effects of passing a high-frequency alternating current through a tissue are governed by the following equation which is a modification of Ohm's Law presented earlier in this chapter[7]:

$$Q = 0.24 \times I^2 \times R \times T$$

Q = quantity of heat in gram calories
I = current intensity
R = electrical resistance of the tissue
T = time of current flow in seconds

Solving the above thermal heating equation using conditions common to modern electrosurgery, i.e., a 500 mA current passed through a tissue with a resistance of 100 ohms for 1 second, we obtain:

$$6 \text{ calories} = 0.24 \times 0.5 A^2 \times 100 \text{ ohms} \times 1 \text{ second}$$

One calorie will heat 1 cm³ of water 1°C. Therefore, under the conditions given in the above equation, if the current is distributed over 1 cm³ of tissue, the tissue will undergo only a 6°C temperature rise. However, if the same amount of current is passed through 0.1 cm³ of tissue, a 60°C temperature rise will occur in the tissue. Both the amount of current and the area through which the current is flowing are important in determining the thermal effects of an electric current. Current density is of key importance in determining the thermal effects of an alternating current.

DESIRED ELECTROSURGICAL EFFECTS

Depending on the waveform, current density and whether arcing occurs between the electrode and the tissue, three different types of electrosurgical effects are obtained (Table 3.6).

Desiccation

Desiccation occurs when the temperature within cells is slowly raised to less than 100°C. Water evaporates from the cells and proteins coagulate. This results in hemostasis both from the drying of blood and tissue and to direct

Table 3.6

Different Types of Electrosurgical Effects

Effect	Arcing	Mechanism of Damage
Desiccation	No	Protein coagulation and dehydration of cells
Cutting	Yes	Vaporization of cells
Spray Coagulation	Yes	Protein coagulation and vaporization of cells

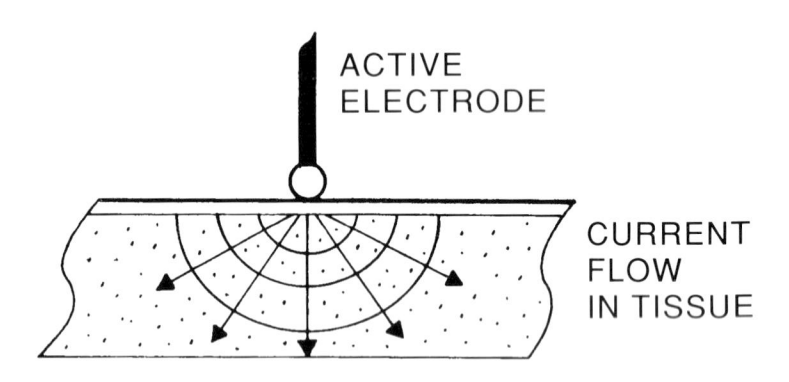

Figure 3.15. Desiccation of tissue occurs upon direct contact with a large electrode.

contraction of small blood vessels that leads to their closure. Desiccation occurs under conditions of low current density as when an electrode is placed in direct contact with tissue, generally under conditions of high current. Since current flows directly from the electrode to the tissue, arcs do not form (Figure 3.15). Under the conditions that allow electrosurgical desiccation to occur, temperature increases in tissues away from direct contact with the electrode are a function of the square of the distance from the electrode.[6] This means that irreversible tissue damage can occur distant to the actual site of electrode contact.

Electrosurgical Cutting

The physical process by which electrosurgical cutting occurs is thought to be identical to that by which CO_2 lasers cut tissue. Cutting occurs when the temperature within tissues rises high enough and rapidly enough that explosive vaporization of water occurs. Only a small proportion of total cellular water must evaporate for rupture of the tissues to occur. With both CO_2 lasers and electrosurgical cutting currents, the temperature within tissues reaches over 100°C within micro- to milliseconds. Under these conditions, superheating of the water within the tissues occurs so that the pressure within the tissues can reach several hundred atmospheres. This results in the formation of highly disruptive shock waves within the tissues that are thought to help "tear the tissues apart".

Electrosurgical cutting occurs only under conditions of extremely high current density. The very high current densities are required to raise the temperature within tissues rapidly and high enough for explosive vaporization to occur. In order to obtain the high current densities required for electrosurgical cutting, the current must be confined to an extremely small cross-sectional area. A number of investigators have observed that this occurs only when the current is confined to arcs traveling between the active electrode and the tissue (Figure 3.16).

Arcs occur when the electric field between 2 electrodes or the electrode and tissue becomes strong enough to ionize the particles in the intervening space. When this happens, light is given off and current is carried through the space between the 2 electrodes or the electrode and tissue (Figure 3.17). Since arcs are a mandatory part of electrosurgical cutting, factors that enhance the formation of arcs will facilitate cutting. Arcs are facilitated by the presence of a vapor (steam) envelope around the electrode which can become ionized in the electric field. The steam envelope is generated by the vaporization of water within the tissues during the cutting process. Therefore, for efficient electrosurgical cutting, it is important that the electrode be moved slowly but continuously through the tissue being cut. This allows cutting to be mediated by arcs traveling through the steam envelope which develops between the electrode and the tissue. Moving the electrode too quickly collapses the steam

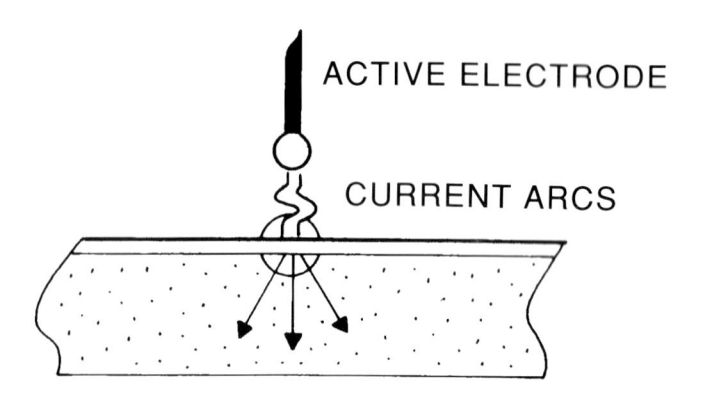

Figure 3.16. Electrosurgical cutting occurs as current arcs between the electrode and the tissue.

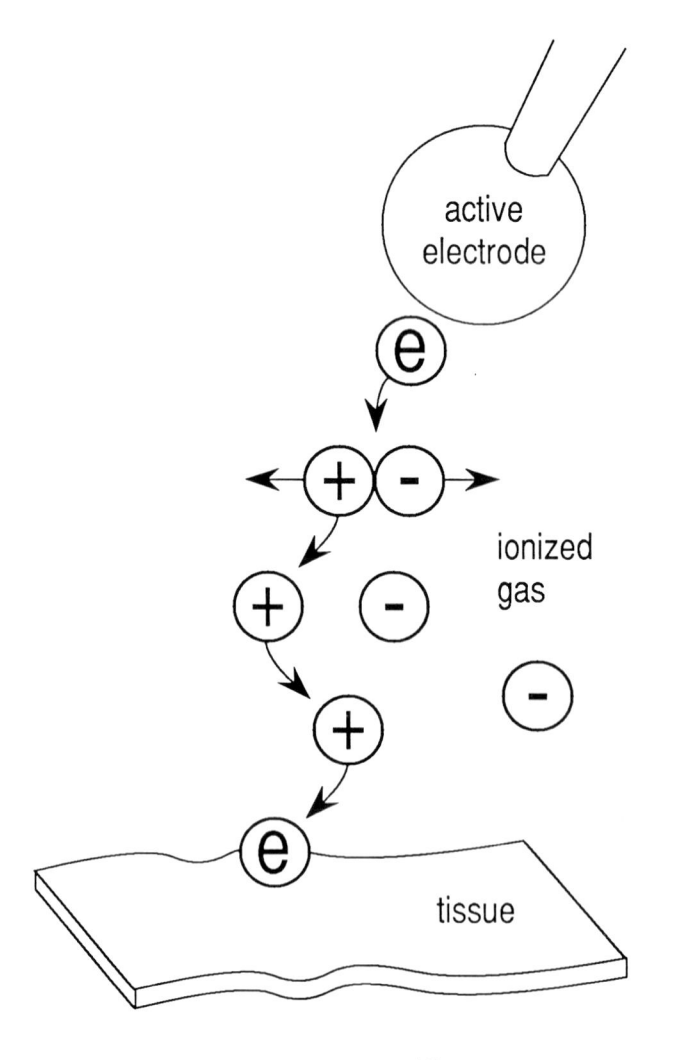

Figure 3.17. Arcs develop when the electrical field is strong enough to ionize gases and allow electrons to move from the electrode to the tissue along the charged molecules.

PRINCIPLES OF ELECTROSURGERY

envelope and places the electrode in direct contact with the tissue. Since the cross-sectional area of the electrode is much greater than an electrical arc, cutting is inhibited under these conditions. The requirement for a steam envelope for efficient electrosurgical cutting also explains why a continuous sinewave current is such an efficient cutting current. Since the current is continuous, the ionized envelope does not have a chance to break down between cycles. This facilitates the formation of repetitive arcs which follow the same path.

When current is carried in an arc between an electrode and a tissue, the equations describing the temperature rise that occurs in tissues adjacent to the site of the impact of the arc are different than those used to describe the temperature rise in tissues in direct contact with a much larger electrode. Under the conditions of electrical arcing, the temperature increases in tissues away from the site of the arc are inversely related to the fourth power of the distance.[1] In practice, this means that the extent of tissue damage is very limited during electrosurgical cutting.

Table 3.7

Factors That Promote Arcing

Moving electrode slowly but continuously to maintain steam envelope.

Continuous sinewave current.

Clean, shiny electrodes.

Spray Coagulation

Spray coagulation differs significantly from electrosurgical cutting. Coagulation is favored when high voltage, interrupted waveforms are used. The higher voltages of coagulating as compared to cutting waveforms allow arcs to form between the electrode and tissue in the absence of a steam envelope. This results in significantly more tissue disruption and charring than does electrosurgical cutting. Since the coagulating waveform is highly interrupted, any steam envelope that forms after an arc dissipates before the next cycle.[8] This means that the arcs strike the tissue in a truly random fashion which insures that electrosurgical cutting does not begin. Spray coagulation is used for producing hemostasis and for destroying lesional tissue but is not the preferred method for excising tissues that need to be examined histopathologically.

REFERENCES

1. Pearce, J. *Electrosurgery*. Wiley Medical, New York, 1986.
2. AAMI American National Standard. *Safe Current Limits for Electromedical Apparatus*. Association for the Advancement of Medical Instrumentation, Arlington, VA. ANSI/AAMI ESI-1985, 1985.
3. Adelson, L. and Hirsch, C.S. Physical agents in causation of injury and disease. In *Pathology,* 7th ed. W.A.D. Anderson and John M. Kissane, eds. Mosby, St. Louis, pp. 227-231, 1977.
4. Davis, J.H. and Abbott, W.E. The pathology of thermal burns--changing concepts: A review of literature since 1945. *Surgery* 40:788-806, 1955.
5. Moritz, A.R. Thermal injury. *Am. J. Pathol.* 23:915-941, 1947.
6. Hoenig, W.M. The mechanism of cutting in electrosurgery. *IEEE Trans. Biomed Eng.* BME-22:58-62, 1975.
7. Binder, S.A. Applications of low and high voltage electrotherapeutic currents. In *Electrotherapy*. Steven J. Wolf, ed. C. Livingstone, New York, 1981.
8. Kelly, H.A. and Ward, G.E. *Electrosurgery*. W.B. Saunders, Philadelphia and London, 1932.

CHAPTER 4

EQUIPMENT FOR THE LOOP EXCISION PROCEDURE AND ELECTROSURGICAL SAFETY

There are a number of items, in addition to those routinely used for colposcopy, that are required to perform loop excision and fulguration procedures (Table 4.1). At the beginning of this chapter it must be stressed that

Table 4.1

Equipment Required for the Loop Excision Procedure

Electrosurgical generator (ESU).

Wire loop and ball electrodes.

Disposable electrode handle and patient return electrode.

Nonconductive, coated speculum suitable for smoke evacuation.

Smoke evacuator.

Colposcope equipped for low magnification (4-7.5x) and complete colposcopy procedure tray.

Dental-type syringe with 27 gauge needle and two 1.8 ml ampules of 2% xylocaine with 1:100,000 epinephrine.

Strong aqueous Lugol's solution.

Monsel's gel.

Twelve inch needle holder and 00 Vicryl Suture material together with a vaginal pack.

---

electrosurgery as applied to the treatment of lower genital tract diseases is a new and rapidly developing technique and that a large number of electrosurgical generators and loop electrodes are currently being produced. We have not used many manufacturers' products. The intent of this chapter is to review briefly some of the equipment which we have used extensively or have observed in use. Our intention is not to provide an exhaustive listing of every available electrosurgical device. Neither inclusion nor exclusion of any instrument in this section should be construed as indicating the authors' endorsement or disapproval of a particular piece of equipment.

Electrosurgical Generators Suitable for Excision/Fulguration

Solid-state electrosurgical generators (ESU) that are suitable for loop excisions are produced by several companies in the United States and Western Europe. There are a number of factors which need to be considered when selecting an ESU for excision/fulguration (Table 4.2).

Table 4.2

Desirable ESU Features

Safety Features

Isolated circuitry.
Return electrode alarm.
Audible indicator when active.

Performance Features

60 watts in both cutting and coagulation mode.
Blended waveform.
Digital power meter.
Foot pedal control.
Rapid start capacity.

The two most important of these features are that the ESU allows the procedure to be performed safely and that it produces sufficient power with a correct type of cutting waveform so that the excised tissue is acceptable for histopathological analysis.

Patients may be burned unintentionally with an electrosurgical current in several ways (Table 4.3). The first is at the active electrode. If an injury occurs due to the patient coming into contact with an activated electrode, this is referred to as an "unintended burn". These burns generally occur due either to operator error or to the patient moving unexpectedly during the procedure. Although,

EQUIPMENT FOR THE LOOP EXCISION PROCEDURE

Table 4.3

> **Sites of Unintentional Burns**
> At the active electrode.
> "Alternate site" burns.
> Under the return electrode.

for the most part, unintended burns are not affected by ESU design, certain safety features such as an audible indicator of when the ESU is activated, may help to prevent them from occurring.

The second site of unintended burns has been termed "alternate site burns". Alternate site burns are produced when an alternative pathway from patient to ground develops through a small contact point at a site other than the return electrode. Under these conditions current division can occur so that the electrical current no longer flows between the active electrode and the patient return electrode, but instead follows an "alternate pathway" from the active electrode to a ground. If the region of contact between the patient's body and this alternate pathway to ground is small, a burn can develop at the site of contact with the alternate pathway.

The majority of ESUs produced in the United States and Western Europe now include a type of circuitry termed "isolated circuitry" which significantly reduces the risk of "alternate site burns". Isolated circuitry can be thought of as a mechanism by which the ESU detects when a significant portion of the electric current is no longer returning to the ESU via the patient return pad, but instead is passing directly to ground. When such an unsafe situation exists, the isolated circuitry inactivates the ESU. Generators which lack isolated circuitry are generally referred to as ground referenced ESUs. In our opinion, ground referenced ESUs should not be used for the loop procedure, since they are inherently less safe than ESUs incorporating isolated circuitry technology.

The third type of unintended patient burns occurs under the return electrode (grounding pad). These burns occur either due to a manufacturing defect in the pad or to a pad not remaining in full contact with the patient. As explained in Chapter 3, the reason an electrosurgical effect occurs at the active electrode, but not at the patient return electrode, is there is a high current density at the active electrode and a low current density at the return electrode. When there is a defect in the patient return electrode or when the electrode does not remain in full contact with the patient, the current density can increase under the return electrode and result in a patient burn (Figure 4.1).

We consider only ESUs that incorporate some form of alarm that will indicate when the patient return electrode has not been connected to the ESU to be safe for electrosurgery. Most ESUs meet this requirement by incorporating a "cord fault alarm" that inactivates the ESU or alerts the user when the return electrode is not plugged into the machine. In addition to this "basic cord fault" type alarm, some ESUs have more elaborate warning indicators to alert the clinician of an unsafe patient return pad (see section Electrode Handles and Patient Return Electrodes).

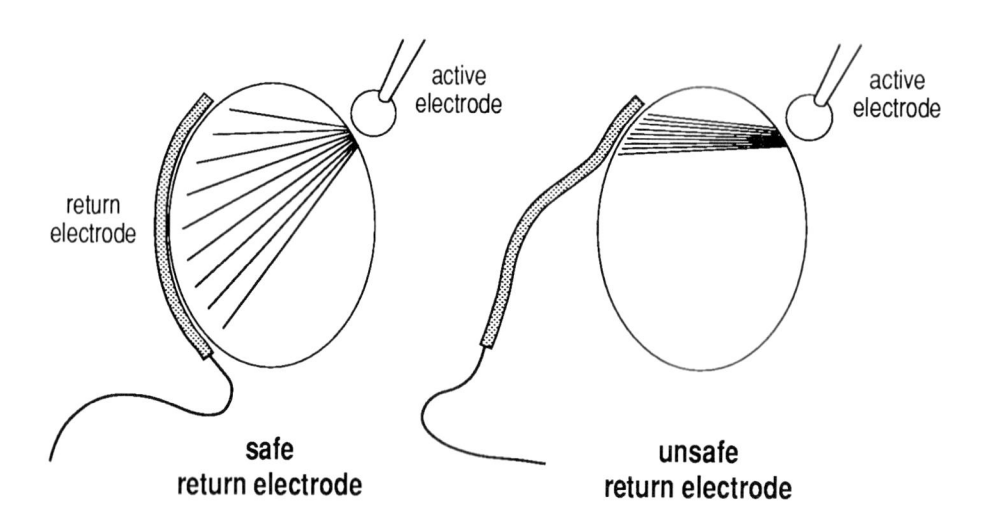

Figure 4.1 Return electrode burn. A) Safe condition with low current density under the return electrode. B) Unsafe condition with a high current density under the return electrode.

The other major consideration in choosing an ESU should be the power specifications of the particular unit and its performance. To date, all the large published series using large loop electrodes for loop excision have utilized electrosurgical generators that are relatively high-powered and capable of producing different types of blended current. These generators have been suitable for a variety of applications including those conducted in an operating room or a cystoscopy suite. In the published series, the ESUs have been operated in a blended cutting mode. The blended mode is a low-voltage, high-current waveform that is designed to provide rapid cutting with a moderate amount of hemostatic effect. Using this waveform, electrosurgery can be performed with a minimal amount of bleeding and yet the specimens produced have limited thermal damage allowing for histopathological analysis (see

Chapter 12). Most high quality ESUs have the capacity to produce a blended current.

Another feature of ESUs suited for loop excision is that they are designed to have a "rapid start" capacity. The "rapid start" capacity is achieved by microprocessor controlling the power output of the ESU which allows it to vary. This insures that electrosurgical cutting commences as soon as the loop electrode is activated and appears to reduce significantly the amount of thermal damage that is produced in a specimen. A number of ESUs have incorporated "rapid start" capacity into their design.

Another important feature of an ESU used for loop excision is that its coagulation mode produces a fulguration-type coagulation current that is powerful enough to insure hemostasis if significant bleeding occurs.

When considering ESUs, it is important to select a unit capable of producing at least 60 watts of power in the cutting mode and 60 watts of power in the coagulation mode. Although many ESUs can produce up to 300 watts of power, these high outputs are not necessary for the loop excision and, in fact, should not be used at high power outputs since that will cause too much thermal damage.

We prefer a unit with a digital power read out. This allows the excision to be performed at a specific power setting and allows precise control of the cutting process. Units in which power is controlled with knobs scaled 1-10 are more difficult to use since power output is usually not linear, e.g., a setting of 3 may equal 30 watts power output whereas a setting of 4 may produce 53 watts output. In addition, the actual power provided to the tissue at a given setting may vary from unit to unit. Therefore, these units require more clinical trial in arriving at acceptable cutting conditions. We also prefer units that allow the use of a foot pedal to activate the electrode, since this allows more precise control of the active electrode.

Generators should meet the American National Standard HP-18 for Electrosurgical Devices as opposed to being merely U.L.-approved for hospital use. This standard was designed specifically to "establish minimum safety and performance requirements for electrosurgical systems".[1] The American National Standard for Electrosurgical Devices HP-18 is endorsed by both the American National Standards Institute and the American Association of Medical Instruments which are nonprofit organizations interested in developing standards for medical instrumentation. We strongly feel that any ESU used for loop excisions of the cervix should meet this standard. This standard requires that safe grounding be used and that there be some form of return electrode monitoring system .

ELECTROSURGERY FOR HPV-RELATED DISEASES

Loop and Ball Electrodes

Loop electrodes specifically designed for electrosurgery can be purchased in a variety of sizes and styles. The original loop electrodes described by Prendiville were hemispherical and had an insulated T-shaped cross bar (Figure 4.2).

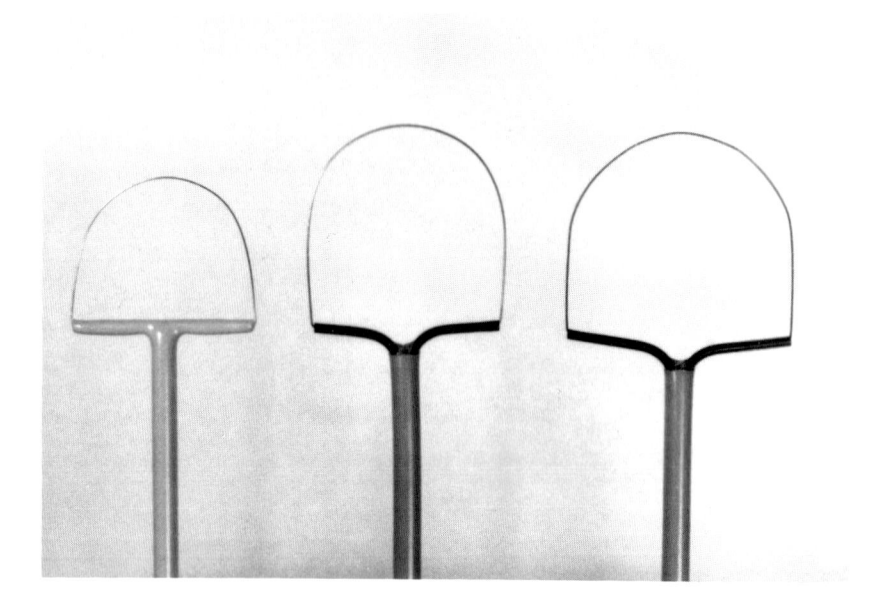

Figure 4.2. Large loop electrodes originally described by Prendiville. These electrodes range in size from 2.2 cm to 2.5 x 2.5 cm.

Caution

Unless the operator is careful, it is very easy to excise much more tissue than is desired. This is particularly a problem with the larger electrodes such as the 2.5 x 2.5 cm loop. The operator must guard against performing an inadvertent cone biopsy or complete trachelectomy when the intent was to excise a CIN to a depth of 0.6 to 0.8 cm.

The Prendiville-type large loop electrodes were fabricated of 0.20 mm, hard, stainless steel wire (Ormiston, London) and were made in a range of sizes from 1 cm wide by 1 cm deep to 2.5 cm wide by 2.5 cm deep. Although electrodes of this design are currently available in the U.S. from several manufacturers we do not recommend their use for loop excisional procedures on the cervix since it is easy to inadvertently excise far too much cervical tissue using these large electrodes. Figure 4.3 shows the relationship between a 2.0 x 2.5 cm loop electrode and a small nulliparous cervix. It is easy to visualize how inadvertently pushing the electrode too deeply into the cervix could result in almost totally removing the cervix.

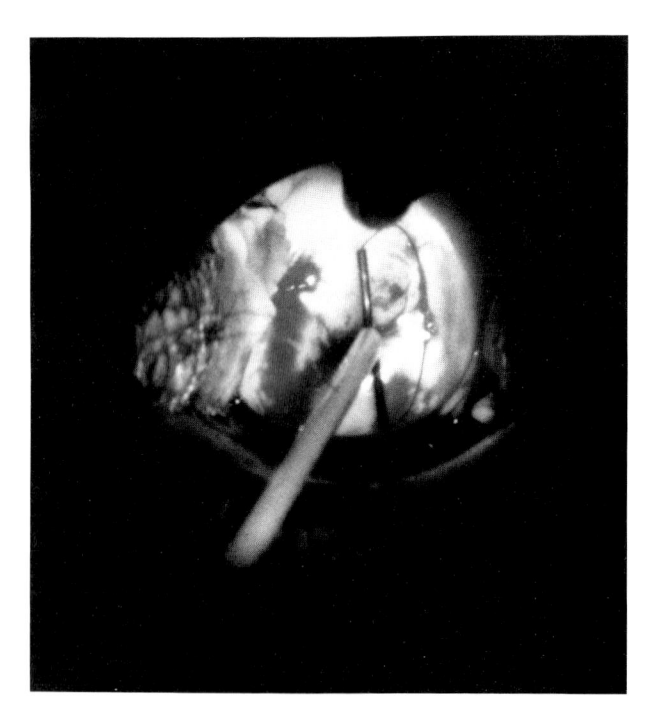

Figure 4.3 Relationship between 2.0 x 2.5 cm loop electrode and a small cervix.

In order to prevent the inadvertent excision of too much cervical tissue, we introduced the concept of using shallow electrodes designed to limit the amount of tissue that can be excised in a single pass (Figure 4.4). With the shallow loop electrodes, the depth of the excision is preset by the depth of the electrode selected. For example, when a 0.8 cm deep electrode is selected, the maximum depth of tissue that can be excised with a single pass is approximately 0.7 cm because the insulated cross bar at the base of the electrode will serve as a stop and prevent deeper penetration. Figure 4.5 compares the shallow loop electrode with the original Prendiville-style electrode. The concept of designing the loop electrode in such a way as to reduce the potential for inadvertently excising too much tissue has been adopted by a number of equipment manufacturers. Both disposable and non-disposable electrodes with the shallow loop design are currently available.

ELECTROSURGERY FOR HPV-RELATED DISEASES

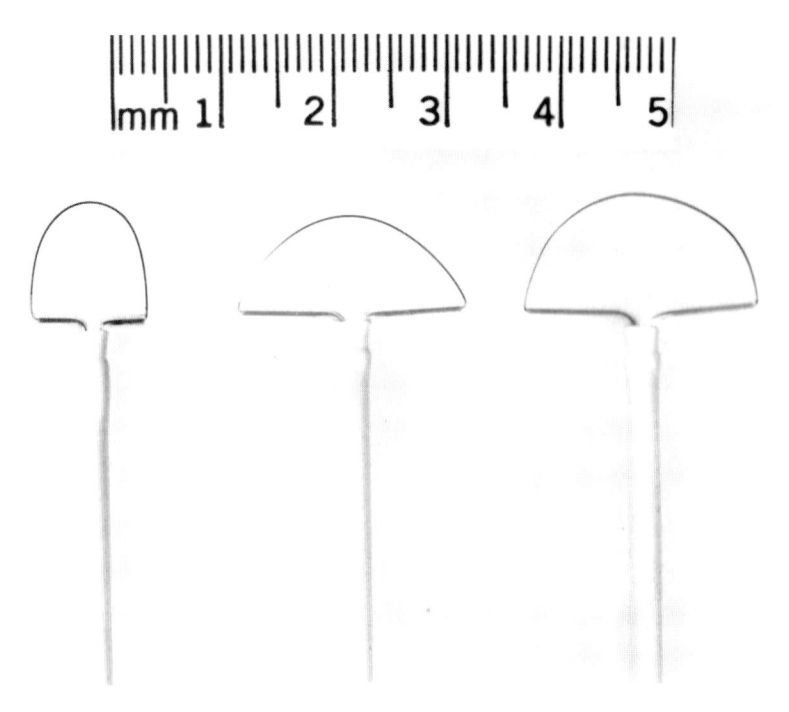

Figure 4.4. Shallow large loop electrodes. These electrodes were designed to limit the amount of cervical tissue that can be excised in a single pass and measure 1.0 or 2.0 cm in width but are only 0.8 or 1.0 cm deep. *(Electrodes courtesy of CooperSurgical, Inc.)*

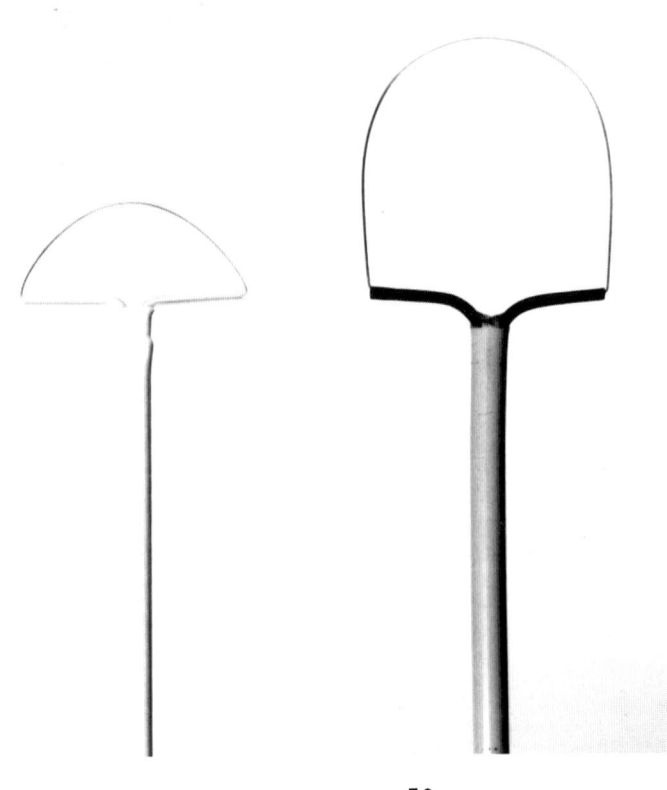

Figure 4.5 Comparison of shallow loop electrode and original large loop electrode. The large loop electrode measures 2.5 cm in depth by 2.0 cm wide whereas the shallow electrode measures 0.8 cm in depth by 2.0 cm wide.

EQUIPMENT FOR THE LOOP EXCISION PROCEDURE

Another style of electrode that effectively limits the amount of tissue that is excised in a single pass incorporates a movable T-shaped guide. With these electrodes, the amount of tissue that can be excised is limited by the setting at which the guide bar is placed. One of the advantages of this style electrode is that a wide range of depths can be set with only a single electrode. Disposable U-shaped electrodes with guides are currently available in the U.S. as well (Figure 4.6).

In the United Kingdom true loop-shaped disposable electrodes that are quite flexible are used by a number of clinicians (Figure 4.7). Although highly flexible electrodes are not commonly used in the U.S. and Canada, in England they are widely used and specialized excision techniques have been developed to maximize their effectiveness and to emphasize their "floppiness". We personally have difficulty in maintaining an even depth of excision using these electrodes since they tend to drag as they are pulled through the cervix.

Non-disposable wire loop electrodes can be purchased. We have been able to use non-disposable electrodes for 10 - 25 procedures, provided care is taken during the cleaning procedure. Ball electrodes used for cauterization can be used many more times (up to 100 in our experience). The use of non-disposable electrodes reduces the cost per excision when compared to the use of both a disposable wire loop and disposable ball electrode. If non-disposable

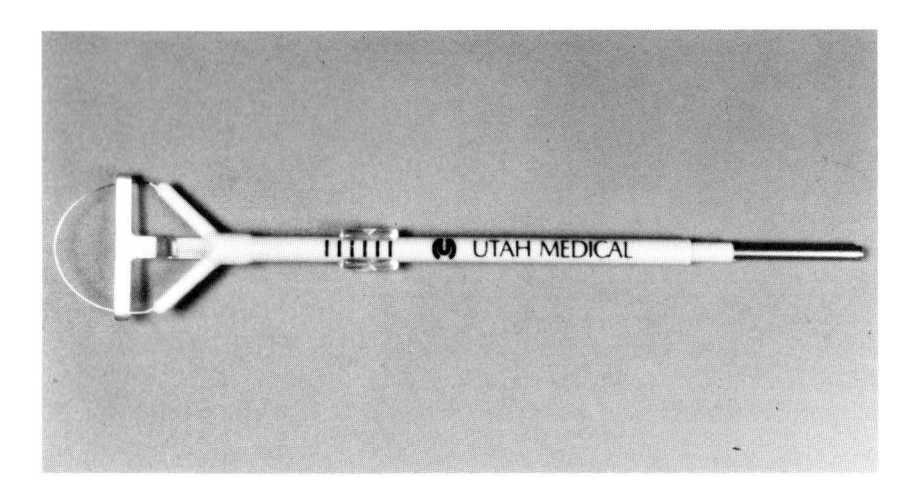

Figure 4.6. Variable depth U-shaped disposable electrode. These electrodes have a T-shaped bar that can be adjusted to limit the amount of tissue that is excised in a single pass. *(Electrode courtesy of Utah Medical Products, Inc.)*

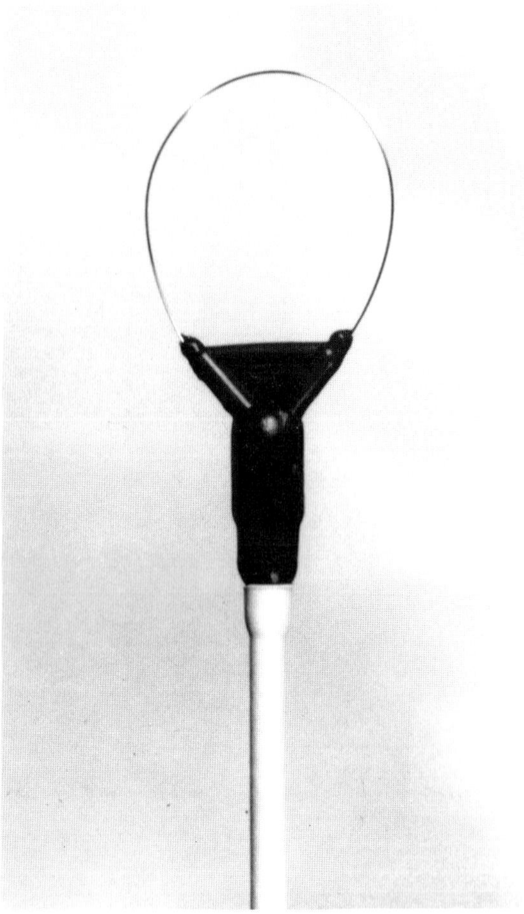

Figure 4.7. True loop style electrode of the type commonly used in the United Kingdom.

electrodes are used for the loop excision, it is very important that they be cleaned and sterilized correctly. Not only must all charred tissue be removed from the electrode surface but all the carbonized residue must be removed down to bright, shiny metal. In our clinic, we clean the electrodes by first soaking them in a strong detergent solution to loosen the char. We then use a soft "pot scrubber" type of cleaning pad (Scotch Brite™) to scrub the carbonized layer away from the wire. Electrodes can then be cold sterilized by soaking in a glutaraldehyde-containing sterilizing solution such as Cidex as described on the package insert. Some non-disposable electrodes (and also some disposable types) can be steam autoclaved.

In contrast to non-disposable electrodes, disposable electrodes are extremely convenient and eliminate the need to scour the char from the wire and sterilize the electrode. The use of disposable electrodes will also reduce variations in power requirements and thermal damage that sometimes occur when electrodes are reused repetitively. The principal disadvantage of disposable electrodes is their cost.

EQUIPMENT FOR THE LOOP EXCISION PROCEDURE

Different styles of loop electrodes are generally used for treating HPV-associated diseases of the vulva, vagina, perianal area and penis (see Chapter 9). For these sites we prefer to use a square or rectangular electrode rather than a true loop or radius electrode. The flat edge of the square or rectangular electrodes allows finer control of the depth to which a particular lesion is being excised compared to the standard loop electrode. It also allows the stalk of small condylomata to be excised without penetrating into the adjacent skin. We utilize either 1.0 x 1.0 cm square electrodes (Figure 4.8) or 1.0 x 0.4 cm rectangular electrodes (Figure 4.9) for removing condylomata. For most cases, we prefer the 1.0 x 0.4 cm electrode since there is less potential for inadvertently excising too much tissue. The 1.0 x 1.0 cm square electrodes are chiefly used for excising the endocervical canal when an electrosurgical loop excisional cone biopsy is performed (see Chapter 7).

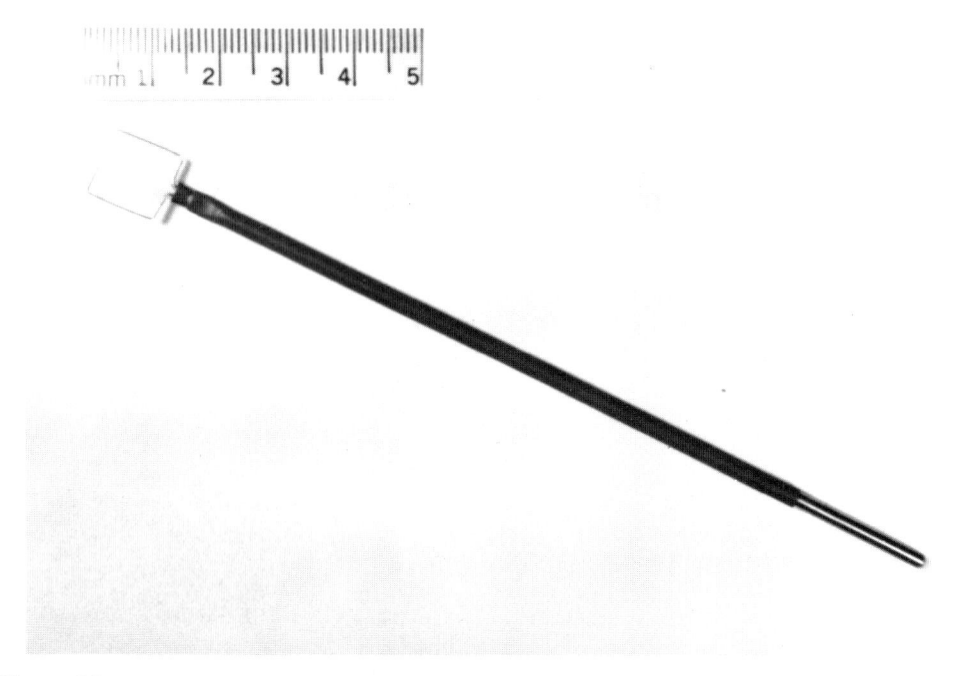

Figure 4.8. 1.0 x 1.0 cm square loop electrode used for electrosurgical cone biopsies and treating large external condylomata.

Small 1.0 cm in width by 0.4 cm in depth rectangular electrodes with short shafts can also be used for excising vulvar intraepithelial neoplasia (VIN) and vaginal intraepithelial neoplasia (VAIN) lesions or can be used any time it is important for the operator to control the depth of the excision more precisely (Figure 4.9) (see Chapter 10).

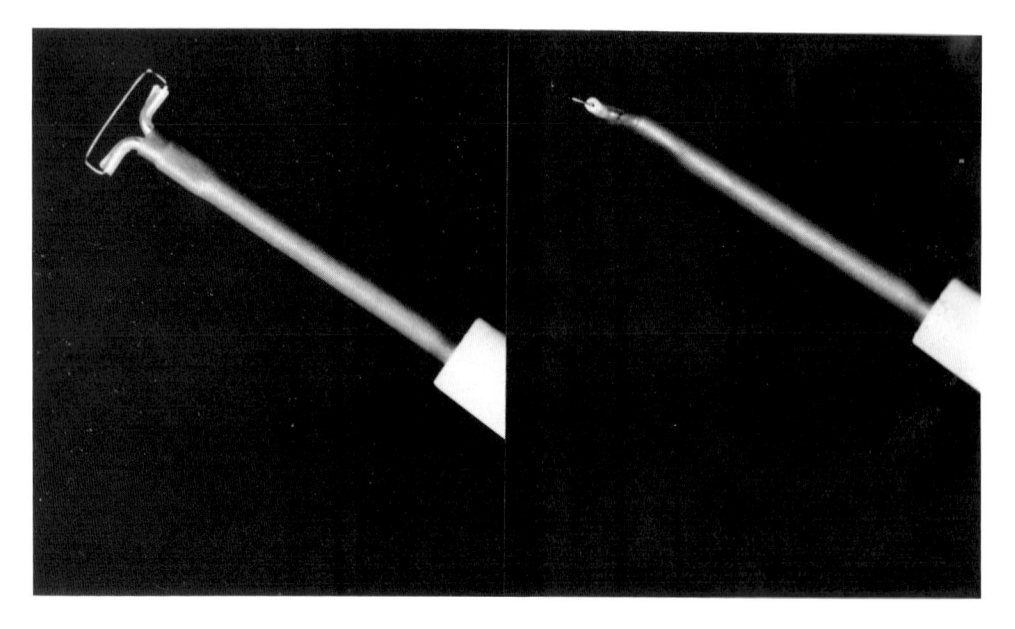

Figure 4.9. Shallow electrode for excising external anogenital lesions. *(Electrode courtesy of CooperSurgical, Inc.)*

Standard ball electrodes that generally measure either 3.0 mm or 5.0 mm in diameter (Figure 4.10) are used for fulguration (coagulation) in order to stop bleeding or to destroy lesional tissue. Ball electrodes are sold in both disposable and non-disposable forms.

We also frequently use needle electrodes. These are sold as very small diameter wires (microneedles) and larger diameter wires (macroneedles) (Figure 4.11). When used with either pure cutting current or a blended cutting current, microneedles are useful for excising vulvar lesions and performing cone biopsies. When used with coagulation current, macroneedles are superb for fulgurating (coagulating) small amounts of lesional tissue. The macroneedles can be used to apply direct coagulation current to a more localized area than with the 3 mm ball electrodes and are useful for stopping significant bleeding and destroying large condylomata.

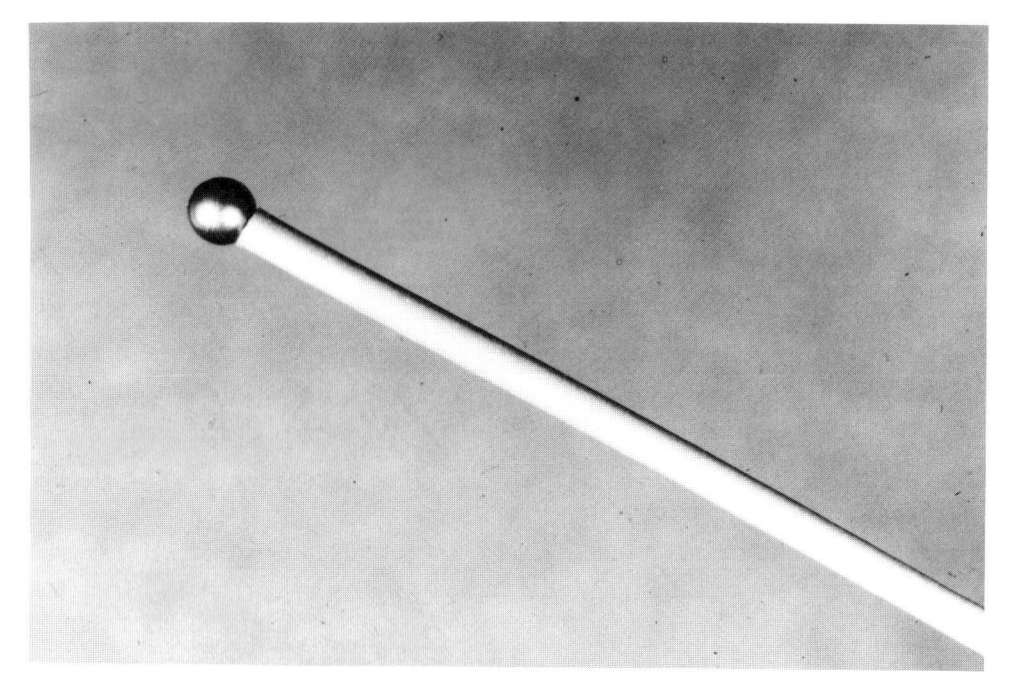

Figure 4.10. Ball electrode used for fulguration (coagulation) in order to stop bleeding or destroy lesional tissue.

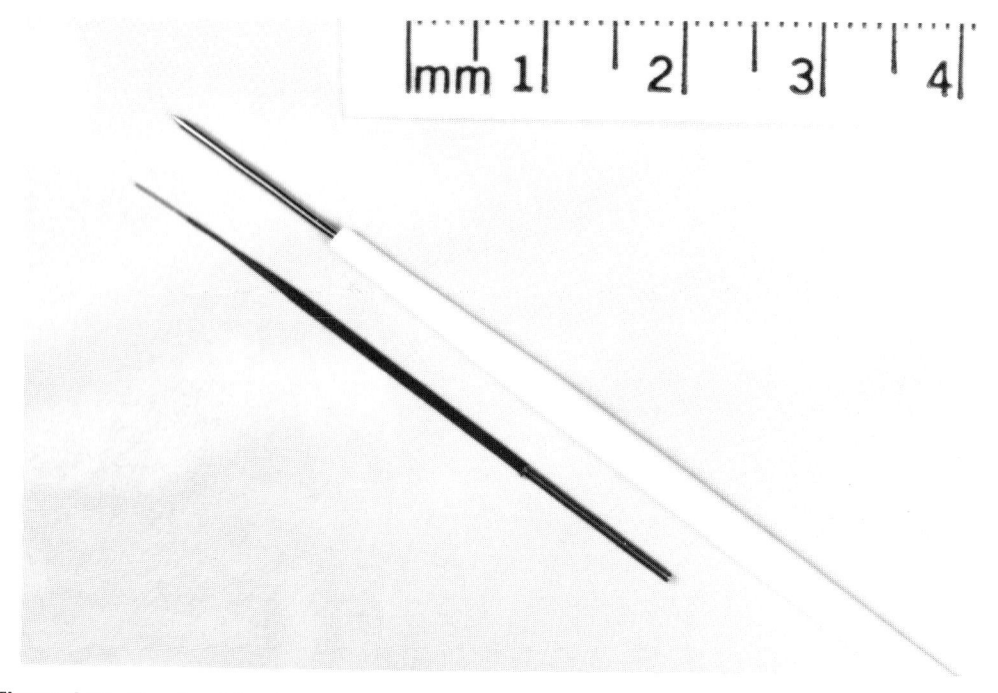

Figure 4.11. Needle style electrodes. These can be either thick macroneedle style electrodes or thin microneedle style.

Speculums, Vaginal Wall Retractors and Smoke Evacuators for Electrosurgery

It is important that a speculum of an adequate size to allow complete visualization of the cervix be used when performing the loop excision. Because there is the potential for contact between a metal speculum and an active electrode which will transmit a strong electric "shock" to the unanesthetized vagina, we recommend that nonconductive speculums be used for the procedure. Nonconductive speculums are sold in a variety of styles and include standard metal speculums that have been coated with a nonconductive material as well as specially designed plastic speculums (Figure 4.12).

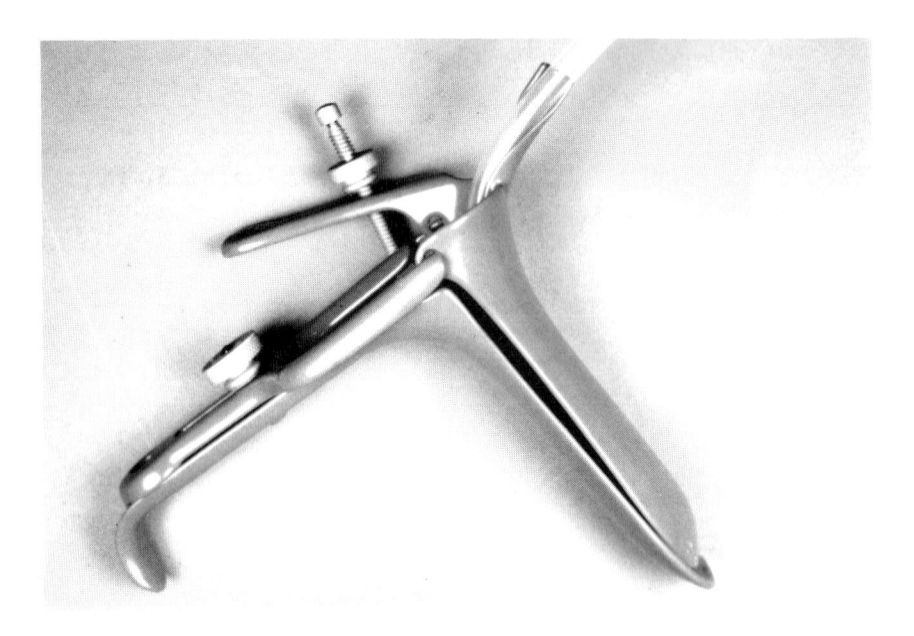

Figure 4.12. Specially coated, nonconductive speculum adapted for use with a smoke evacuator which prevents inadvertent shocks to the vagina. *(Speculum courtesy of CooperSurgical, Inc.)*

One word of caution about plastic speculums: The standard, disposable, clear plastic speculum frequently used in clinics and emergency rooms should not be used since they have a tendency to close inadvertently. If this happens during the procedure, undesired consequences could occur. If plastic speculums are used, we suggest that only speculums designed specifically for performing cervical loop electrosurgical procedures, which have a strong locking mechanism, be used.

EQUIPMENT FOR THE LOOP EXCISION PROCEDURE

The speculum used for loop excisions must be equipped for use with a smoke evacuator. A smoke evacuator is required for safely performing loop excisions. Unless a smoke evacuator is used, the operator will be unable to visualize the electrode during the procedure and there is a risk of inadvertently excising too much tissue or contacting the vaginal wall with the electrode. The smoke evacuator should be capable of removing particles at least as small as 0.1 micron in diameter (Figure 4.13). Removal of smoke from the vagina is best accomplished by using a speculum with a smoke evacuator tube built directly into it or by using a disposable plastic tube that is backed with adhesive tape and can be applied temporarily to a standard speculum. Smoke evacuators adequate for laser surgery are adequate for electrosurgery.

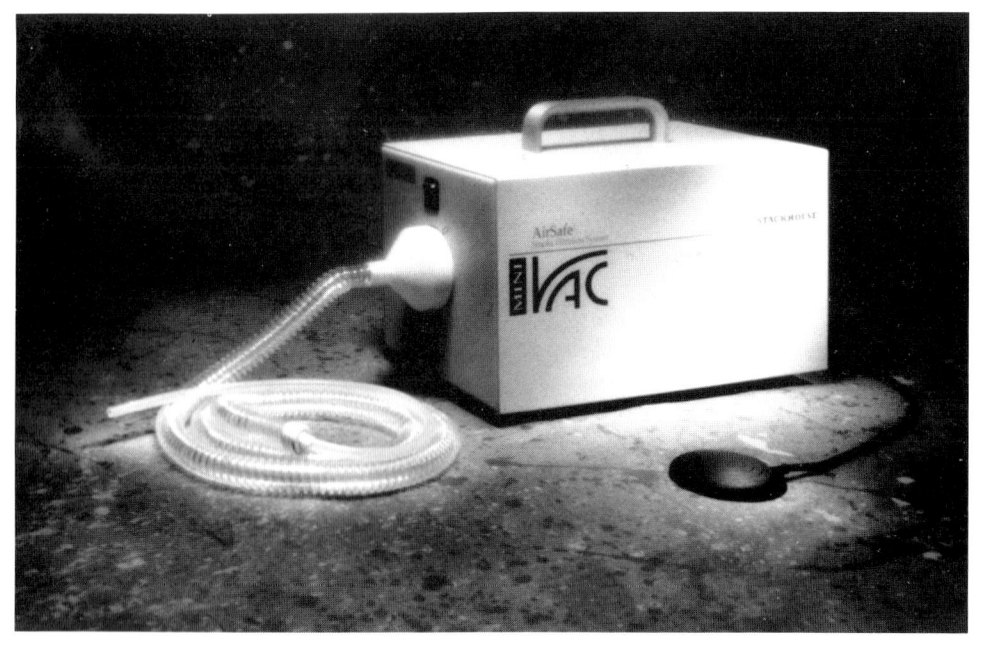

Figure 4.13 Smoke evacuator. A smoke evacuator is a requirement for loop excision of the cervix and is strongly recommended when performing electrosurgical fulguration procedures. *(Photograph courtesy of Cabot Medical Corp.)*

Recently some electrosurgical generators specifically designed for loop excision have incorporated smoke evacuators as an integral part of the generator (Figure 4.14).

ELECTROSURGERY FOR HPV-RELATED DISEASES

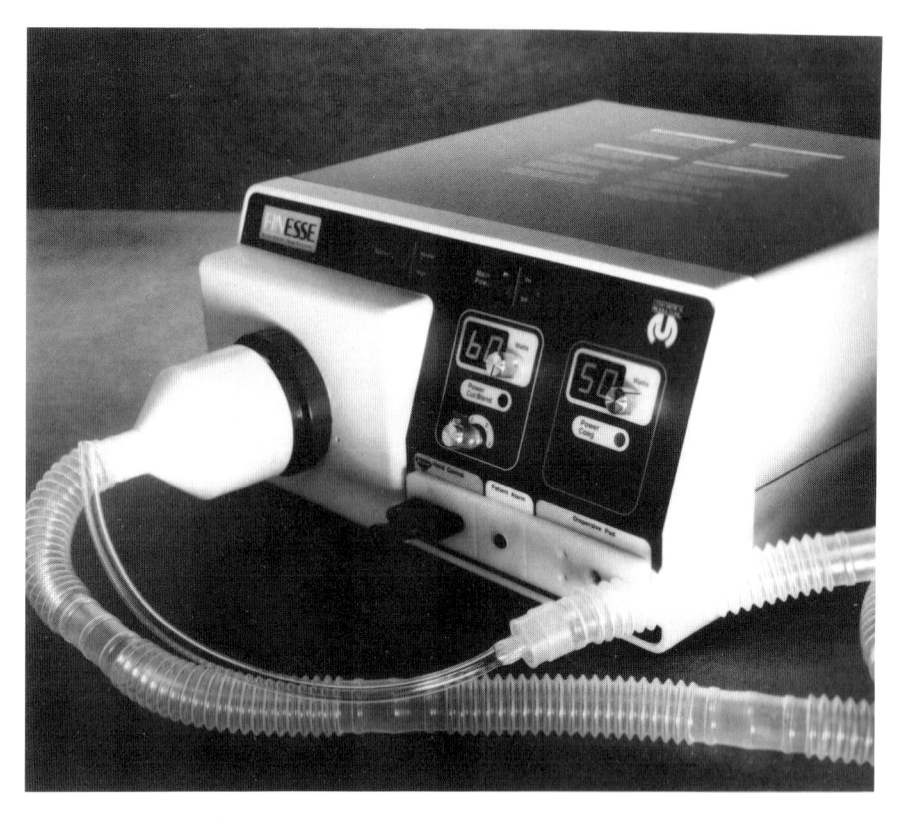

Figure 4.14. Electrosurgical generator that incorporates a smoke evacuator directly into the generator. *(Photograph courtesy of Utah Medical Products, Inc.)*

Another problem which frequently arises when performing electrosurgery on the cervix is the prolapse of the vaginal side walls into the field of view so the cervix cannot be visualized completely. This is particularly a problem in older patients who have had multiple pregnancies and who have considerable vaginal laxity. We frequently use an insulated vaginal wall retractor (Figure 4.15) in these patients to retract the vaginal sidewalls and to obtain an unobstructed view of the cervix. Another approach to this problem is to use two carefully inserted, moistened, wooden tongue blades between the cervix and the sides of the speculum.

Local Anesthesia for Electrosurgery

In the majority of cases, ectocervical loop excisions can readily be performed in the office but require anesthesia. In Prendiville's original description of the procedure, local anesthesia was obtained by infiltrating 5-10 ml of 3% prilocaine hydrochloride with 0.03% octapressin into the cervical stroma to produce an intracervical block. In the United States most clinicians use 2% xylocaine with 1:100,000 epinephrine to obtain an intracervical block.

EQUIPMENT FOR THE LOOP EXCISION PROCEDURE

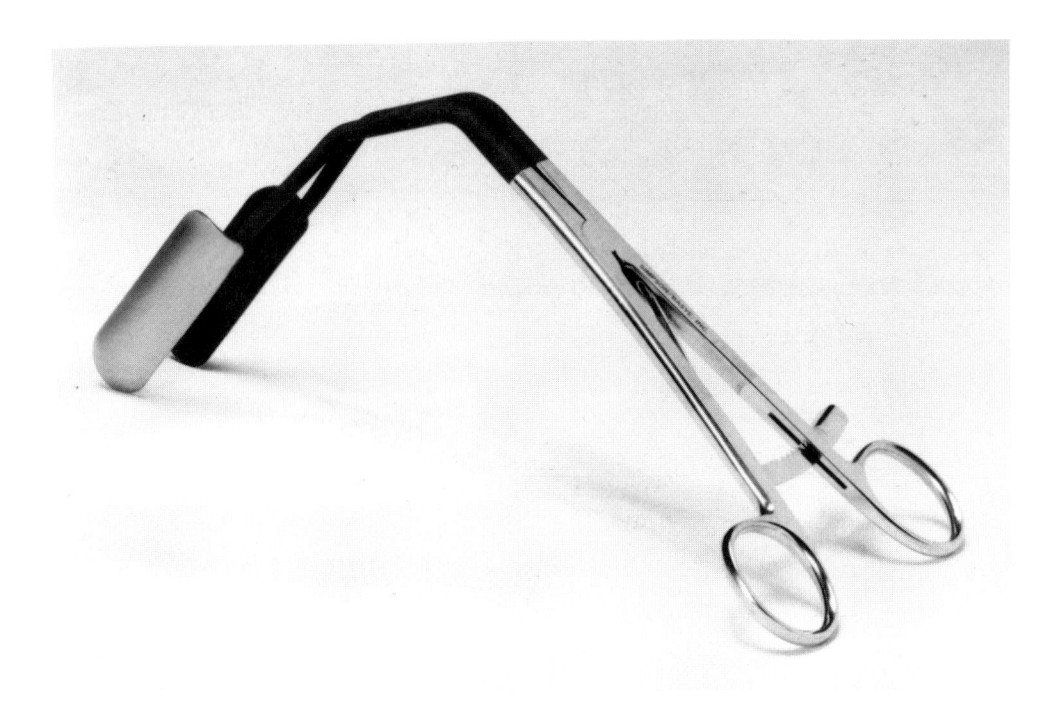

Figure 4.15. Nonconductive vaginal retractor used to retract the vaginal sidewalls while working on the cervix. *(Photograph courtesy of Simpson/Basye, Inc.)*

There are a number of techniques that can be used for injecting the local anesthetic into the cervix. Some clinicians prefer to use a 5 or 10 cc Luer-Lok syringe equipped with a 25 or 27 gauge spinal needle. We have found two problems with this approach. The first is that it is quite difficult to push the plunger and expel the anesthetic when this combination is used. The second is that the spinal needle tends to bend excessively before entering the cervix and, when it does enter, it tends to penetrate too deeply. Although the excessive bending of the spinal needle can be overcome by using a needle extender on the syringe and a shorter needle, we prefer to use a reusable metal dental aspirating syringe and prefilled, 1.8 ml ampules of anesthetic solution (Figure 4.16).

A variety of different formulations of anesthetic, including 1% or 2% xylocaine solutions with or without epinephrine, can be purchased in prefilled ampules to fit these syringes. A standard 27 gauge 1.5 inch dental needle can be used with the dental syringe. In most cases there is no problem in reaching the cervix with the needle. A reinforced, 8.5 cm long, 27 gauge needle which fits on the dental syringe and was designed specifically for injecting the cervix can also be used (Figure 4.16). In our opinion dental syringes equipped with either style needle are much more convenient and easier to use than Luer-Lok

ELECTROSURGERY FOR HPV-RELATED DISEASES

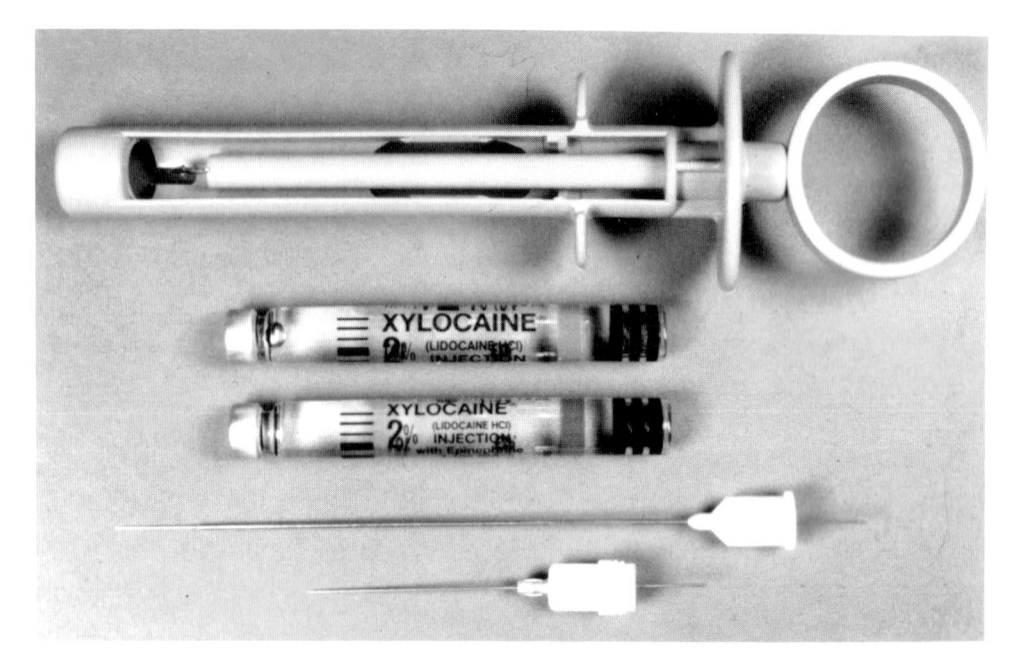

Figure 4.16. Dental aspirating syringe with prefilled ampules of 2% xylocaine with and without 1: 100,000 epinephrine. Both the standard 1.5 inch and a specially designed 8.5 cm extended 27 gauge needle are shown. *(8.5 cm extended needle courtesy of Euro-Med, Inc.)*

syringes and spinal needles. Recently, a new type of syringe specifically designed for injecting the cervix has been developed that uses standard 1.5 inch, 27 gauge dental needles and 1.8 ml prefilled ampules. This syringe is longer than the standard dental syringe which makes it easier to inject the cervix and is designed to deliver a measured amount of anesthesia (Figure 4.17). Dental syringes, modified dental-type syringes, needles and prefilled ampules of anesthesia can be obtained from dental supply houses and companies specializing in electrosurgical equipment.

Electrode Handles and Patient Return Electrodes

Two types of electrode handles are available for electrosurgery. Both types are disposable, pencil-type handles into which the loop electrodes are inserted (Figure 4.18). The difference between the two types of electrode handles is that a control switch for activating the electrode and selecting cutting and coagulating current is incorporated into some electrode handles whereas

EQUIPMENT FOR THE LOOP EXCISION PROCEDURE

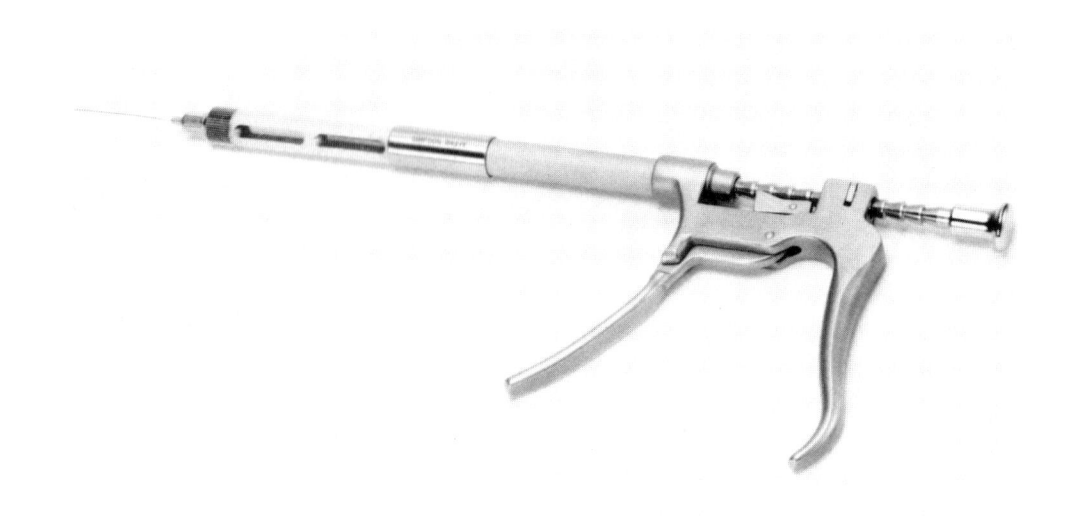

Figure 4.17. Special syringe designed specifically for injecting the cervix that utilizes dental needles and prefilled cartridges of anesthesia. *(Photograph courtesy of Simpson/Basye, Inc.)*

others lack such switches and are designed to be used with a footswitch connected to the ESU. We prefer to use a footswitch to activate the electrode, since the hand switched electrodes are more difficult to control.

The use of a high quality, patient return electrode is much more important in performing a safe electrosurgical procedure than is commonly recognized. Prior to the development of gel-type adhesives for attaching return electrodes to patients, electrosurgical burns beneath improperly attached return electrodes were common. A wide variety of styles of disposable (single use) patient return electrodes which have excellent adhesive properties are now readily available. In general, the stickier the return electrode pad is, the less likely it is to become detached during an electrosurgical procedure. For the loop excision, we attach the patient return electrode to the patient's thigh (Figure 4.19). This reduces the flow of the electrosurgical current through vital structures in the thorax and abdomen.

A safety feature that has been designed into some ESUs and return electrodes is the use of a special monitoring circuit which detects when a patient return electrode has become partially detached from the patient and inactivates the ESU before a burn can develop under the return electrode. Such monitoring

ELECTROSURGERY FOR HPV-RELATED DISEASES

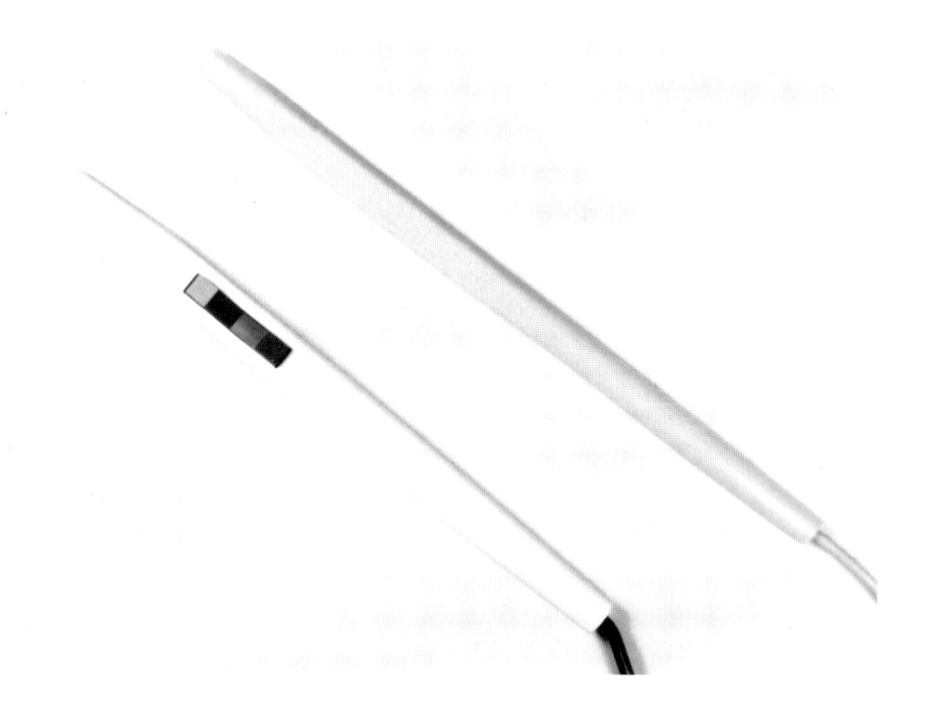

Figure 4.18. Pencil-type electrode handles. The one on the left incorporates a control switch for activating the electrode whereas the one on the right is designed to be used with a footswitch.

circuits add an extra margin of safety to electrosurgical procedures but are more expensive than standard patient return electrodes. Since loop excisions are generally performed under local anesthesia and employ relatively low power settings for short periods of time, it seems unlikely that significant burns would have a chance to develop under a partially detached return electrode before the patient becomes aware of pain at the site.

Monsel's Paste or Gel

At the end of the loop procedure we routinely pack the crater base with Monsel's paste or gel. Monsel's paste is made by allowing Monsel's solution (ferric subsulfate) to evaporate until it becomes a thick yellow paste which has the consistency of Dijon mustard. Prepared Monsel's gel is commercially available in the United States as part of a loop excision "prep kit" (Figure 8.2).

EQUIPMENT FOR THE LOOP EXCISION PROCEDURE

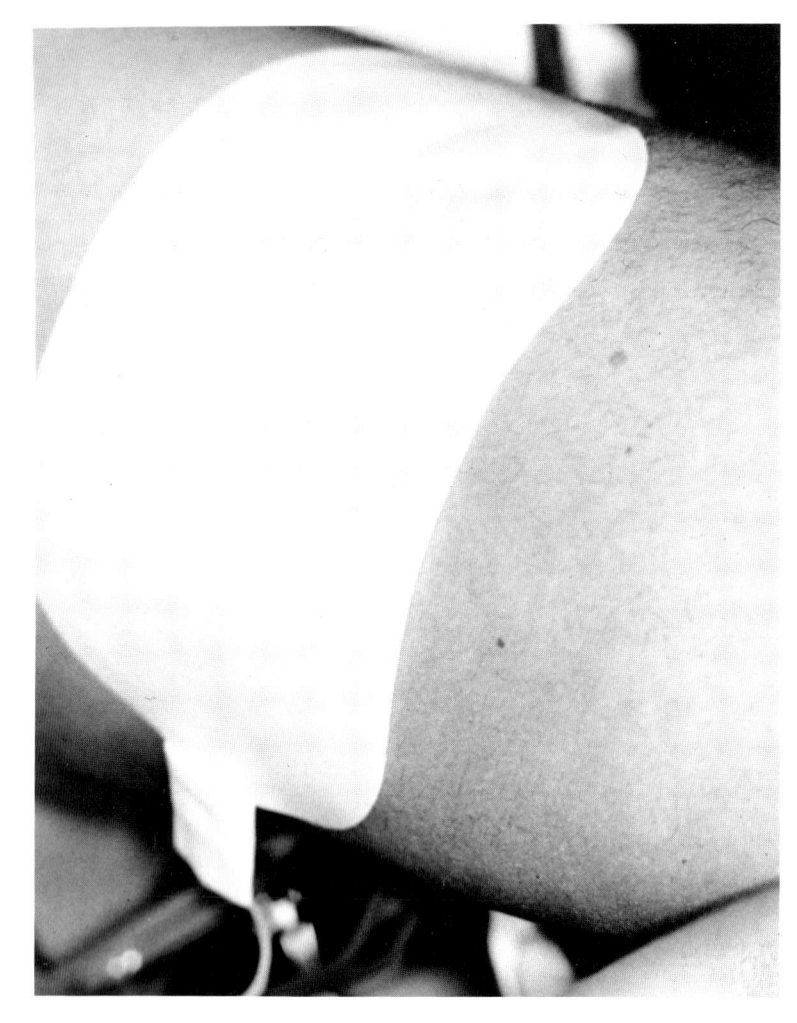

Figure 4.19 Patient return electrode. For electrosurgery the patient is grounded by attaching the patient return electrode to the thigh.

REFERENCES

1. AAMI American National Standard. *Safe Current Limits for Electromedical Apparatus.* Association for the Advancement of Medical Instrumentation, Arlington, VA. ANSI/AAMI ESI-1985, 1985.

ELECTROSURGERY FOR HPV-RELATED DISEASES

CHAPTER 5

DEVELOPMENT OF LOOP EXCISIONAL PROCEDURES

Electrosurgery in the form of excision/fulguration provides the clinician with a new and powerful technique for managing patients with cervical intraepithelial neoplasia (CIN) and other HPV-related lesions. Since this technique utilizes modern electrosurgical generators and thin wire loop electrodes to excise CIN lesions in their entirety, it offers a number of advantages over conventional, conservative therapies for the treatment of CIN (Table 5.1).

Table 5.1

Advantages of Electrosurgical Loop Excision

It is excisional as opposed to ablative and provides a tissue specimen for histological assessment.

It allows for the diagnosis and treatment of selected patients at a single visit.

It is fast and relatively easy to perform and learn.

It utilizes relatively inexpensive equipment.

The most important of these advantages is that electrosurgery provides a tissue specimen for histopathological assessment. This allows the pathologist to confirm the colposcopist's clinical impressions in every case and protects against the inadvertent ablation of an invasive cancer. The generation of a complete tissue specimen for histopathological assessment also allows for both diagnosis and management of selected patients to be performed in a single visit saving both the patient and the clinician significant time. Because of these advantages, electrosurgery has rapidly been adopted in Europe and the U.S. as the preferred method for treating precancerous and other HPV-related lesions of the cervix and other organs.

DEVELOPMENT OF ELECTROSURGERY—HISTORICAL ASPECTS
Studies Using Electrocautery to Treat Cervical Diseases

Electrocautery has been used since the early 1900s to treat cervical disease. Until 1928, electrocautery was used primarily as a method for treating chronic cervicitis or as a "prophylactic" measure for preventing the subsequent development of cervical cancer (Table 5.2). In 1906, Hunner reported on the use of electrocauterization as a means of preventing cervical cancer.[1] He treated 2,895 patients with "chronic cervicitis" using cervical cauterization and did not detect a single case of cervical cancer in this group of patients during the subsequent follow-up. Similarly, Huggins as well as Pemberton and Smith, reported that "prophylactic" electrocautery reduced the incidence of cervical cancer.[2,3] These results were widely interpreted as indicating that cauterization of chronic cervicitis and ectropion prevented the development of cervical cancer by eliminating both the cells and the infections from which cancers developed.

Because of these studies, electrocautery was frequently used throughout the 1930s and 1940s to "prophylactically" ablate the transformation zone in post-partum patients. The studies were relatively primitive epidemiologically but their strength was that they included large numbers of women who were

Table 5.2

Electrocautery as Prophylaxis for Cervical Cancer

Study / Year	# of Pts.	# of Cancers Observed
Hunner / 1906	2,895	0
Huggins / 1929	2,985	0
Pemberton and Smith / 1928	1,408	0
Peyton / 1963	10,500	0
Bouda / 1965	94,072	2

followed for relatively long periods of time after treatment. In a much larger series of patients treated by "prophylactic" cervical electrocautery, published in 1963 by Peyton and Rosen, it was reported that of 10,500 patients who underwent cervical electrocauterization before the age of 45, not a single case of cervical cancer was detected on follow up.[4] Similarly, Bouda and Dohnal presented a series of 94,072 patients who had undergone electrocauterization of cervix.[5] Only two cases of cervical carcinoma were subsequently detected in this population. Since the incidence of cervical cancer in the United States and Western Europe was approximately 44 per 100,000 women aged 20 years or older at this time, the finding of virtually no invasive cervical cancers in this large group of women convincingly demonstrated a reduction in the incidence of cervical cancer in women whose transformation zone was "prophylactically" ablated. "Prophylactic" ablation of the transformation zone as a cancer preventive measure is no longer advocated. However, it should be pointed out that "prophylactic" ablation of the transformation zone was justified at the time of these early studies because cervical cancer was the most frequent malignant neoplasm in women and there were no screening methods to detect its precursors.

These studies provided the basis for electrosurgical treatment protocols for CIN lesions that eventually led to the development of the loop excisional procedures since they clearly demonstrated that electrosurgery could be performed on the cervix with few complications.

Hyams' "Hot Wire" Cone Biopsies

The early electrocautery treatment protocols utilized resistance-type ball electrodes similar to soldering irons. As electric current flows through this type of electrode, they become "red hot". The electrodes can then be used to char or cauterize tissue but no tissue is obtained for pathological assessment. In 1928, Hyams introduced the concept of using electrosurgery to remove a core of endocervical tissue in patients with chronic cervicitis.[7,8] This tissue core could be examined histologically to rule out cervical cancer precursor. The electrode developed by Hyams for "hot wire" cone biopsy was triangular-shaped (Figure 5.1). To perform a cone biopsy, the electrode was inserted into the endocervix and rotated 360 degrees to remove a cylinder of endocervical tissue. For this procedure, the patient was grounded by putting a 6 inch square return electrode on her stomach with a wet sandbag placed on top of the electrode. The patient would apply pressure to the bag with both hands maintaining contact with the electrode. An anesthetic of crystalline cocaine hydrochloride was placed in the cervical canal.

Improvements were subsequently made in the electrode to allow the excision of wider portions of the exocervix and to reduce the amount of thermal artifact in the specimens.[9,10] Despite these improvements in electrode design, there remained a number of disadvantages to the Hyams' cone biopsy technique which prevented its use by most clinicians. One of the major disadvantages was that the specimens obtained with this method usually had extensive thermal artifact. This precluded complete histological assessment. In many cases invasive carcinoma could not be ruled out. The extensive thermal artifact was due to the relatively primitive design of the electrosurgical generators and electrodes used at that time.

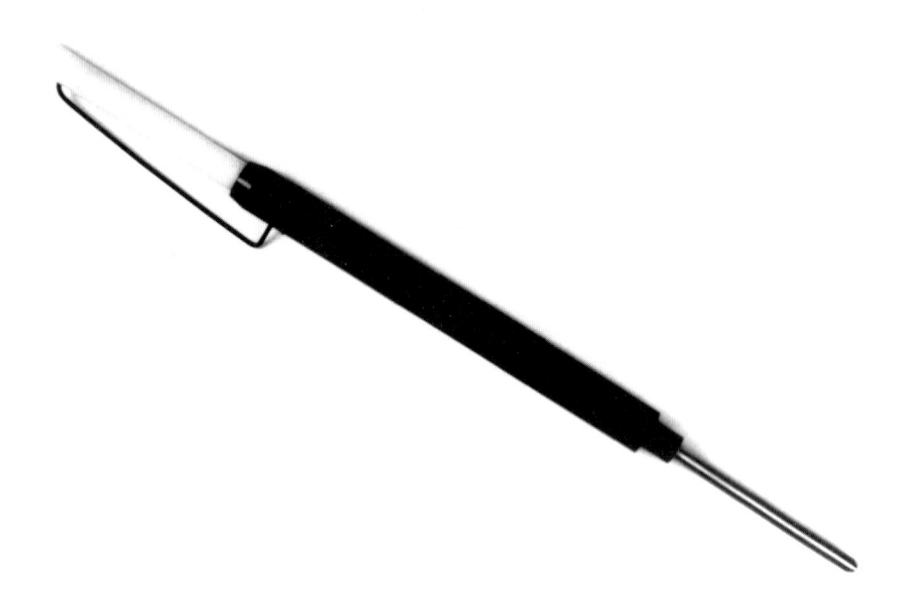

Figure 5.1. Hyams' style electrode for performing "hot wire" cone biopsies. Although the base and cross-bar are insulated, this type of electrode produces excessive thermal damage in the excised tissue.

Another problem with the "hot wire" cone biopsy was that many patients experienced severe post-conization bleeding 10-14 days after the procedure had been performed. Bleeding appeared to coincide with sloughing of the thick, cauterized eschar from the endocervical canal and was occasionally catastrophic, requiring emergency surgery and blood transfusions.[11] Patients who underwent electroconization also frequently complained of a profuse vaginal discharge. This, in turn, required daily douching and the use of intravaginal antibiotics. The other major problem with this technique was the high rate of cervical stenosis. This was especially a problem in patients over the age of 40. Because of these problems, "hot wire" cone biopsies fell into disfavor in the early 1950s, and most clinicians returned to the use of cold knife cone biopsies.

Recently Boulanger and co-workers published a comparative study of "hot wire" conizations using triangular electrodes and cold knife conizations.[12]

This study was performed between 1984 and 1988 and involved 38 patients in the cold knife group and 88 patients in the "hot wire" conization group (Table 5.3).

Although the frequency of perioperative and postoperative hemorrhage after "hot wire" conization was lower in this recent series than in the series performed in the 1930s to 1950s, there still were occasional cases in which the pathological specimen was considered to be inadequate secondary to extensive thermal damage.

Table 5.3

Comparison of Different Modalities of Conization

Method	Perioperative Bleeding	Postoperative Bleeding	Inadequate Specimen	Cervical Stenosis
Cold Knife	22%	7%	0%	0%
"Hot Wire"	7%	3%	1%	4%

Electrocautery for the Treatment of CIN

When Pap smears began to be used for the widespread detection of cervical cancer and its precursors, few therapeutic options existed for treating the cervical cancer precursors (CIN) that were detected by cytological screening programs. Either a hysterectomy or a cone biopsy was performed in almost all cases. Both of these surgical approaches had obvious disadvantages including the loss of reproductive capacity after hysterectomy, and the complications of bleeding, stenosis, and infertility after cone biopsy. Because of these problems, clinicians searched for ways to non-surgically (conservatively) manage cervical cancer precursor lesions. The earlier studies using electrocautery to ablate the transformation zone "prophylactically" led Paul Younge who was working at the Free Hospital for Women in Boston in the 1940s, to investigate the efficacy of electrosurgical ablation as a treatment modality for CIN.[13] Younge's series consisted of 43 patients with biopsy-proven carcinoma *in situ* (CIN 3) who either presented an unacceptable surgical risk for undergoing hysterectomy or cone biopsy or had refused surgical

ELECTROSURGERY FOR HPV-RELATED DISEASES

treatment of their cervical lesions. Because these women could not undergo standard therapy, Younge used fulguration applied with ball style electrodes and Bovie-type electrosurgical generators to destroy the CIN lesions (Figure 5.2).

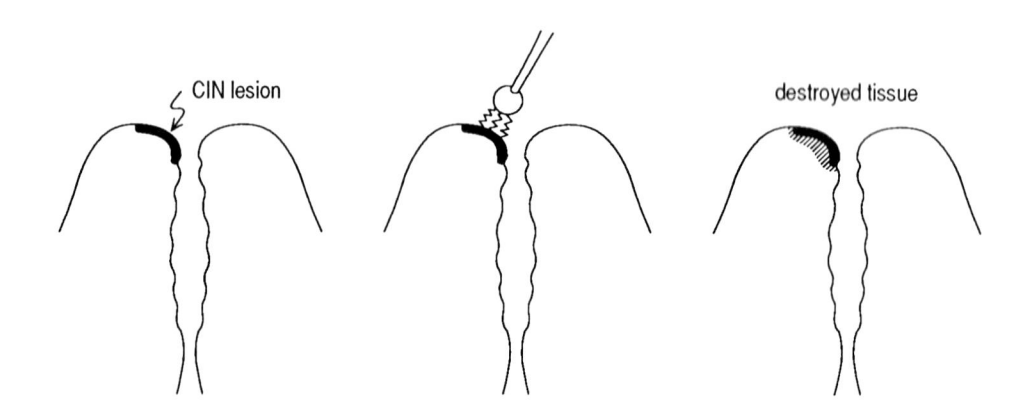

Figure 5.2. Use of a ball type electrode to electrocoagulate (fulgurate) a CIN lesion.

Sixteen of these patients who had been treated with fulguration were followed for 5-12 years. Of these sixteen, four had persistent/recurrent disease detected 1-14 months after fulguration and subsequently underwent hysterectomy or radiation therapy. Twenty-seven of the patients were followed for 16 months to 4.5 years and ten of these patients later were treated either by a hysterectomy or radiation for persistent/recurrent carcinoma *in situ*. Younge found that when carcinoma *in situ* involved both the glands and the surface of the cervix, the failure rate of fulguration was 63%. In contrast, when only the surface was involved, the failure rate was 15% (Table 5.4). This difference apparently reflected the capacity of electrosurgical generators (ESUs) and electrodes used at that time to coagulate effectively to the base of the glands, and may also have been effected by extension of disease into the endocervix in the patients with gland involvement since disease extending into the endocervical canal is quite difficult to treat with electrocautery.

The excellent results in patients with limited disease led Younge to suggest that selected patients with carcinoma *in situ* who desired to maintain their reproductive function be offered electrocauterization (fulguration) as an alternative to hysterectomy or cone biopsy. This early study also assessed the effects of electrocautery on pregnancy and observed that 6 of the 29 patients whose carcinoma *in situ* was cured by electrocautery went on to become pregnant.

Table 5.4

Results of Electrocautery for Treating CIN

Extent of CIN (Carcinoma *in situ*)	Failure Rate
Surface Involvement Only	15%
Gland Involvement	63%

The first prospective use of fulguration (electrocautery) to ablate CIN was not published until 20 years after Younge's original study (Table 5.5). In 1968, Richart and Sciarra published a study of 170 patients with CIN who were treated with fulguration rather than undergoing cone biopsy or hysterectomy.[6] The ablations were performed on an out-patient basis without local anesthesia using an older model Bantam Bovie Electrocoagulation Unit. All 170 patients

Table 5.5

Electrocautery and Fulguration as a Treatment for CIN

Study / yr	Electrocautery (EC) or Fulguration (F)	# of Pts.	Success Rate
Younge / 1949	F	43	68%
Richart / 1968	F	170	89%
Ortiz / 1973	EC	148	92%
Schuurmans / 1984	EC	413	86%
Chanen / 1985	F	1,734	98%
Deigan / 1986	EC	724	89%

had histologically diagnosed CIN and were followed for 12 to 16 months after fulguration. Although all grades of CIN were included in this series, only 3%

of the women had CIN 3 (Table 5.6). Sixty-seven percent had CIN 1. A single application of fulguration produced a success rate of 89% in these patients. The success rate increased to 95% after two applications of fulguration. Although the number of patients with CIN 3 was small in this series, it appeared that fulguration was not very effective in these patients (Table 5.6).

Table 5.6

Effectiveness of Fulguration for Treating CIN

Cytologic Diagnosis	# of Pts.	% Response
CIN 1	114	88%
CIN 2	51	98%
CIN 3	5	60%

Since the prospective study of Richart and Sciarra was published, a number of other studies[6,13-17] have confirmed that fulguration or electrocautery for CIN has an excellent therapeutic success rate (Table 5.5). However, despite the effectiveness of electrocautery and fulguration for treating CIN, there were a number of drawbacks that greatly reduced its appeal (Table 5.7).

One significant problem with electrocautery and fulguration was that cervical stenosis often occurred after treatment. This was such a problem in older women that it was suggested that they were contraindicated as a treatment modality in women over 40 years of age.[18] Perhaps the most significant drawback was that the ESUs available in the 1960s produced significant galvanic contractions of the uterus resulting in severe corpus pain. In addition, smoke evacuators were not available and the smoke produced by this procedure was quite offensive to both the patients and the staff. Significant post-cauterization bleeding was an infrequent complication. Sufficient bleeding to result in hospitalization occurred in only one patient in the series of Richart and Sciarra. This is a surprise, considering the high frequency of post-treatment bleeding after "hot wire" conizations.

Table 5.7

> **Disadvantages of Electrocautery and Fulguration for CIN as Practiced in the 1960s and 70s**
>
> Recessed squamocolumnar junction in 70% of patients.
>
> Frequent cervical stenosis in patients over 40 yrs.
>
> Causes significant corpus pain.
>
> Not effective for CIN 3.

In the early 1970s, cryosurgery became widely available. Because of problems associated with electrocautery and electrosurgery, these modalities became unpopular in North America and Europe. The one place fulguration continued to be used was in Australia where William Chanen popularized the use of a technique that he termed "radical electrocoagulation diathermy" for treating CIN.[16,19] Radical diathermy is a fulguration technique that utilizes ball-type electrodes to ablate the superficial portions of CIN lesions. This superficial fulguration is then combined with deep desiccation that is achieved by inserting needle electrodes 1.5 cm into the cervical stroma to produce extensive necrosis (Figure 5.3).

Radical electrocoagulation diathermy, as practiced by Chanen, had a spectacular success rate. In one series of 1734 patients published in 1985[16], Chanen reported a success rate of 98% for this technique although it should be noted that this number indicates only the percentage that did not have to undergo cone biopsy or hysterectomy and that the success rate for a single treatment was slightly lower (96%). Despite this success rate, there were a number of drawbacks to this technique (Table 5.8).

Because of the extensive necrosis obtained by inserting needle electrodes 1.5 cms into the cervical stroma and the requirement for cervical dilation to reduce the incidence of cervical stenosis, it was necessary to perform this procedure under general anesthesia. Another problem was in the majority of patients (60%), radical diathermy drove the squamocolumnar junction deep into the endocervical canal. This prevented complete colposcopic evaluation of the patient in the event of subsequent atypical smears.

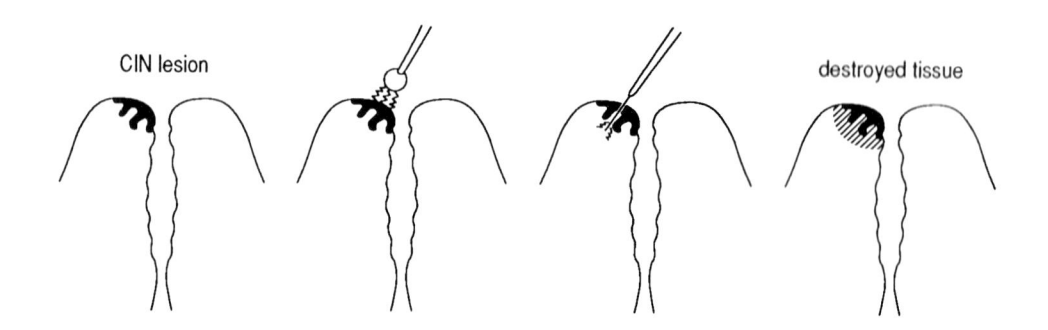

Figure 5.3. Radical diathermy. The procedure destroys tissue by a combination of deep desiccation and superficial fulguration.

Serious post-treatment bleeding and cervical stenosis were relatively infrequent after radical electrocoagulation diathermy. More recently, Chanen published a modification of his technique that allows it to be performed on an out-patient basis.[19] The results with the modified technique appear also to be excellent, although broad clinical experience with the modified technique is limited.

Table 5.8

Disadvantages/Complications of Radical Electrocoagulation Diathermy

Requires general anesthesia and cervical dilatation.

Recessed squamocolumnar junction in 60%.

Cervical stenosis in 0.5%.

Serious secondary hemorrhages in 1.4%.

DEVELOPMENT OF LOOP EXCISIONAL PROCEDURES

Early Studies Using Thin Wire Loop Electrodes to Diagnose CIN

The use of thin wire loop electrodes to excise CIN is conceptually a totally different therapeutic approach than ablating CIN by fulguration. Although both approaches use electrosurgical generators and high-frequency alternating currents, in one, a specimen is made available for histopathologic analysis whereas in the other, the lesional tissue is destroyed.

Dermatologists have used wire loop electrodes and small electrosurgical generators to excise dermatological lesions for many years. Because the lesions removed are generally very small, this procedure is easy, safe, and generally produces cosmetically acceptable results. The first person to apply this technology (wire loop electrode) to the cervix was Raoul Palmer in France. After the Second World War, Palmer began using rounded wire loop electrodes no greater than 6 mm. in diameter to treat cervical lesions.[20] These loop electrodes were essentially a dermatological loop electrode that was placed on a longer insulated shaft to allow the electrode to be used through the vaginal speculum (Figure 5.4).

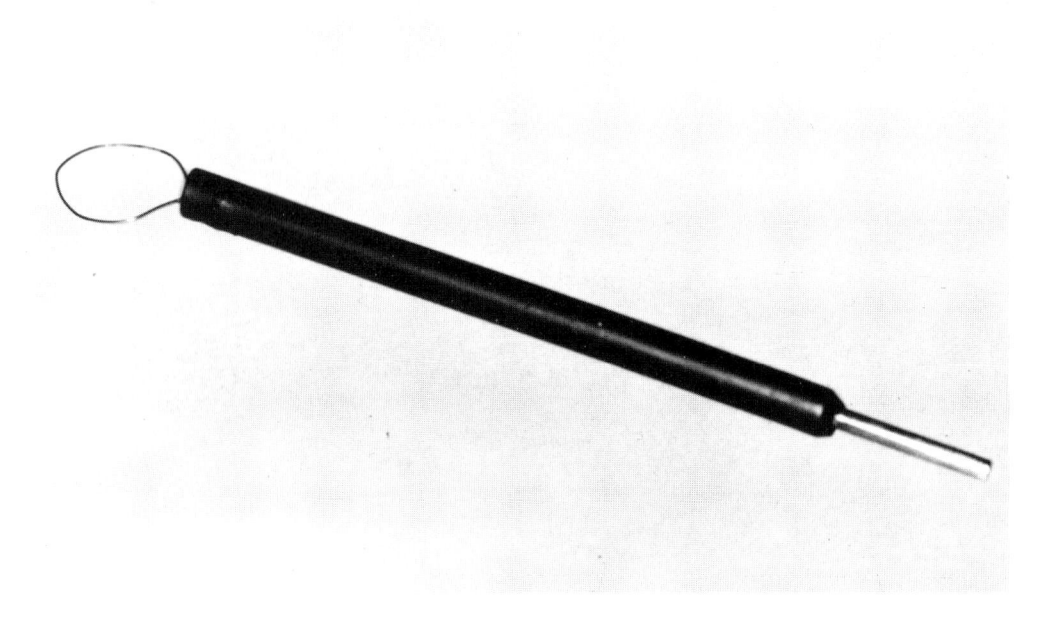

Figure 5.4. Loop electrode of the type used by Palmer. The circular loop is made of thick wire and inserted into an extended shaft.

ELECTROSURGERY FOR HPV-RELATED DISEASES

Although Palmer experimented with these electrodes for a variety of conditions, for the most part they were used to treat cervicitis and polyps. The usefulness of the electrodes was limited by their small size and primitive design which incorporated very thick wire. This caused extensive thermal injury and precluded them from being used to take cervical biopsies. Because of the rounded design, it was hard to excise cervical tissue to an even depth. In addition, it was almost impossible for the pathologist to orient the "shavings" in any meaningful manner to allow pathological interpretation, since the excised tissue had rounded edges and varying thicknesses.

Rene Cartier, who was a student of Palmer, became interested in using these wire loop electrodes (i.e., diathermy loop) both as biopsy instruments and as a therapeutic technique for CIN[21,2] (diathermy = electrosurgery, see Chapter 3). Cartier, who is still practicing pathology and colposcopy in Paris, was concerned, at the time, that the standard cervical biopsy, taken with biopsy forceps, often lacks sufficient depth for the pathologist to rule out stromal invasion that might arise from CIN that had extended into endocervical glands. He decided to use loop electrodes to obtain large cervical biopsies. To allow better orientation of the excised tissue during histological processing, Cartier designed a rectangular, as opposed to a circular, loop electrode (Figure 5.5).

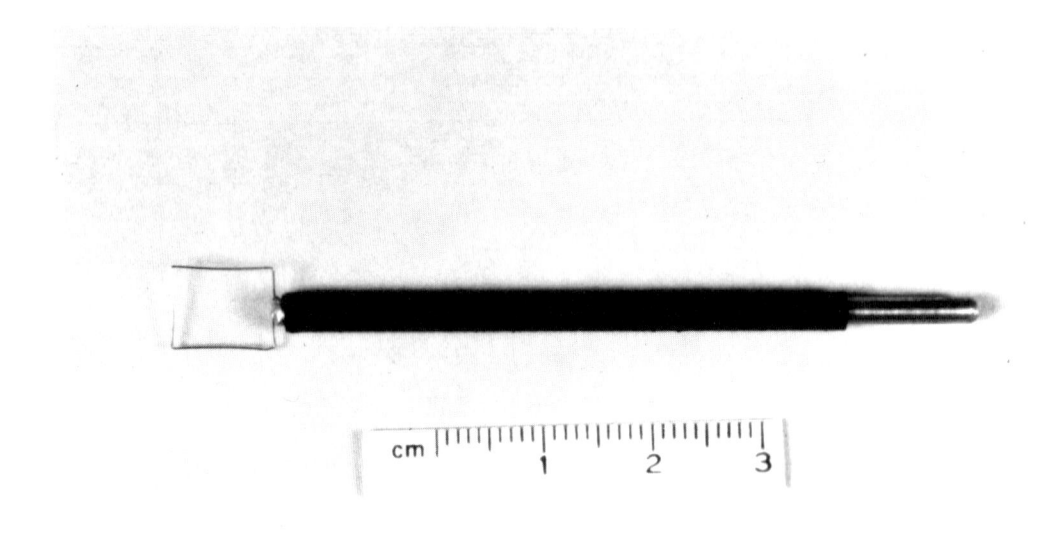

Figure 5.5. Diathermy loop electrode used by Cartier for taking large cervical biopsies. The rectangular electrodes measured approximately 7 mm square and had uninsulated bases.

Because of the hemostatic effects of the electrosurgical current, Cartier found that large biopsies could be obtained using these electrodes with a minimum of bleeding. The early rectangular Cartier electrodes measured 5 mm to 7 mm in width and were generally 7 mm deep. They were fabricated of a narrower gauge wire than used by Palmer to reduce the amount of thermal damage in the excised tissues. Using these electrodes, Cartier could readily obtain a deep cervical biopsy that could easily be oriented for pathological examination and had a minimal amount of thermal damage. In his textbook of colposcopy, Cartier lists his indications for using the diathermy loop electrode for cervical biopsy as including any situation in which it is necessary to obtain a wide and deep biopsy that can be oriented correctly (Table 5.9).

Table 5.9

Cartier's Indications for "Diathermy Loop" Biopsy

Rule out invasive or microinvasive cancer in larger lesions where it is necessary to excise through a large amount of necrotic tissue.

Patients with probable carcinoma where deep biopsies are needed to detect invasion.

Any lesion where there is a thick squamous epithelium such as a condyloma.

CIN where there is probable deep gland involvement.

Fibrotic cervices where forceps might skip, such as in previously treated patients.

Prendiville and co-workers published a study in 1986 comparing the size and quality of biopsies obtained with Cartier's wire loop "diathermy" electrodes to those obtained using a standard Yeoman's rotating biopsy forceps (Table 5.10).[23]

The size of biopsies obtained electrosurgically was significantly greater than that obtained with biopsy forceps (Table 5.10). More importantly, there were no significant differences in the extent of tissue artifacts in the two types of cervical biopsies. Although the electrosurgically obtained biopsies often had considerable thermal damage that obscured the cytological details of the surface epithelium, in biopsies obtained with the forceps, the surface epithelium was often stripped away from the underlying stroma. In terms of accuracy of diagnosis, Prendiville concluded that the larger biopsies obtained with the wire loop electrodes should allow a more accurate diagnosis to be made. There are a number of disadvantages to this technique, however, which tempered its acceptance (Table 5.11).

Table 5.10

Punch Biopsy vs. "Diathermy Loop" for Cervical Biopsy

Instrument	Mean Depth (mm)	Mean Length (mm)	Artifact Score (0-4)
Biopsy Forceps	1.5	2.9	1.3
Diathermy Loop	3.3	5.9	1.7

Table 5.11

Diathermy Loop Electrodes Compared to Biopsy Forceps for Cervical Biopsies

Provide wider, deeper cervical biopsies allowing more accurate diagnosis.
Increased patient discomfort—requires local anesthesia.
More bleeding from biopsy site.
Requires more time to perform.

Unless local anesthesia is used, wire loop biopsies are painful. Although local anesthesia can readily be obtained by injecting xylocaine solution into the biopsy site, this is time consuming and also causes patient discomfort. Another problem is that bleeding often occurs from the biopsy site despite the fact that an electrosurgical current with its attendant hemostatic effects is used. In many patients it is necessary to coagulate (fulgurate) the biopsy crater to achieve hemostasis.

DEVELOPMENT OF LOOP EXCISIONAL PROCEDURES

Electrosurgery for the Treatment of CIN

Cartier also developed the concept of using loop electrodes (diathermy loops) for the therapeutic excision of CIN. Cartier felt that diathermy loop excision was an especially good procedure for treating young women who wanted to preserve their fertility.

Using the small rectangular loop electrodes that he had designed, CIN lesions had to be removed in multiple sections (often referred to as "strip-mining") (Figure 5.6).

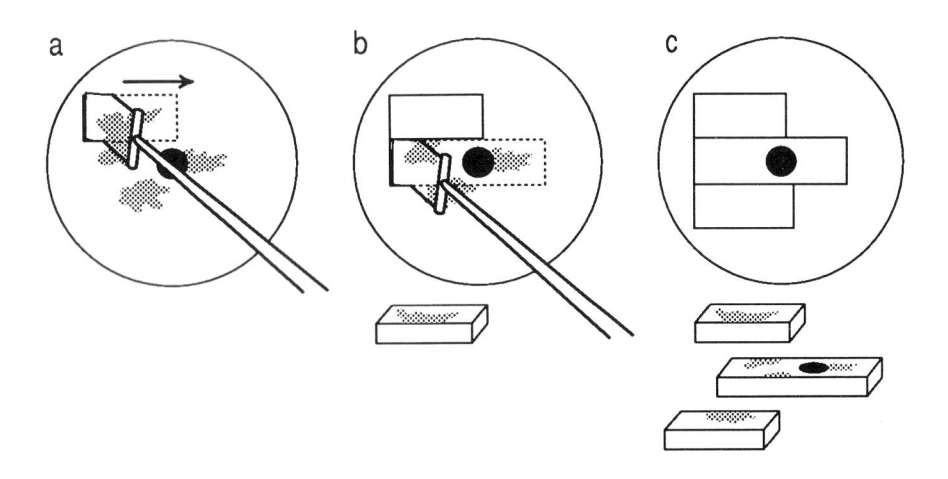

Figure 5.6. Use of small rectangular loops to remove CIN in multiple strips.

The diathermy loop excision procedure that Cartier developed was designed strictly for ectocervical lesions which met the criteria in Table 5.12.

Because multiple strips were removed with this procedure, Cartier advocated the use of detailed drawings to show the location of the individual strips. In addition, the strips were processed by the pathology laboratory in such a way that their orientation and the status of the margins of surgical excision could be assessed (Figure 5.7).

ELECTROSURGERY FOR HPV-RELATED DISEASES

Table 5.12

Cartier's "Diathermy Loop" Excision of CIN

The squamocolumnar junction was on the ectocervix or at the external os.

The os was sufficiently wide so that stenosis does not develop after excision.

Lesions did not extend onto the vagina.

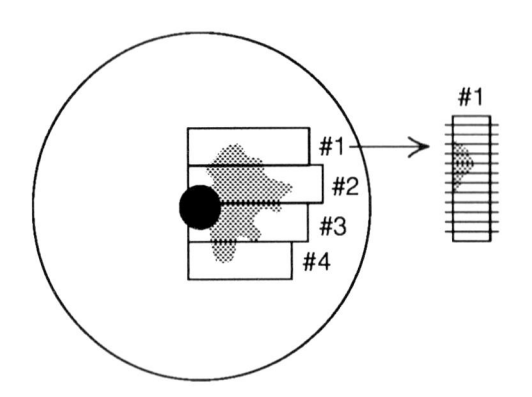

Figure 5.7. Diagram of the type used by Cartier to designate location of each of the excised strips (Modified from ref. 21.)

Cartier presented the method for "diathermy loop" excisions of CIN at the IV World Congress on Colposcopy and Cervical Pathology in the early 1980s[22] and numerous people took his methods back to their laboratories and tried them. In general, Cartier's method of "diathermy loop" excision was found be unacceptable by most colposcopists for the routine treatment of CIN. The major disadvantages of this technique were the time required to excise the lesional tissue in strips and the time required to make the complex drawings and maintain the orientation of the small strips of tissue through pathological examination. The loops designed by Cartier were an improvement over those of Palmer since they were fabricated from a thinner, higher quality steel and produced less thermal damage in the excised tissue. However, many pathologists still felt that the potential for thermal damage precluded using these loops as a diagnostic procedure when invasive cancer was suspected. It should be pointed out that there were large differences in the results obtained with

DEVELOPMENT OF LOOP EXCISIONAL PROCEDURES

different batches of loops. The loops used by Cartier were prepared in his hospital machine shop and were made of 0.2 mm steel. Since the loops were not commercially available, other colposcopists had to have them fabricated in their local machine shops, and the loops they obtained were generally inferior to those used by Cartier and caused more extensive thermal damage.

Although many colposcopists tried and discarded Cartier's method, Prendiville continued to experiment with this technique and made a number of modifications in the design of the electrodes which made them much more acceptable.[24] The wire loop electrodes were widened to 2 cm. This increased width is important because it allows many CINs to be excised in a single pass. The wire loop electrodes also were made deeper and were given an insulated base. This insured that electrosurgical arcing did not occur between the base of the electrode and the epithelial surface and reduced thermal damage to the excised tissue (Figure 5.8).

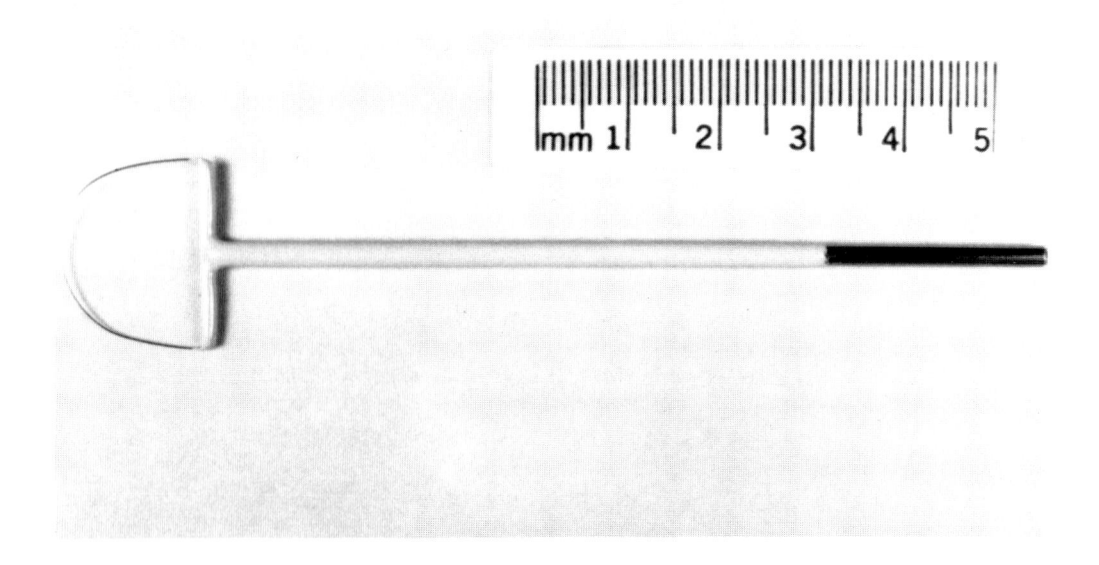

Figure 5.8. Large wire loop electrode with insulated base.

Another modification was to use sophisticated, modern electrosurgical generators (ESU) for the procedure. The ESU that Prendiville used was a solid state unit capable of producing a blended current combining hemostatic effects with excellent cutting characteristics. One of the problems with the earlier Cartier technique was that bleeding occurred during the procedure due to the use of a continuous sinewave cutting current. Although a sinewave current produces good electrosurgical cutting (see Chapter 3), it produces a minimal

ELECTROSURGERY FOR HPV-RELATED DISEASES

amount of hemostasis. The use of a modern ESU that produced a blended waveform reduced the amount of bleeding that occurred during the procedure and made it more acceptable for outpatient use. Prendiville termed his modification of Cartier's technique "Large Loop Excision of the Transformation Zone (LLETZ)" and in 1989, he published the first series of patients with CIN treated with large loop excision.[24] Using the large loop electrodes, many CIN lesions and atypical transformation zones can be excised in a single pass (Figure 5.9).

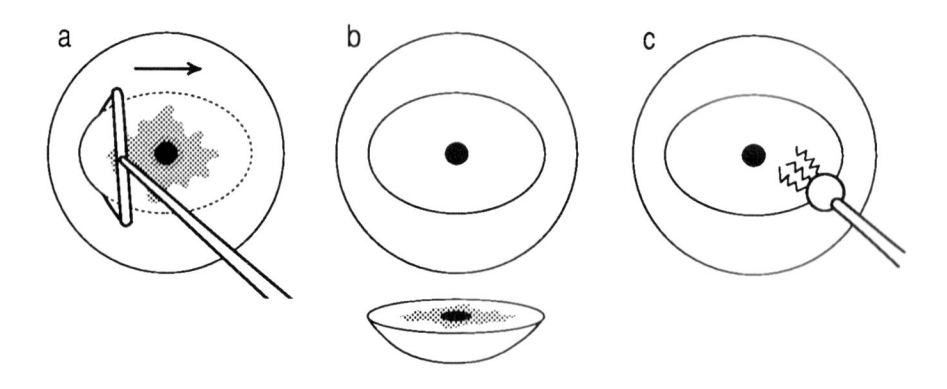

Figure 5.9. Excision of a CIN lesion using a large loop electrode.

In Prendiville's initial study, 102 women with CIN were treated with loop electrosurgical excision and were followed for at least 12 months. A high degree of success was reported. Only three of the patients had an abnormal cervical cytology (moderate or severe dysplasia) post-treatment for an overall success rate of 97%. The complications of the loop excision procedure are given in Table 5.13.

Although no cases of cervical stenosis occurred, in 7% of the patients the squamocolumnar junction was recessed to such an extent that it could not be visualized colposcopically. The most important complication of the procedure was perioperative and postoperative bleeding (Table 5.13). Four patients required hospitalization in order to control bleeding. Two patients developed significant bleeding during the procedure and two developed significant bleeding postoperatively. In addition to these four patients, nine additional patients developed postoperative bleeding at 8-21 days. These patients were diagnosed as having secondary infection and were treated with broad spectrum antibiotics. Many of the patients that developed perioperative/postoperative bleeding were thought to have a pre-existing cervicitis. Exclusion of these patients might have reduced the frequency of bleeding.

The method described by Prendiville for excising CIN had a number of advantages over ablative procedures. A pathological specimen was produced which could be used to confirm the colposcopist's clinical impression and, more importantly, to insure that a colposcopically inapparent invasive cancer was not inadvertently ablated. The fact that the entire lesion was available for histopathological assessment also allowed selected patients to be diagnosed and treated in a single setting, the so-called "See and Treat" approach. Other advantages of LLETZ were that it was rapid, easy to perform, easy to learn and required relatively inexpensive equipment.

Table 5.13

Complications of "LLETZ"	
Recessed squamocolumnar junction	7%
Significant perioperative bleeding requiring hospitalization	2%
Significant postoperative bleeding requiring hospitalization	2%
Postoperative bleeding insufficient to warrant hospitalization	9%

Because of the obvious advantages of the loop excisional procedure using the large loop electrodes, it was quickly adopted by many of the colposcopy centers in the United Kingdom. A number of large clinical series have now been published from the U.K. For the most part, these studies have shown excellent overall success rates and very acceptable complication rates. The results of treatment of more than 2,000 women with loop excision have now been published (Table 5.14).

The study of Murdoch *et al.* from the National Health Service colposcopy clinic at Gateshead, England presents their experience with 600 patients with CIN treated by loop excision.[28] The cervical lesions in this group of patients were relatively heterogeneous. Patients with ectocervical CIN that fulfilled the standard criteria for conservative management were treated by the technique originally described by Prendiville. The study also included a large number of patients with CIN that extended into the endocervical canal who required a "loop diathermy cone biopsy" (see below, Loop Diathermy Cone Biopsy). A smaller group of patients included in this study received loop excision of the central area of a lesion that was combined with laser ablation of the peripheral extensions of CIN into the vaginal fornices. Eradication of CIN was achieved with a single treatment in 96% of the cases.

Table 5.14

Studies Investigating Electrosurgery for CIN

Author / Year	# of Pts.	Length of Follow-up	Failure Rate
Prendiville / 1989	101	12 mos.	3%
Whiteley / 1990	80	6 mos.	5%
Luesley / 1990	557	6 mos.	4%
Bigrigg / 1990	1,000	3 mos.	4%
Murdoch / 1990	600	3 mos.	4%
Wright / 1992	157	6 mos.	10%

The largest of the published series is that of Bigrigg *et al.* from Birmingham.[27] This series presents their experience using loop excisions to treat 1,000 patients with an abnormal Pap smear referred to a National Health Center colposcopy center. Ninety percent of the patients were managed using a "See and Treat" protocol in which a loop excision was performed as both a diagnostic and therapeutic procedure on the first visit to the clinic. Although Bigrigg reports an excellent overall response rate for loop excision, with 96% of the patients having a normal Pap smear at their follow-up visits, there are a number of other findings in this study that need emphasis. The first is that 23% of the patients treated under the "See and Treat" protocol were subsequently found to have no CIN in their excised specimens. A second finding was a 0.3% incidence of colposcopically unexpected invasive squamous cell carcinomas and a 0.9% incidence of colposcopically unexpected microinvasive carcinoma in the excised specimens.

Recently, we compiled our treatment results after loop excision with the large loop in 157 patients with CIN.[29] All patients were suitable for conservative management and were followed for at least 6 months (Table 5.15).

Table 5.15

Results of Treatment of CIN with Loop Excision

Diagnosis	# of Pts.	Patients Free of Disease at First Follow-up* #	%
CIN 1	82	79	96%
CIN 2	34	30	88%
CIN 3	41	33	81%
Total	157	142	90%

* Follow-up ranged from 6-12 months.

Although this series is smaller than those from the United Kingdom, it is the first experience from North America with loop excision of CIN. In our hands, the overall failure rate of a single treatment after 6 to 12 months of follow-up was 10%. When stratified on the basis of lesional grade, a failure rate of only 4% was found in patients who were being treated for CIN 1 whereas patients with CIN 3 had a 19% failure rate. However, many of the patients with CIN 3 in this series had previously failed either cryotherapy or laser ablation. When the patients were stratified as to whether they were undergoing loop excision for recurrent/residual or primary CIN, a treatment failure rate of only 6% was found in patients being treated for the first time (Table 5.16).

These results are similar to those of the larger series from the United Kingdom. Similar complication rates were also noted in our series and in the series from the United Kingdom (see below).

Table 5.16

Treatment Results by Primary vs Residual Disease After Cryosurgery or Laser Ablation Therapy

	# of Pts.	Patients Free of Disease at First Follow-up* #	%
Primary Disease	141	132	94%
Residual Disease+	16	10	62%

* Follow-up ranged from 6-12 months.
+ Patients that previously failed laser ablation or cryosurgery for CIN

Electrosurgical Cone Biopsies

Together these studies clearly indicate that the loop excision procedure is a safe and highly effective treatment for patients with CIN lesions that fulfill the standard criteria for conservative management, i.e., lesions that can be visualized colposcopically in their entirety and have a negative endocervical curetting. Recently, Mor-Yosef and co-workers described a modification of Prendiville's basic technique that allows large loop electrodes to be used to perform cone biopsies in patients with CIN that extends into the endocervical canal.[30] In this modification, called "loop diathermy cone biopsy", the same electrodes as those used by Prendiville are utilized but much more tissue is excised than in the standard "LLETZ" (Figure 5.10).

In the original description of "loop diathermy cone biopsy" no follow-up of the patients was presented but the complication rate of the procedure appeared to be significantly less than that of cold knife cone biopsies (Table 5.17). Although over 80% of patients undergoing loop diathermy cone biopsies had the procedure performed while under general anesthesia, in other patients the procedure was safely and comfortably performed using local anesthesia.

DEVELOPMENT OF LOOP EXCISIONAL PROCEDURES

Loop Excision Procedure
"LLETZ" or "LEEP"

Monaghan's Loop
Diathermy Cone Biopsy

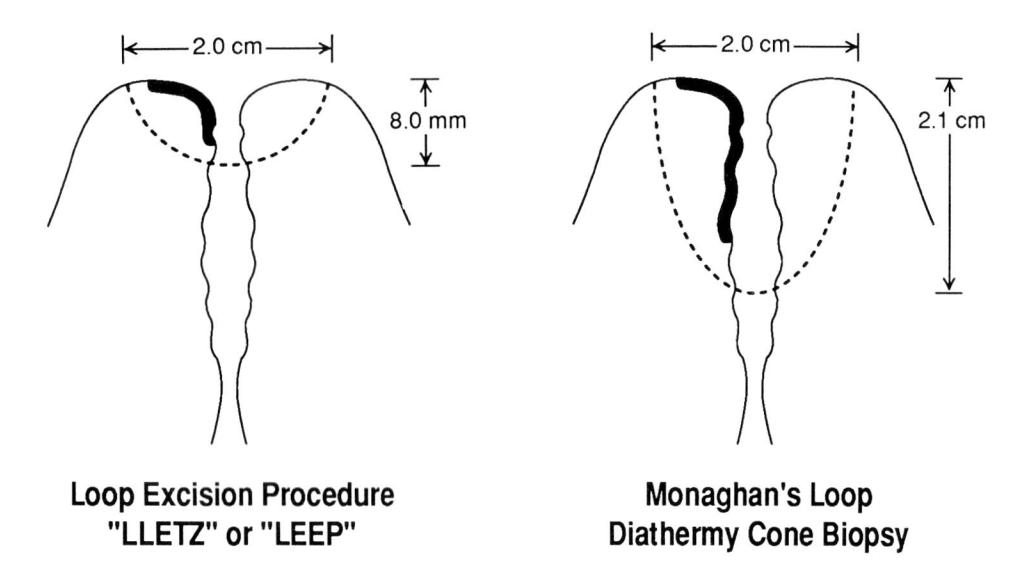

Figure 5.10. Comparison of the amount of tissue excised by "LLETZ" and loop diathermy cone biopsy.

Table 5.17

Complications of Cold Knife Cone Biopsies and Loop Diathermy Cone Biopsies

Type of Biopsy	Perioperative Bleeding	Postoperative Bleeding	Length of Cone
Cold Knife Cone	6%	8%	24.7 mm
Loop Diathermy Cone	2%	6%	20.2 mm

Recently we have performed cone biopsies electrosurgically on an outpatient basis using local anesthesia. In our procedure we use a combination of the shallow, large loop electrodes and a 1 x 1 cm rectangular loop electrode to excise lesions extending into the endocervical canal. We have found this technique useful for patients who have CIN extending into the endocervical canal but in whom there is a low suspicion of invasive cervical cancer. The typical patient that is treated with this approach on an outpatient basis is one in whom CIN extends up to 7 mm into the endocervical canal but in whom the upper limit of the lesion can be identified (although incompletely visualized) by careful inspection with an endocervical speculum. These patients do not have cytologic findings suggestive of invasive squamous cell carcinoma or a glandular neoplasm. In the latter cases we perform either a traditional cold knife conization or an electrosurgical needle electrode conization.

REFERENCES

1. Hunner, G.L. The treatment of leucorrhea with the actual cautery. *J.A.M.A.* 46:191-192, 1906.
2. Huggins, R.R. Problems associated with the cervix. *Am. J. Obst. & Gynec.* 17:589-596, 1929.
3. Pemberton, F.A. and Smith, G.V. The early diagnosis and prevention of carcinoma of the cervix: A clinical pathologic study of borderline cases treated at the Free Hospital for women. *Am. J. Obst. & Gynec.* 17:165-176, 1929.
4. Peyton, F.W. and Rosen, N.A. Cervical cauterization and carcinoma of the cervix. *Am. J. Obst. & Gynec.* 86:111-119, 1963.
5. Bouda, V.J. and Dohnal, V. Zur frage der krebsprophylaxe durch elektro koagulation bei ektopie und umwandlungszone. *Geburtsh. u. Frauenh.* 25:1186-1194, 1965.
6. Richart, R.M. and Sciarra, J.J. Treatment of cervical dysplasia by outpatient electrocauterization. *Am. J. Obst. & Gynec.* 101:200-205, 1968.
7. Hyams, M.N. A new instrument for excision of the diseased endocervix with surgical diathermy. *N.Y. State J. Med.* 28:646-648, 1928.
8. Rosen, R.J. and Wulff, G.J.L. Three hundred cases of extensive conization of the cervix. *Am. J. Obst. & Gynec.* 37:849-855, 1939.
9. Crossen, R.J. Wide conization of the cervix. *Am. J. Obst. & Gynec.* 57:187-206, 1949.
10. Bushnell, L.F. Prevention of complications in cervical conization. *Am. J. Obst. & Gynec.* 22:190-198, 1963.
11. Sze, E. H. M., Rosenzweig, B.A., Birenbaum, D.L., Silverman, R.K. and Baggish, M.S. Excisional conization of the cervix uteri: A five-part review. *J. Gynec. Surg.* 5:325-341, 1989.
12. Boulanger, J.C., Vitse, M., Lavallard, C., Levet, S. and Deparis, A. Comparative study of the treatment with CO_2 laser and electroresection using a diathermy loop for cervical dysplasia. Rev. fr. *Gynecol. Obstet.* 79:797-803, 1984.
13. Younge, P.A., Hertig, A.T. and Armstrong, D. A study of 135 cases of carcinoma *in situ* of the cervix at the Free Hospital for women. *Am. J. Obst. & Gynec.* 58:867-895, 1949.
14. Ortiz, R., Newton, M. and Tsai, A. Electrocautery treatment of cervical intraepithelial neoplasia. *Obstet. & Gynec.* 41:113-116, 1973.
15. Schuurmans, S.N., Ohlke, I.D. and Carmichael, J.A. Treatment of cervical intraepithelial neoplasia with electrocautery: Report of 426 cases. *Am. J. Obst. & Gynec.* 148:544-546, 1984.
16. Chanen, W. Symposium on cervical neoplasia III. Electrocoagulation diathermy. *Coloposcopy & Gynecologic Laser Surgery* 1:281-284, 1984/1985.

17. Deigan, E., Carmichael, J.A., Ohlke, D. and Karchmar, J. Treatment of cervical intraepithelial neoplasia with electrocautery: A report of 776 cases. *Am. J. Obst. & Gynec.* 154:255-259, 1986.
18. Richart, R.M. and Townsend, D.E. Outpatient therapy of cervical intraepithelial neoplasia with cryotherapy or CO_2 laser. In *Advances in Clinical Obstetrics and Gynecology*. H.J. Osofsky, ed. Williams and Wilkins, Baltimore. pp. 235-246, 1982.
19. Chanen, W. The efficacy of electrocoagulation on diathermy performed under local anesthesia for the eradication of precancerous lesions of the cervix. *Aust., N.Z. J. Obst. & Gynec.* 29:189, 1989.
20. Cognies, J. La biopsie exerese a l'anse diathermique don les lesions epitheliales de Museau de Tanche (theses). Paris, 1955.
21. Cartier, R. *Practical Colposcopy*, ed 2. Laboratoire Cartier, 20 Rue des Cordelieres, Paris, 1984.
22. Cartier, R., Sopena, B. and Cartier, I. Use of the diathermy loop in the diagnosis and treatment of lesions of the uterine cervix (abstract). Proceedings of the International Federation for Cervical Pathology and Colposcopy, 1981.
23. Prendiville, W., Davies, R. and Berry, P.J. A low voltage diathermy loop for taking cervical biopsies: A qualitative comparison with punch biopsy forceps. *Br. J. Obst. & Gynec.* 93:773-776, 1986.
24. Prendiville, W. and Cullimore, N.S. Large loop excision of the transformation zone (LLETZ). A new method of management for women with cervical intraepithelial neoplasia. *Brit. J. Obst. & Gynec.* 96:1054-1060, 1989.
25. Whiteley, P.F. and Olah, K.S. Treatment of cervical intraepithelial neoplasia: Experience with the low-voltage diathermy loop. *Am. J. Obst. & Gynec.* 162:1272-1277, 1990.
26. Luesley, D.M., Cullimore, J. and Redman, C.W.E., *et al.* Loop diathermy excision of the cervical transformation zone in patients with abnormal cervical smears. *Brit. Med. J.* 300:1690-1693, 1990.
27. Bigrigg, M.A., Codling, B.W., Pearson, P., Read, M.D. and Swingler, G.R. Colposcopic diagnosis and treatment of cervical dysplasia at a single clinic visit. *Lancet* 336ii:229-231, 1990.
28. Murdoch, J.B., Grimshaw, R.N. and Monaghan, J.M. Loop diathermy excision of the abnormal cervical transformation zone. *Int. J. Gynec. Cancer* 1:105-111, 1991.
29. Wright, T.C., Gagnon, M.D., Richart, R.M. and Ferenczy, A. Treatment of cervical intraepithelial neoplasia using the loop electrosurgical excision procedure. *Obst. Gynec.* 79:173-178, 1992.
30. Mor-Yosef, S., Lopes, A., Pearson, S. and Monaghan, J.M. Loop diathermy cone biopsy. *Obst. Gynec.* 75:884-886, 1990.
31. Luesley, D.M, McCrum, A., Terry, P.B., Wade-Evans, T., Nicholson, H.O., Mylotte, M.J., Emens, J.M. and Jordan, J.A. Complications of cone biopsy related to the dimensions of the cone and the influence of prior colposcopic assessment. *Brit. J. Obst. & Gynec.* 92:158-164, 1985.

ELECTROSURGERY FOR HPV-RELATED DISEASES

CHAPTER 6

THE ETIOLOGY OF EPITHELIAL CANCER AND PRECURSOR LESIONS IN THE LOWER MALE AND FEMALE ANOGENITAL TRACT

From recent studies, which will be outlined in this chapter, it is apparent that the vast majority, if not all, cervical squamous cell carcinomas and adenocarinomas and their precursors are causally related to infection by human papillomavirus (HPV). It is assumed that the same relationship holds true for neoplasms of the vagina, vulva, perineum, perianal, and penile epithelia but less data has been accumulated for these lesions, so proof of this relationship is largely speculative in non-cervical sites.

EPIDEMIOLOGY OF CERVICAL CANCER

The traditional risk factors for the development of cervical cancer are relatively well known and are given in Table 6.1.[1-3] The abundant

Table 6.1

Risk Factors for Development of Cervical Cancer

- Early age at first intercourse
- Early age at first pregnancy
- Low socioeconomic class
- Multiple sexual partners
- Association with "high risk" male
- Cigarette smoking
- Herpes simplex virus
- Antibodies against HSV

observational and epidemiological data which has accumulated over the past hundred years suggest that cervical cancer and its precursors are largely sexually transmitted diseases (Table 6.2). These data include the observations

Table 6.2

> ### Cervical Cancer as a STD
>
> More common in sexually active than in celibate women.
> Higher incidence in incarcerated women and prostitutes.
> Risk related to number of sexual partners.
> Risk related to sexual history of mate.
> Almost never occurs in virgins.

that cervical cancer is seen more often in sexually active women than in celibate women, that it is seen more often in incarcerated women and prostitutes than in controls, and that a woman's risk of developing cervical cancer is related to the number of male sexual partners she has had or the number of sexual partners that her male partner or partners have had. In addition, it was reported that subsequent spouses of a man whose first wife died of cervical cancer are at greater risk of developing cervical cancer than are appropriately chosen controls. As cervical cancer is almost never seen in virginal women, the logical conclusion from these data was that cancer of the cervix was sexually transmitted, with the male partner serving as a vector.

Infectious Agents Previously thought to Cause Cervical Cancer

As a result of these epidemiological observations, investigators have focused at one time or another on most sexually transmitted diseases as etiologic agents for cervical disease (Table 6.3). Each of these agents, when examined, bore a statistically significant relationship with cervical neoplasia. As investigators delved more deeply into the putative etiologic relationships between these sexually transmitted diseases and cervical neoplasia, it became obvious that statistical associations represented associations between sexually transmitted diseases and number of sexual partners rather than cause and effect.[4] Moreover, there was no compelling data to favor one STD over another as an etiologic agent for cervical cancer until investigators reported that there was a correlation between the presence of antibodies to HSV-2 and the risk of developing cervical neoplasia. These data produced extremely good

Table 6.3

Agents Previously Thought to Cause Cervical Cancer

Chlamydia
Herpes simplex virus
Trichomonas vaginalis
Chronic infections
Syphilis
Sperm

correlations between HSV-2 antibodies and cervical neoplasia and, in studies controlled for other factors—including age at first intercourse, age at first pregnancy, number of pregnancies, and number of sexual partners—HSV-2 was found to be significantly associated with cervical neoplasia.[5-7] This led many investigators to speculate that HSV was an etiological agent for squamous cell cancer of the cervix. The suggestion was further supported by *in vitro* studies, in which it was found that attenuated HSV-2 could transform normal cells to neoplastic cells and by studies in which it was reported that portions of the HSV genome could be found in cervical neoplasia.[8,9]

Despite the multiple lines of evidence suggesting that HSV-2 was etiologically important in cervical neoplasia, other authors suggested that these were largely statistical artifacts and that an etiological relationship had, in fact, not been demonstrated convincingly. More importantly, in certain epidemiological studies in which rigorous controls were used, HSV appeared not to be an important factor for increasing the relative risk of developing cervical cancer.[10] The finding of HSV-2 genome in cervical cancer was potentially the most important of all these observations, but it now appears, in the light of a more thorough understanding of the molecular technology which was used at that time, that the finding was spurious and may have represented non-specific hybridization under conditions of low stringency. HSV is now widely believed not to be an etiological agent in cervical neoplasia.

Associations Between HPV and Cervical Cancer

Meisels *et al.* and others were the first to present evidence that human papillomavirus (HPV) could be found in presumed cervical cancer precursors (Table 6.4).[11-13] This was followed shortly by papers by Jensen *et al.* in which

Table 6.4

Studies Associating HPV with Cervical Cancer	
Meisels *et al.* (1977)	Detected "koilocytes" in both CIN and condyloma acuminata and suggested association with HPV.
Hills and Laverty (1979)	Identified HPV in dysplasia by electron microscopy.
Jensen *et al.* (1980)	Detected HPV capsid antigen in CIN.
zur Hausen *et al.* (1983)	Cloned HPV DNA from cervical cancer.

it was reported that HPV capsid antigen could be identified by labeled antibodies in a high proportion of early presumed cervical cancer precursors.[14] Subsequently, in 1983, zur Hausen and associates were able to clone HPV DNA from cervical cancers.[15,16]

HUMAN PAPILLOMAVIRUSES
Classification of Papillomaviruses

Papillomaviruses are obligatory, intranuclear, double stranded, DNA tumor viruses that contain approximately 7800-7900 base pairs of genomic DNA (Table 6.5). They are generally found as a non-enveloped virion, surrounded by an icosahedral capsid. The classification of papillomaviruses is based on the species they infect and on their DNA base pair sequence, as determined by hybridization homology under appropriate conditions of ionic strength and temperature. These viruses are widely distributed in the animal kingdom and appear to be highly species specific. The human papillomaviruses are epitheliotropic and are highly tissue specific as well.[17,18]

HPVs are named by number and are numbered according to order of discovery. If two viruses share less than 50% sequence homology based on DNA hybridization, they are classified as different viral types. Minor variations in DNA base pair sequence have been used to describe sub-types as well, although the degree of relatedness required for a sub-type has not precisely been defined. More than 65 HPVs have now been identified. Of these, more than 22 different types infect the male and female lower genital tract (Table 6.6).

Table 6.5

Characteristic Features of HPV

Double stranded DNA tumor virus with 7.8-7.9 kb genomic DNA as a non-enveloped virion.

Icosahedral capsid.

Classification based on species specificity and DNA base pair sequence.

Epitheliotropic and tissue specific.

HPV Genomic Organization

An increasingly large number of papillomaviruses, including multiple human types, have been sequenced completely. Their genomic organization appears to be highly conserved and similar (Figure 6.1).[19] The viral genome can, in general, be divided into three regions. A regulatory region, which is generally referred to as the "long control region" or the "upstream regulatory region" (URR), contains many of the regulatory elements of the genome. The URR lies between the other two regions. The late region encodes the structural proteins which are required for viral encapsulation. The early region encodes proteins which are required for the assembly of infectious viral particles, controls the replication of viral DNA, and, in some viral types, encodes for proteins which have transforming properties.

The term "open reading frame" (ORF) is used for those areas of the viral genome which do not contain stop codons and hence are potentially transcribable. These may be thought of as viral genes. The late region contains two large open reading frames, referred to as L1 and L2. L1 encodes for the virus' major capsid protein and appears to be highly conserved. The L2 ORF encodes for a minor capsid protein which varies significantly among different HPV types. The L1 and L2 ORFs appear to be highly sensitive to differentiation-dependent signals which are derived from the host cells. As viral replication is dependent on terminal differentiation of epithelial cells, capsid proteins are most commonly found in those lesions which are highly differentiated and in which viral replication is taking place.[14] They are

ELECTROSURGERY FOR HPV-RELATED DISEASES

Table 6.6

Principal Anogenital Human Papillomaviruses

HPV Type	Disease Association	Oncogenic Association
6	Condyloma acuminatum Low-grade neoplasia Laryngeal papillomas	Rarely malignant
11	Condyloma acuminatum Low grade neoplasia Laryngeal papillomas	Rarely malignant
16	CIN 1-3 Bowenoid papulosis Bowen's disease Cervical, vulvar and anal cancers	Malignant
18	CIN 3; rarely CIN 1-2 Cervical cancers	Highly malignant
31	CIN 1-3, cancers	Malignant
33	CIN 1-3, cancers	Malignant
35	CIN 1-3, cancers	Malignant
39	Bowenoid papulosis	Rarely malignant
41	Condyloma and cutaneous flat warts	Benign
42	Flat condyloma Bowenoid papulosis	Benign
43	Low-grade neoplasia	Benign
44	Condyloma acuminatum	Benign
45	Condyloma/CIN/cancers	? Highly malignant
51	CIN 1-3, cancers	Malignant
52	Condyloma acuminatum CIN 1-3, cancers	Malignant
53	Genital HPV	?
54	Genital HPV	?
55	Genital HPV	?
56	Condyloma/cancers	? Highly malignant
57	Genital HPV	?
58	Genital HPV	?

uncommonly found in high-grade CIN lesions in which differentiation is minimal or in invasive cancers in which viral replication seldom, if ever, takes place.

The early region of HPV contains five different ORFs which are designated E1, E2, E4, E6, and E7. The E4 ORF appears to encode for a structural protein, but its precise role is not known. The E4 protein is, however, a major protein found in HPV 1 induced plantar warts and its mRNA is the major RNA in condylomata acuminata induced by HPV 11.

The E1/E2 encoded proteins are key regulatory proteins for papillomaviruses. Two proteins encoded for by the E2 ORF have been well studied and their functions include both transactivation and transrepression of DNA transcription. These proteins appear to "control" the replication of the E6/E7 ORF. Inactivation of E1/E2 releases transcriptional control of E6 and E7 resulting in increased production of the E6/E7 proteins. The E6/E7 proteins of certain HPV types can cause cellular transformation in *in vitro* model systems.[20,21]

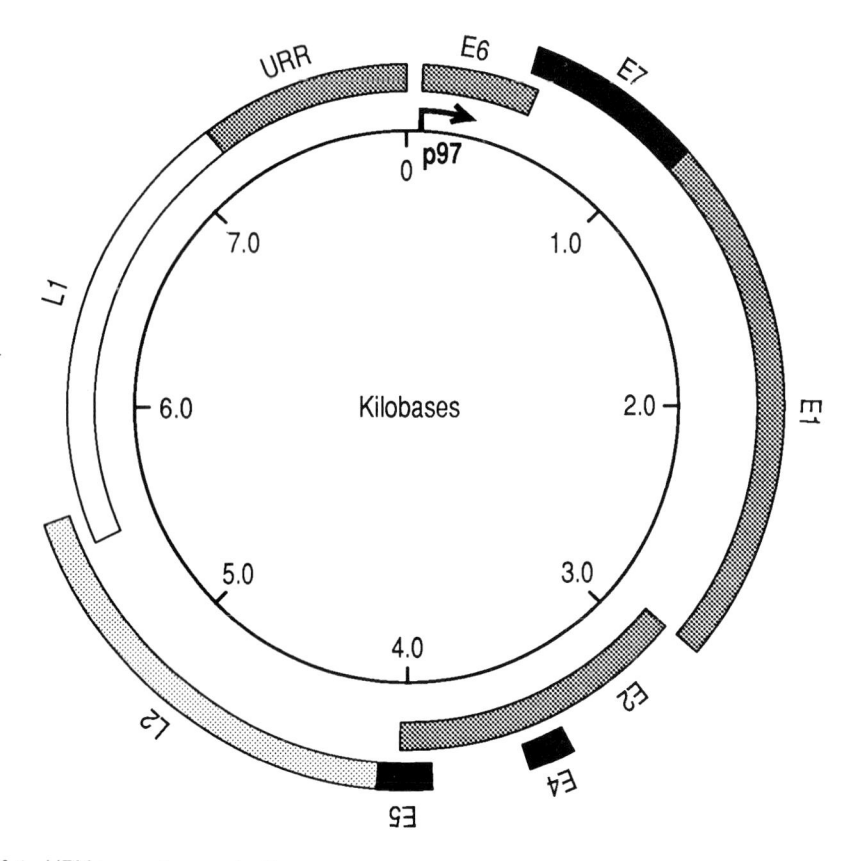

Figure 6.1. HPV genomic organization.

THE PATHOGENESIS OF CIN

The initial step in an HPV infection appears to be infection of either basal or parabasal cells which are capable of mitotic division.[22] The infectious particle, which is known as a complete virion, consists of a core of DNA surrounded by a protein coat. For an active infection to take place, the virus must have access to the generative compartment of the epithelium. This is thought to be the principal reason why the transformation zone is so susceptible to infections by HPV. In this region of the cervix the squamocolumnar junction constantly exposes basal and parabasal cells to the environment. In addition, in the immature portion of the transformation zone, the thin, replicating epithelium commonly contains generative compartment cells at the surface which are potential targets for HPV infection and replication.

Types of HPV Infections

A number of different replicative states appear to be possible for HPV. These include latent infection, productive infection, and the inclusion of an integrated virus in the host chromosomal DNA (Table 6.7).[23] Latent

Table 6.7

Replicative States of HPV

Replicative State	State of DNA
Latent infection	(?)Episomal
Productive infection	Episomal
Integrated virus	Integrated into host DNA

infections are thought to contain viruses in the generative compartment of the epithelium in the form of circular, extra-chromosomal DNA (Table 6.8). These units, referred to as episomes, are thought not to be functional and to replicate only once during every cell cycle. Single copy virus is beneath the level of sensitivity of commonly used tests for identifying DNA in tissue

Table 6.8

> **Latent Infections**
>
> Viral infections that cannot be identified histologically.
> Can only be detected by molecular methods.
> Thought to contain single copy episomal DNA in basal cells.

sections. Therefore, it is impossible to identify episomal HPV DNA in individual cells or to know which cells are actually infected and contain latent virus. As the virus is not functionally active during its latent phase, it is believed that cells containing latent virus do not contain any of the classical cytopathogenic effects (CPE) of HPV and that they cannot be identified under the light microscope as being infected. The only way latently infected cells can be histologically identified as containing HPV is when the state of the virus changes and viral replication occurs accompanied by typical HPV CPE. The conditions which favor latency over a productive infection are not known, but an immunological role is almost certainly important, as evidenced by the commonly made observations that pregnancy may be associated with a finding of clinically visible and histologically identifiable HPV-related lesions which commonly disappear post-partum and then recrudess during a subsequent pregnancy.[24] It is extremely difficult, if not impossible, to correlate latently infected cells with so-called subclinical HPV infections, and it is necessary to distinguish between viral latency and subclinical disease. It is possible that a latently infected cellular population may be detected through screening of populations or individuals for HPV DNA, but recent studies have suggested that a high proportion of patients who are clinically negative with normal Pap smears yet have detectable HPV DNA may, in fact, harbor productive lesions which are simply too small to be detected. Thus, many questions regarding latency and its influence on disease states remain open.

Subclinical Infections

Patients with subclinical infections are generally defined as patients in whom, on routine clinical examination, no lesion is found yet who, under magnification with cervicography or colposcopy, have a putative HPV-related lesion (Table 6.9).[23] Putative subclinical lesions can be confirmed by biopsy

Table 6.9

> *Subclinical Infections*
>
> Lesions that can only be detected with magnification.
> Histologically demonstrate HPV-related features.
> Frequently overdiagnosed.

and histological identification of HPV-related cytopathic effects in the lesional tissue. The concept of subclinical infection is very poorly defined, and some rigor needs to be introduced due to the casual fashion in which the term subclinical infection is currently being used. It is our experience that many of the so-called subclinical infections are, in fact, morphological variants of normal and that many people who are said to have an HPV infection do not have patients' diseases but only clinicians' or pathologists' diseases. In order to ascertain that a presumed abnormality is truly HPV-related, it is essential that it contain cells with the typical cytopathogenic effects associated with HPV or, in the absence of such changes, that HPV DNA be identifiable using *in situ* hybridization or some other technique which will unambiguously detect HPV DNA at the individual cell level. It is our experience, based on our consultation material, that a high proportion of patients who are said to have subclinical HPV are, instead, suffering from histological over-diagnosis of tissue changes which mimic HPV but are not HPV-related. The classical examples of such over-diagnosis are immature transformation zone epithelium, examined as a result of colposcopic or cervicographic screening, and micropapillomatosis labialis (MPL), the symmetrical finger-like projections not uncommonly seen on the medial aspect of the labia or around the introitus or hymeneal ring.[25,26] Both the immature T-zone and micropapillomatosis contain alterations which are easy to mistake for HPV-related changes. In the immature T-zone repair is the rule, and mitotically active cells which vary in size, shape, and staining and have changes in chromatin distribution patterns are not infrequently seen (Figure 6.2). These histologic changes are, however, the hallmarks of repair, and the

THE ETIOLOGY OF EPITHELIAL CANCER

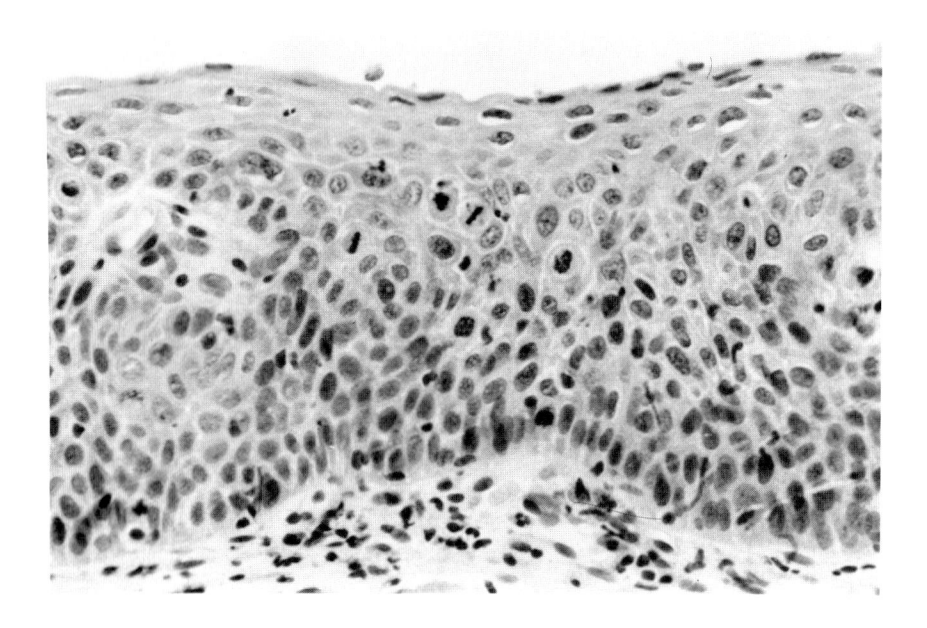

Figure 6.2. Immature T-zone with reparative changes. Immature T-zone changes that are sometimes difficult to distinguish from CIN both on colposcopy and histology.

other features associated with HPV infection, such as significant pleomorphism, koilocytosis, and multinucleation, are generally absent. Similarly, MPL is commonly misdiagnosed as being HPV-related because the pathologist is not familiar with the microanatomy of the epithelium around the introitus (Figure 6.3). In MPL, the epithelium is commonly papillary, generally contains mild variation in the size, shape, and staining of the nuclei, and the cells commonly contain a small, perinuclear halo. Multinucleation, significant cytological atypia, and true koilocytes are absent, however, and serve to distinguish the true HPV-related lesion from non-HPV-related micropapillomatosis.

Productive Infections

Productive HPV lesions require an epithelium in which differentiation is taking place, as there are host and cellular feedback controls on viral replication which must be overcome before new virus can be produced. Evidence suggests that some of these factors reside on chromosome 11 but that there are humoral factors as well.[28,29] When HPV replicates, the infection is referred to as a

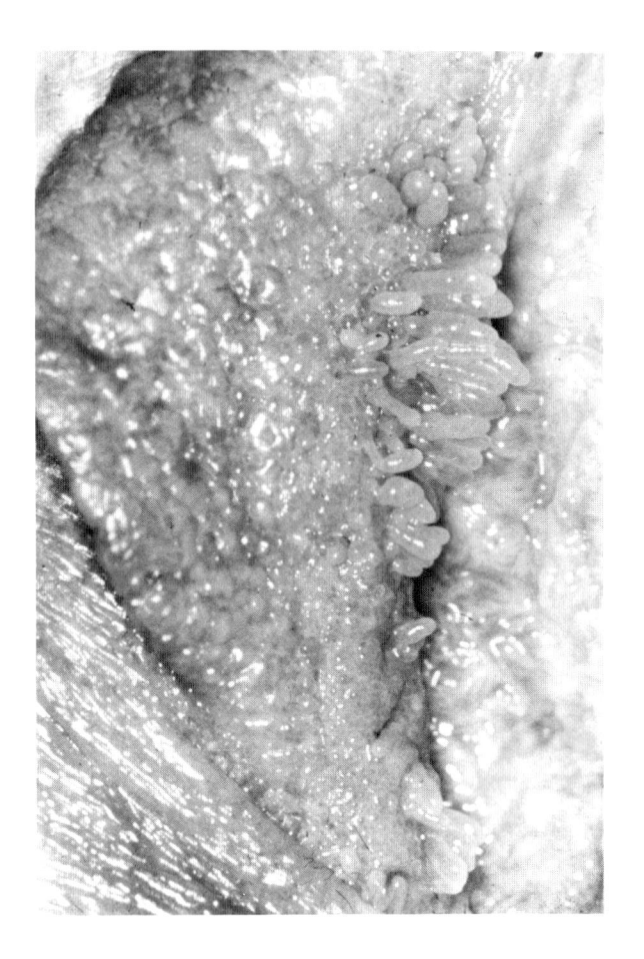

Figure 6.3. Micropapillomatosis labialis. These lesions occur at the introitus and are frequently misdiagnosed as condylomata accuminata. (Reprinted with permission from ref. 27)

productive infection, and it generally results in the formation of large numbers of new viral particles. There is evidence to suggest that early in the development of a lesion the number of viral particles which is produced is significantly greater than that which occurs in older lesions in which viral assembly is significantly down regulated, commonly to a level of only 10-25% of that in the initial infection. DNA replication generally begins in the parabasal and early intermediate cell layers where the early portions of the genome are most active. This is followed in the upper, intermediate, and superficial cell layers by significant capsid protein production and the formation of the complete virion, the infectious particle, in the superficial layers. These changes can readily be appreciated in stains for capsid antigen, which are generally found only in the upper half of the epithelium, and by stains for viral DNA which begin to accumulate in the upper two thirds.[14] Recent *in situ* hybridization studies demonstrating messenger RNA, rather than DNA, have shown that the virus is actively producing message and that, presumably, DNA

THE ETIOLOGY OF EPITHELIAL CANCER

replication has begun even in the basal cells in productive infections.[30] However, the quantities of DNA which are produced are insufficient for the level of sensitivity of the commercially available DNA *in situ* hybridization techniques.

Histological Hallmarks of an HPV Infection

Human genital tract epithelia which are productively infected by HPV always contain the typical cytopathogenic effects (CPE) of HPV, and these effects are a *sine qua non* for the diagnosis of an HPV-related lesion. In the absence of CPE, an etiology other than HPV should be considered. The cytopathogenic effects of HPV appear to be related, in productive infections, principally to the effects that HPV replication has upon the conduct of mitosis and the mitotic spindle. During cellular replication, the amount of DNA in the nucleus doubles during the S-phase in preparation for mitosis. In the immediately premitotic cell, a tetraploid quantity of DNA is present in the nucleus, and all 46 chromosomes have replicated preparatory to being divided between two daughter cells. During the normal conduct of mitosis, the equal division of the diploid chromosome set takes place in a regular fashion producing two daughter cells with nuclei, each of which contains a diploid amount of DNA and the normal complement of chromosomes. However, in HPV-infected cells in the productive phase of viral replication, a significant number of cells do not complete mitosis in a normal fashion. The DNA doubles but cytokinesis does not occur, and the cell that should produce two daughter cells, instead, becomes a binucleated cell or a cell with a single tetraploid nucleus. In subsequent cell divisions, the same mitotic errors may occur so that multinucleation and ploidy levels as high as 32X may be found in productively infected lesions.[31]

Any significant change in ploidy level is accompanied by cytological atypia.[32] The normal diploid cell is the benchmark and contains a nucleus with a uniformly distributed chromatin pattern, a thin uniform nuclear membrane, and, except under conditions of repair, regeneration or severe inflammation, a uniformity which is widely recognized by pathologists and cytologists as indicating normalcy (Figures 6.4 and 6.5). All productive HPV infections of lower genital tract epithelia are accompanied by polyploidy, that is, an increased amount of DNA which occurs in multiples of the normal set, i.e., tetraploid, octoploid, hexadecaploid, etc.[31] Polyploidy is always accompanied by cytological atypia, and this atypia must be present in order to make a diagnosis of an HPV-related lesion.

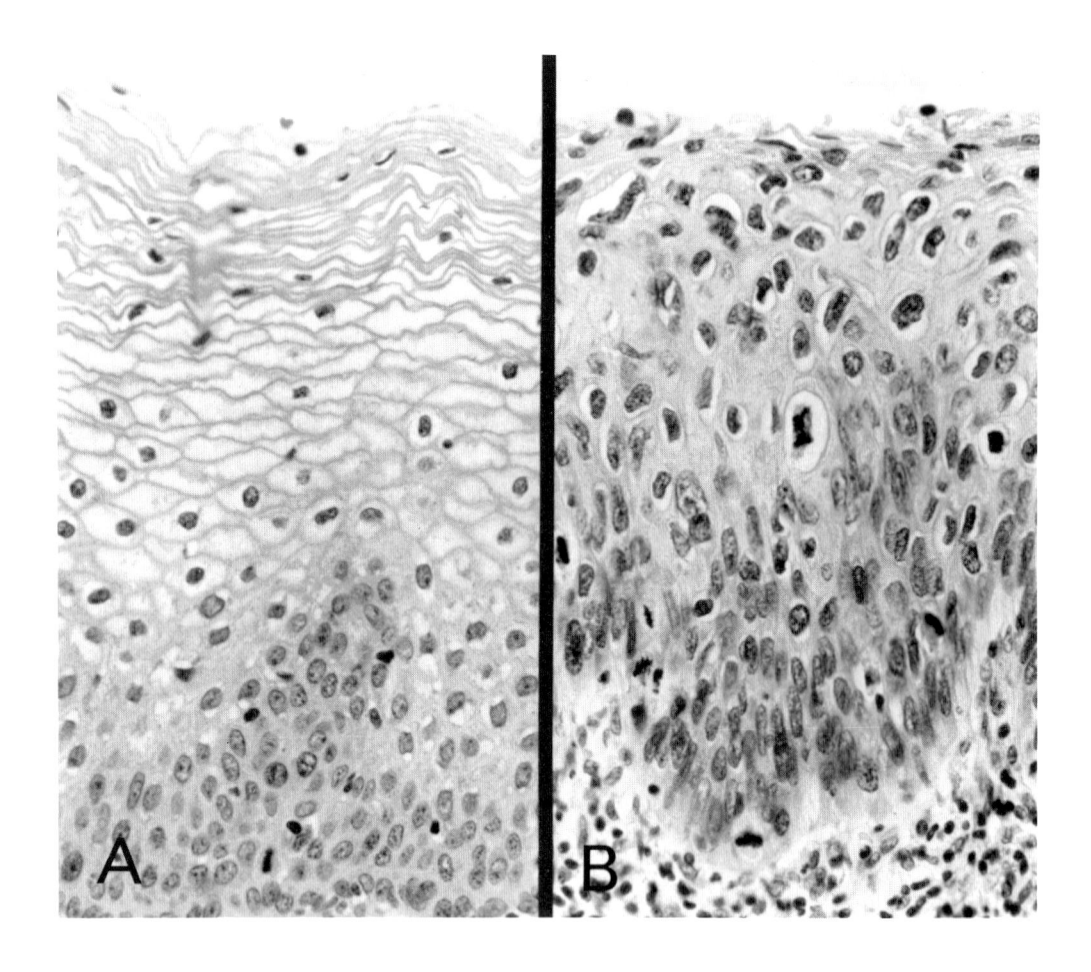

Figure 6.4. Normal squamous epithelium of cervix compared to a CIN lesion. A) Normal squamous epithelium. B) Classic cytopathogenic effects (CPE) associated with productive HPV infection. These include nuclear atypia, hyperchromaticity, perinuclear halos, and multinucleation.

Polyploidy is the histologic hallmark of a productive HPV infection. At the cytological level, it has now been reported by several groups, using modern molecular techniques to define HPV-related infections and distinguish them from other changes such as repair and inflammation, that cytological atypia is the only criterion which is reproducibly correlated with an HPV infection.[33] They further point out that a perinuclear halo is the least specific criterion and that for a koilocyte to be identified as being related to HPV, not only must perinuclear halos be found, but they must be found in a cell which contains a nucleus which is cytologically atypical (Figure 6.6). Therefore, it is extremely

THE ETIOLOGY OF EPITHELIAL CANCER

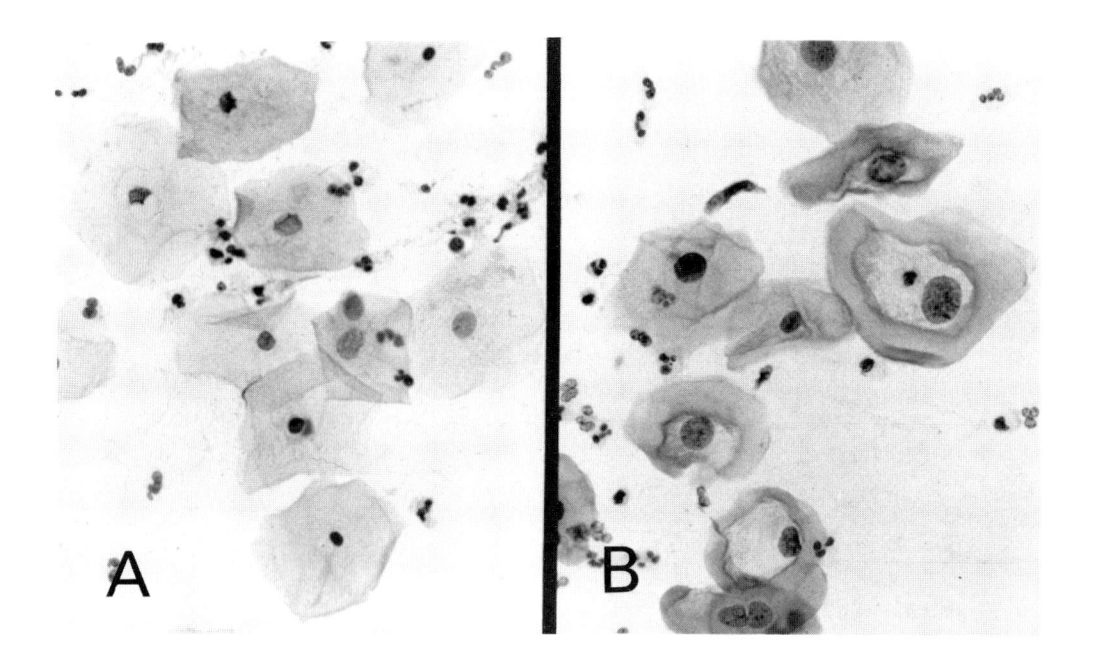

Figure 6.5. Normal exfoliated superficial squamous cells compared to CIN lesion detected on Pap smear. A) Normal superficial squamous cells. B) Superficial squamous cells with HPV cytopathogenic effects exfoliated from a CIN 1 lesion and detected on a Pap smear.

important that the pathologist use strict criteria for the diagnosis of HPV-related lesions cytologically and histologically and that the clinician know the criteria that the cytologist or pathologist is using so they can assess the adequacy of the diagnoses which are being rendered. As is apparent from the foregoing

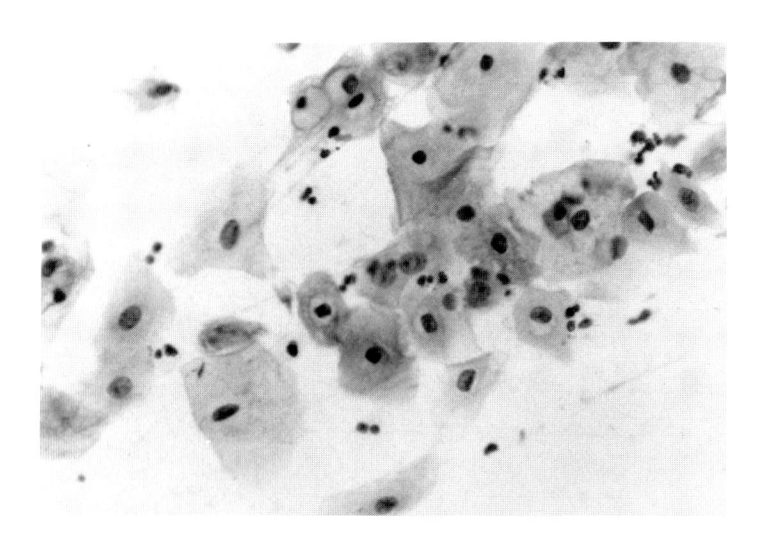

Figure 6.6. Cells that can be mistaken for HPV infected cells on Pap smears unless the criteria of nuclear atypia is strictly adhered to.

ELECTROSURGERY FOR HPV-RELATED DISEASES

discussion, cytological atypia will also be accompanied by multinucleation and by variations in size, shape, and staining of the nucleus and the cytoplasm, a condition referred to as pleomorphism.

In situ Hybridization as a Quality Control of Histologic Diagnosis

One of the ways of verifying the adequacy of the histological criteria used for making a diagnosis of HPV is to apply *in situ* hybridization for HPV DNA to a series of consecutive cases in which an HPV-related diagnosis has been rendered.[34] There have now been several different studies correlating HPV DNA *in situ* hybridization with histological changes and other detection techniques for HPV DNA.[35] A typical CIN 1 lesion in which HPV 16/18 DNA is detected using the technique of *in situ* hybridization (ISH) is shown in Figure 6.7. A comparison of the detection rate of HPV DNA using standard

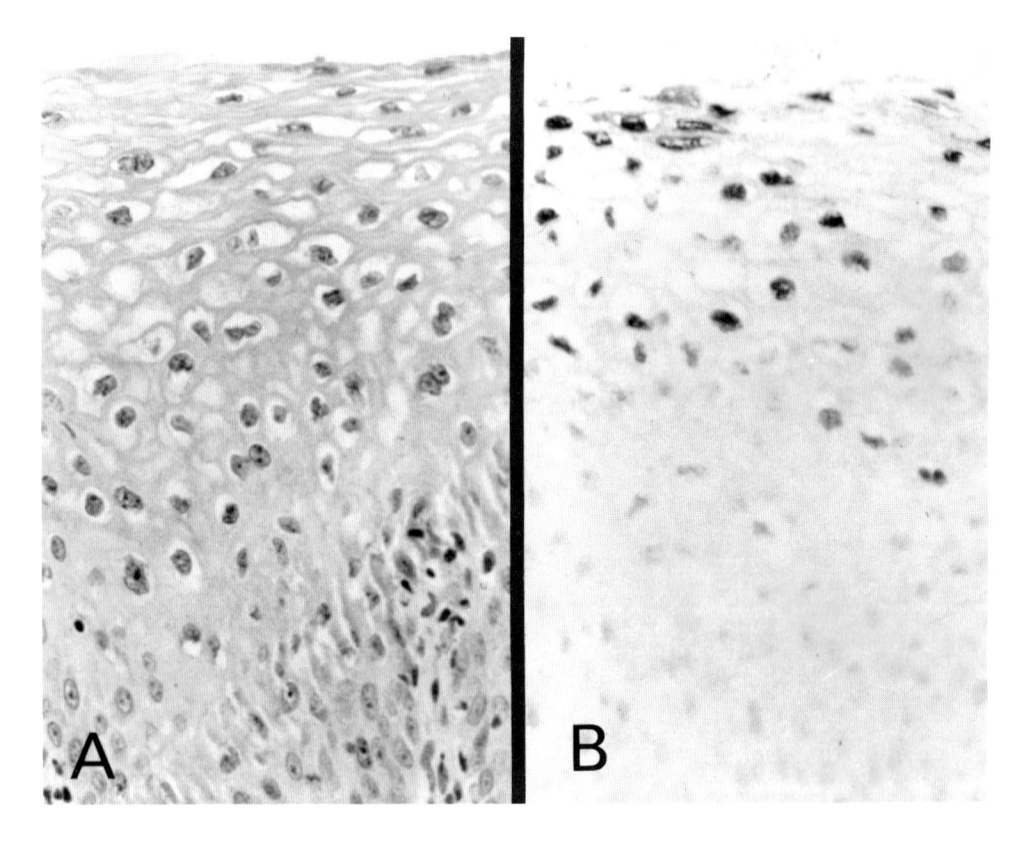

Figure 6.7. *In situ* hybridization of a condyloma acuminatum using probes for HPV 6/11 DNA. The darkly stained nuclei contain HPV 6/11 DNA.

commercially available *in situ* hybridization reagents with published data will provide the pathologist or the clinician with the information required to assess the specificity of histological diagnoses. For example, between 70-80% of CIN 1/condyloma lesions of the cervix will be positive for HPV DNA using the Digene *in situ* hybridization kit (Table 6.10).[34]

Approximately 95% of acuminate warts from the external genitalia will be positive using that kit. If, in a series of consecutive cases examined by *in situ* hybridization, a similar percentage is found, this will lend support to the accuracy of the diagnoses. In contrast, if the positive rate is only 20% or 30%, the assumption can be made that a significant number of the lesions diagnosed as being HPV-related in that group have been over-diagnosed.

Although most of the mitotic figures in productively infected epithelia are normal appearing, there are, in addition, two types of abnormal mitotic figures which are seen, the tripolar mitosis and the tetraploid dispersed metaphase. The significance of this will become apparent in subsequent discussions.

Table 6.10

Use of In Situ Hybridization for Quality Control of Cervical Biopsies

Diagnosis	% HPV (+) By *In Situ* Hybridization
CIN 1	80%
CIN 2/3	67%
Vulvar Condyloma	94%
VIN 2/3	67%

The principal difference in the histological criteria used to make a diagnosis of condylomata acuminata as opposed to flat condyloma differ only in the presence of papillomatosis and extreme acanthosis (proliferation of the spiny layer) in the acuminate warts. Otherwise, the criteria are identical. However, HPV-related lesions of the penis, the perineum, the perianal tissue, and vulvar lesions which have been present for some time may present some diagnostic difficulties due to the down-regulation of viral replication and the relative

ELECTROSURGERY FOR HPV-RELATED DISEASES

absence of the typical cytopathogenic effects which accompany the productive, replicative cycle. Under these circumstances papillomatosis and acanthosis may be present, but cytological atypia, multinucleation, and koilocytosis may be extremely uncommon or inapparent.[36] Histologically, we often diagnose these lesions as having changes suggestive but not diagnostic of a condyloma (Figure 6.8). For lesions of this type at external anogenital sites, *in situ* hybridization may be useful in establishing which lesions are HPV-related. Approximately

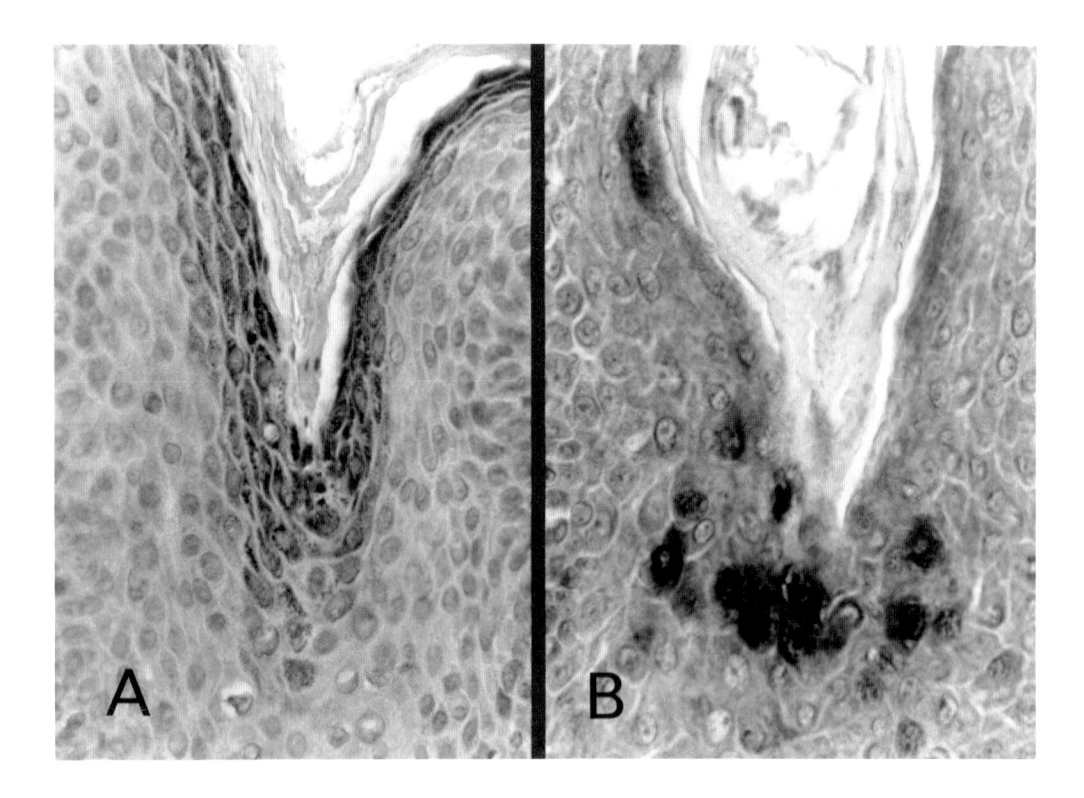

Figure 6.8. Histology of a lesion with features suggestive, but not diagnostic of condyloma. The lesion has acanthosis and focal parakeratosis, but lacks the classic cytopathic effects of an HPV-associated lesion. A) H & E stained section. B) *In situ* hybridization using a 16/18 probe. The dark staining nuclei contain HPV DNA.

50% of the lesions with this histology will be HPV DNA positive by either *in situ* hybridization or using the polymerase chain reaction to detect HPV DNA (Table 6.11).[37] As positivity in acuminate lesions is high (approximately 95%), a negative *in situ* hybridization for HPV DNA, although not completely ruling out HPV as the etiology, certainly makes it less likely.

Table 6.11

HPV DNA In Lesions of External Anogenital Tract			
Histologic Diagnosis	# of Cases	ISH (+)	% PCR (+)
Negative for condyloma	74	3%	6%
Suggestive but not diagnostic of condyloma	22	50%	44%
Condyloma	27	89%	100%

CELLULAR TRANSFORMATION AND NEOPLASIA

The risk of an infected cell undergoing transformation to neoplasia is directly related and, in the aggregate, can be predicted by knowing the type of the HPV which has infected the cell. Three viral groups are generally distinguished—the low or no oncogenic risk viruses, the "high" oncogenic risk viruses, and the intermediate oncogenic risk viruses (Table 6.12).[38,39] The principle representatives of the low or no oncogenic risk group includes 6, 11, 41, 42, 43, and 44. The high oncogenic risk group includes 16, 18, 45, and 56, and the intermediate oncogenic risk group includes 31, 33, 35, 39, 51, and 52.[39]

Table 6.12

Oncogenic Risk Groups of HPV	
"Low" Risk	6, 11, 41, 42, 43, 44
"Intermediate" Risk	31, 33, 35, 39, 51, 52
"High" Risk	16, 18, 45, 56

For all practical purposes, the low oncogenic risk viruses are not associated with high-grade neoplasia. Despite some papers to the contrary, HPV types 6, 11, 41, 42, 43, and 44 are virtually never found in association with cancer except for verrucous carcinomas. Only a handful of cancers which contain HPV type 6 or 11 (other than verrucous carcinomas) have been described, and even some of these are suspect. It is solely the viruses in the high or intermediate oncogenic risk group which play a significant role in producing neoplasia in the genital tract.

Under conditions which have not been defined, cell transformation may occur. This nearly always occurs as a monoclonal event and is hypothesized to be associated with the continued or overproduction of the protein encoded for by the E6/E7 ORF.[40,41] In many cases in which neoplasia has occurred, the virus has been found to have integrated into the host cell chromosome.[42] For integration to occur, the circular DNA genome must be linearized. When the genome is opened, it almost always opens at the E1/E2 open reading frame, inactivating E1/E2 and allowing for the continued or overexpression of the E6/E7 encoded proteins.[43] Alternate mechanisms through which E6 and E7 proteins may be continuously or over produced which do not require integration may occur, but integration appears to play a major role in the production of neoplasia.

It has been reported that E6/E7 encoded proteins share many features with oncoproteins produced by other well-studied oncogenic DNA viruses particularly the adenovirus and the SV40 virus (Table 6.13). The adenovirus produces the E1 proteins and the SV40 virus produces the large T protein. All three oncogenic proteins, E1, large T and E6/E7, share in their ability to bind with two anti-oncogenic proteins which exert negative feedback control on mitosis and to inactivate them (Figure 6.9). The retinoblastoma protein referred to as $p105^{RB}$ and another important cell regulatory protein designated p53 are inactivated by the proteins encoded for by the E6/E7 encoded ORFs.[44-47] In model tissue culture systems, the oncogenic effect of the E6/E7 proteins is dependent upon their ability to bind to $p105^{RB}$ and to p53.[46,47] If the p53 and $p105^{RB}$ binding regions on these proteins are ablated, the transforming effect of E6/E7 is blocked. Binding of E6 to p53 increases the binding of ubiquitin to the E6/p53 complex.[48] The binding of ubiquitin facilitates the degradation of proteins and may result in the clearance of p53 from the cell and subsequent loss of its "tumor suppressor" effect.

The process of transformation of epithelial cells by HPV appears to be more complex than simple interactions between these five proteins. In *in vitro* model systems, the production of E6/E7 proteins will lead to cell immortalization, but complete transformation requires other events. For example, HPV 16 DNA alone does not transform *in vitro* early passage keratinocytes, but does so when introduced into a cell in combination with an activated ras oncogene.[49] Similarly, it has been reported that amplification of the c-myc oncogene is a common event in cervical cancer.[50] This would suggest that there are multiple routes to the development of cervical cancer,

THE ETIOLOGY OF EPITHELIAL CANCER

although it is generally believed that the common denominator for all these routes is the E6/E7 oncoproteins of HPV.

Table 6.13

Transforming Functions

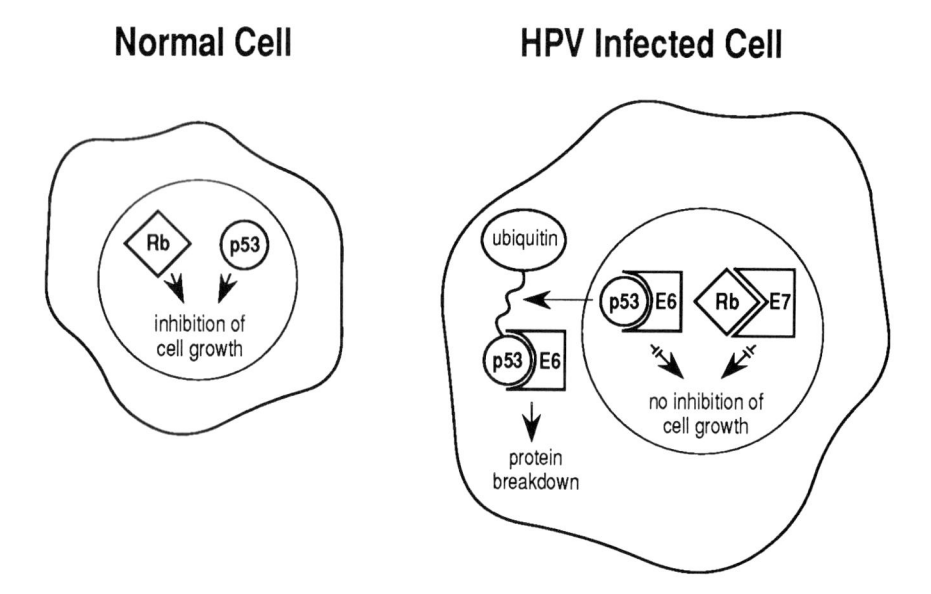

Virus	Binding To: p53	p105^{RB}
HPV	E6	E7
Adenovirus	E1B	E1A
SV40	Large T	Large T

Figure 6.9. Model for the way in which HPV E6/E7 proteins cause unregulated cell proliferation.

Methods for Detecting HPV

A variety of detection techniques for HPV has been described, including the filter *in situ* hybridization (FISH) technique, *in situ* hybridization on tissue sections, the Southern blot hybridization technique, a variety of membrane-binding techniques generally referred to as dot blots or slot blots, and the polymerase chain reaction (PCR) (Table 6.14). Without reviewing the technical aspects of these tests, it is important to note that the FISH technique is generally regarded as being insufficiently sensitive to be useful clinically. The Southern blot, which is generally taken to be the gold standard of HPV DNA detection, is complex, time consuming, expensive, and probably not applicable to clinical testing procedures. The polymerase chain reaction which is being widely used at the research level is incredibly sensitive, able to detect 10 copies of a particular DNA, but is not yet being used for routine clinical samples because of a number of problems including the potential for contamination between samples. The PCR method forms a cornerstone of many recent studies and will probably prove useful in clinical practice in subsequent years. Most HPV DNA detection and typing performed at the clinical level uses one of the dot blot techniques which appear to provide sufficient sensitivity to be clinically useful but not to be so sensitive that it detects levels of viral replication which are not clinically important.

Table 6.14

Tests for Detecting HPV DNA

Method	Advantages	Problems
Southern blot	Gold Standard	Time consuming
Filter *in situ* (FISH)	Easy, Inexpensive	Too insensitive
Dot Blot	Easy, FDA approved	Relatively insensitive
In situ Hybridization	Useful for tissue sections	Requires biopsy
Polymerase Chain Reaction	Inexpensive, Sensitive	May be too sensitive

The ViraPap and ViraType test have been FDA-approved for clinical use and in a number of studies appear to be applicable to certain clinical situations for which viral detection or typing may play a significant role (Figures 6.10, 6.11).

THE ETIOLOGY OF EPITHELIAL CANCER

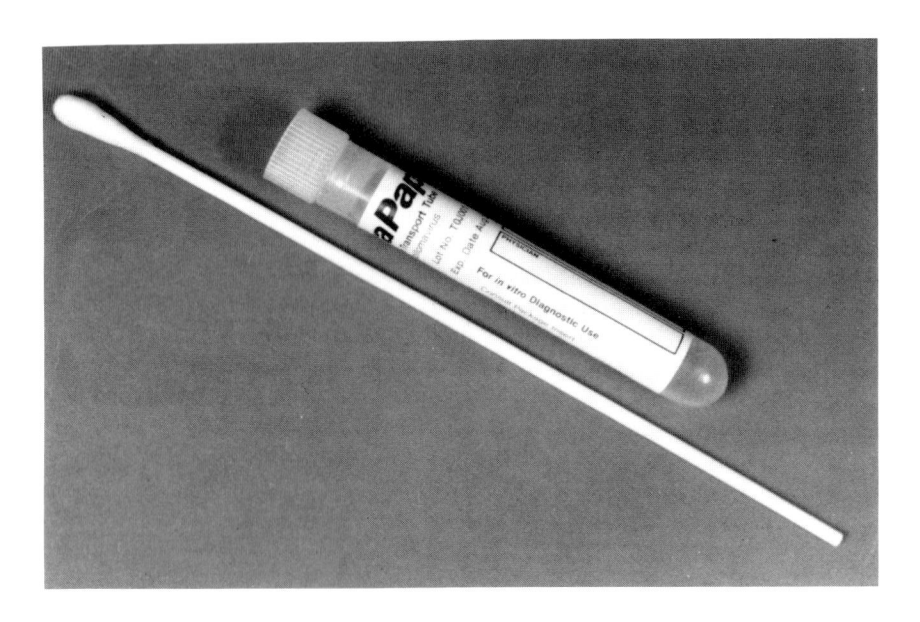

Figure 6.10. ViraPap/ViraType™ Kit for detecting HPV DNA. The ViraPap/ViraType™ collection kit consists of a dacron-tipped applicator stick which is swabbed over the cervix, placed in a transport tube and sent to the laboratory. *(Virapap™ is produced by Digene Diagnostics, Inc.)*

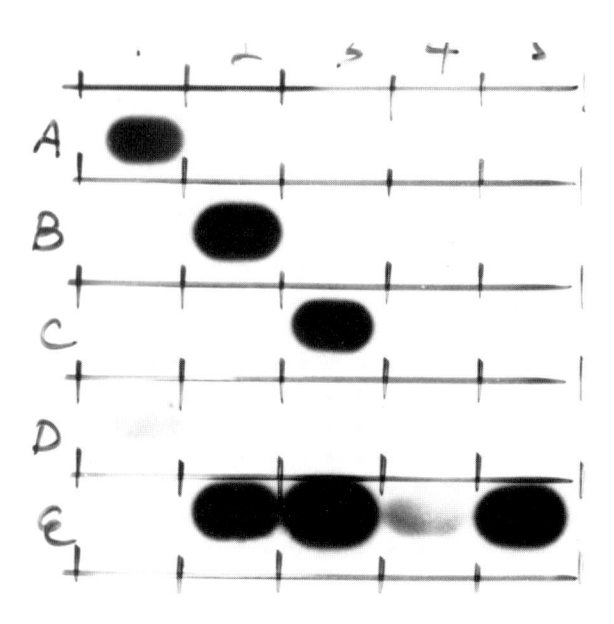

Figure 6.11. In the laboratory the ViraPap™ sample is filtered onto a membrane and hybridized with labeled DNA probes against various types of HPV. Dark staining lanes contain HPV DNA. *(Virapap™ is produced by Digene Diagnostics, Inc.)*

There are several large, ongoing prospective studies of patients who are HPV DNA positive and Pap smear negative, and it would appear from the preliminary data that patients who are HPV DNA positive and type as HPV 16 are at substantially increased risk, when compared to controls, of developing an abnormal Pap smear in the short term. Additional studies will be required to determine whether this is so, but HPV DNA testing may play a significant role in the not too distant future.

For all of these detection techniques, it is critical that the material be collected in an appropriate fashion and analyzed promptly. When exfoliated cells are being collected for analysis, they must be placed in a transport medium, as DNA degradation occurs promptly due to the release of enzymes which degrade it. If the need to detect HPV DNA or to do viral typing is anticipated, transport medium should be obtained from the laboratory and be available in the office. Similarly, if *in situ* hybridization is anticipated, the tissues must be placed in neutral buffered formalin to maximally facilitate the detection of HPV DNA using *in situ* hybridization. Acidic fixatives such as Bouin's or Zenker's solution reduce sensitivity through degradation of the DNA to a level which diminishes the clinical utility of the test.[51] Even in tissues which are fixed in neutral buffered formalin, a prolonged immersion in the fixative will significantly degrade the DNA and decrease the sensitivity of the test. Care should be taken to account for these variables when HPV testing is planned or undertaken.

Histologic Correlates of the Transformation Process

Histologically, lesions which are undergoing transformation from a productive infection to a neoplasm begin as a single cell which, through a series of mitotic cell divisions, develops into a clone of cells which eventually becomes clinically and histologically apparent and, with the passage of time, increases in size and geographic extent.[41] Because this change occurs at the single cell level, it is clearly impossible to distinguish between a flat condyloma and a CIN 1, since at the cytological or histological level the pathologist can not determine whether the single cell event which characterizes the first stages of neoplasia has taken place. When the neoplastic clone has reached such a size as to be detected colposcopically, histologically or cytologically, one can reliably predict that the lesion is a neoplasm rather than a "simple HPV infection." Although it is possible to say that a lesion is a neoplasm, it is impossible to say that it is not. When neoplasia occurs, there is generally a change from a polyploid cellular population to an aneuploid cellular population. Aneuploidy is the hallmark of a truly neoplastic lesion. Aneuploidy is defined as highly abnormal amounts of DNA and highly abnormal chromosome numbers, and it is thought to be a relatively specific criterion of neoplasia in non-endocrine dependent epithelia. Aneuploid cells are generally much more cytologically atypical than diploid or polyploid cells, and this high degree of cytological atypia, which is accompanied by nuclear alterations, including significant chromatin clumping and increased pleomorphism, can be used to identify those cells in which neoplastic transformation has taken place (Figure 6.12). Aneuploidy is also accompanied by changes in the conduct of mitosis, and it is very common to find abnormal mitotic figures (AMFs) in transformed aneuploid epithelial populations. The classical AMFs which are diagnostic of an aneuploid neoplastic lesion include coarsely clumped chromosomes, multipolar mitoses, multigroup mitoses and highly abnormal forms. If such AMFs are found, it is possible to conclude with confidence that the lesion is aneuploid and is a cancer or cancer precursor.

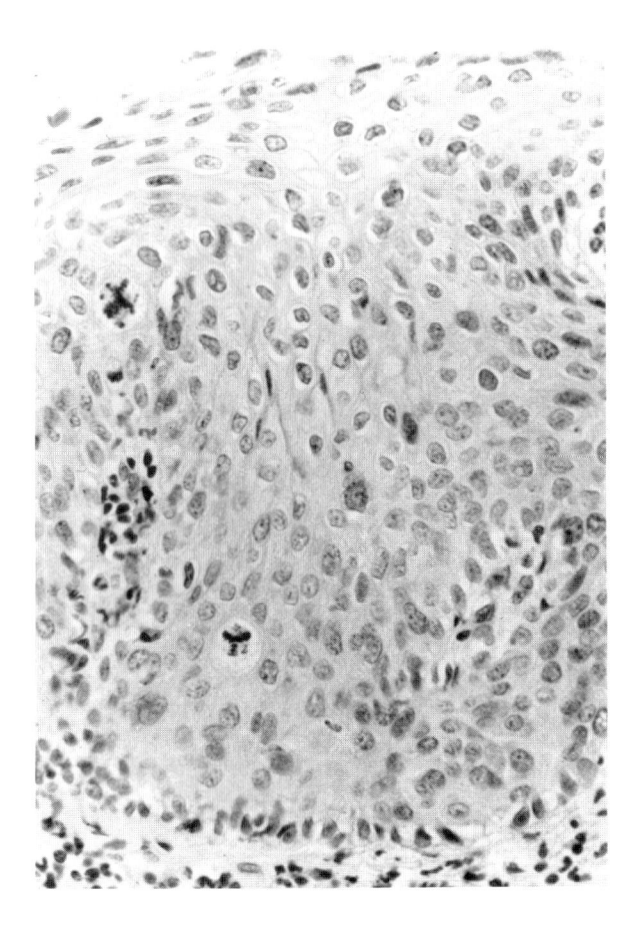

Figure 6.12. Aneuploid lesion that contains abnormal mitotic figures and characteristic nuclear alterations.

Just as it has generally been agreed that it is impossible to distinguish between severe dysplasia and carcinoma *in situ* , so it is now generally agreed that, in the absence of AMFs, it is impossible to distinguish between flat condyloma and CIN. It is fruitless to make such a distinction as it is not only impossible but it is also not a useful clinical distinction.

REFERENCES

1. Franceschi, S., LaVecchia, C. and Decarli, A. Relation of cervical neoplasia with sexual factors, including specific venereal diseases. In *Viral Etiology of Cervical Cancer* , R. Peto and H. zur Hausen, eds. Cold Spring Harbor Laboratory, Cold Spring Harbor, NY, 1986.
2. Hulka, B.S. Risk factors for cervical cancer. *J. Chron. Dis.* 35:3-11, 1982.
3. Brinton, L.A. and Fraumeni, J.F. Epidemiology of uterine cervical cancer. *J. Chron. Dis.* 39:1051-1065, 1986.
4. Munoz, N. and Bosch, F.X. Epidemiology of cervical cancer. In *Human Papillomavirus and Cervical Cancer* N. Munoz, ed. IARC Publications, 1989.
5. Naib, Z.M., Nahmias, A.J., Josey, W.E., *et al*. Genital herpetic infection. Association with cervical dysplasia and carcinoma. *Cancer* 23:940-945, 1969.
6. Park, M., Kitchner, H.C., Macnab, J.C.M. Detection of herpes simplex virus type 2 DNA restriction fragments in human cervical carcinoma tissue. *EMBO J.* 2:1029, 1983.
7. DiLuca, D., *et al*. Simultaneous presence of herpex simplex virus and human papillomavirus sequences in human genital tumors. *Int. J. Cancer* 40:763, 1987.
8. Galloway, D.A. and McDougall, J.K. The oncogenic potential of herpes simplex viruses: Evidence for a "hit" and "run" mechanism. *Nature* 302:21-24, 1983.
9. Frenkel, N., *et al*. A DNA fragment of herpes simplex virus type 2 and its transcription in human cervical cancer tissue. *Proc. Natl. Acad. Sci. USA* 68:3784-3789, 1972.
10. Vonka, V., Kanka, J. and Roth, Z. Herpes simplex type 2 virus and cervical neoplasia. *Adv. Cancer Res.* 49:149-191, 1987.
11. Meisels, A., Fortin, R. and Roy, M. Condylomatous lesions of the cervix: II cytologic, colposcopic and histopathologic study. *Acta Cytol.* 21:379-390, 1977.
12. Meisels, A., Casas-Cordero, M, *et al*. HPV veneral infections and gynecologic cancer. *Pathol. Annu.* 18:277-293, 1983.
13. Hills, E. and Laverty, C.R. Electron microscopic detection of papillomavirus particles in selected koilocytotic cells in routine cervical smears. *Acta. Cytol.* 23:53-56, 1979.
14. Jenson, A.B., Rosenthal, J.D., Olson, C., *et al*. Immunological relatedness of papillomavirus from different species. *J. Natl. Cancer Inst.* 64:495-500, 1980.
15. Gissman, L., Wolnik, L., Ikenberg, H., *et al*. Human papillomavirus types 6 & 11 DNA sequences in genital and laryngeal papillomas and in some cervical cancers. *Proc. Natl. Acad. Sci. USA* 80:560563, 1983.
16. Boshart, M., Gissman, L., Ikenberg, H., *et al*. A new type of papillomavirus DNA, its presence in genital cancer biopsies and in cell lines derived from cervical cancer. *Eur. Mol. Biol. Org. J.* 3:1151-1157, 1984.
17. Wright, T.C. and Richart, R.M. Role of human papillomavirus in the pathogenesis of genital tract warts and cancer. *Gynecol. Oncol.* 37:151-164, 1990.
18. Taichman, L.B. and La Porte, R.F. The expression of papillomaviruses in epithelial cells. In *The Papovaviridae*. P.M. Howley and N.P. Salsman, eds. Plenum, New York, 1987.

19. Broker, T.R. Structure and genetic expression of papillomaviruses. *Obstet. Gynecol. Clin. North Amer.* 14:329-348, 1987.
20. Bedell, M.A., Jones, K.H. and Laimins, L.A. The E6-E7 region of human papillomavirus type 18 is sufficient for transformation of NIH 3T3 and rat 3Y1 cells. *J. Virol.* 61:3635-3640, 1987.
21. Kanda, T., Furuno, A. and Yoshiike, K. Human papillomavirus type 16 open reading frame E7 encodes a transforming gene for rat 3Y1 cells. *J. Virol.* 62:610-613, 1988.
22. Pfister, H. Papillomaviruses: General description, taxonomy, and classification. In *The Papovaviridae*. P.M. Howley and N.P. Salsman, eds. Plenum, New York, 1987
23. Schneider, A. Latent and subclinical genital HPV infections. *Papillomavirus Report*. 1:2-5, 1990.
24. Rando, R.F., Lindheim, S., Hasty, L., *et al.* Increased frequency of detection of human papillomavirus deoxyribonucleic acid in exfoliated cervical cells during pregnancy. *Am. J. Obstet. Gynecol.* 161:50-55, 1989.
25. Bergeron, C., Ferenczy, A., Richart, R.M. and Guralnick, M. Micropapillomatosis labialis appears unrelated to human papillomavirus. *Obstet. Gynecol.* 76:281-286, 1990.
26. Manoharan, V. and Sommerville, J.M. Benign squamous papillomatosis: A case report. *Genitourin. Med.* 63:393-395, 1987.
27. Wright, T.C. and Richart, R.M. Pathogenesis and diagnosis of preinvasive lesions of the lower genital tract. In *Principles and Practices of Gynecologic Oncology*. W.J. Hoskins, C. A. Perez and R.C. Young, eds. J.B. Lippincott, Co., Philadelphia, in press.
28. Stanbridge, E., Der, C.J., Dorsen, C.-J., *et al.* Human cell hybrids: Analysis of transformation and tumorigenicity. *Science*. 215:252-259, 1982.
29. Pater, M., Hughes, G.A. and Hyslop, D.E. Glucocorticoid-dependent transformation by type 16 but not by type 11 human papillomavirus DNA. *Nature (London)* 335:832-834, 1988.
30. Stoler, M.H. and Broker, T.R. *In situ* hybridization detection of human papillomavirus DNA and messenger RNA in genital condylomas and cervical carcinoma. *Hum. Pathol.* 17:1250-1258, 1986.
31. Fu, Y.S., Braun, L., Shah, K.U., *et al.* Histologic, nuclear DNA, and human papillomavirus studies of cervical condyloma. *Cancer* 52:1705-1711, 1983.
32. Fu, Y.S., Reagan, J.W. and Richart, R.M. Precursors of cervical cancer. *Cancer Surv.* 2:359, 1983.
33. Franquemont, D.W., Ward, B.E., Anderson, W.A. and Crum, C.P. Prediction of "high-risk" cervical papillomavirus infection by biopsy morphology. *Am J. Clin. Pathol.* 92:577-582, 1989.
34. Richart, R.M. and Nuovo, G.J. HPV DNA *in situ* hybridization can be used for the quality control of diagnostic biopsies. *Obstet. Gynecol.* 75:223-226, 1989.
35. Willet, G.D., Kurman, R.J. and Reid, R. Correlation of the histological appearance of intraepithelial neoplasia of the cervix with human papillomavirus types. *Int. J. Gynecol. Pathol.* 8:18-25, 1989.
36. Oriel, J.D. Natural history of genital warts. *Br. J. Vener. Dis.* 47:1-13, 1971.
37. Felix, J.F. and Wright, T.C. Comparison of *in situ* hybridization and PCR for detecting HPV in lesions clincially suspicious for condylomata acuminata. In prep., 1991.
38. Reid, R. and Lorincz, A.T. Should family physicians test for human papillomavirus infection? An affirmative view. *Journ. of Fam. Prac.* 32(2):183-188, 1991.
39. Lorincz, A.T., Reid, R., Jenson, A.B., Greenberg, M.D., Lancaster, W. and Kurman, R.J. Human papillomavirus infection of the cervix: Relative risk associations of 15 common anogenital types. *Am. J. Obstet. Gyn.*, in press.
40. zur Hausen, H. Papillomaviruses in human cancer. *Cancer* 59:1692-1696, 1987.
41. Richart, R.M. Colpomicroscopic studies of the distribution of dysplasia and carcinoma *in situ* on the exposed portion of the human uterine cervix. *Cancer* 18:950-954, 1965.

42. Schneider-Maunoury, S., Croissant, O. and Orth, G. Integration of human papillomavirus type 16 DNA sequences: A possible early event in the progression of genital tumors. *J. Virol.* 61:3295-3298, 1987.
43. Cullen, A.P., Reid, R., Campion, M.J. and Lorincz, A.T. An analysis of the physical state of different human papillomavirus DNAs in preinvasive and invasive cervical neoplasia. *J. Virol.* 65(2):606-612, 1991.
44. Barbosa, M.S., Edwards, C., Fisher, C., et al. The region of the HPV E7 oncoprotein homologous to adenovirus E1A and SV40 large T antigen contains separate domains for Rb binding and casein kinase II phosphorylation. *EMBO J.* 9:153-160, 1990.
45 Blume, E. P53: How a tumor suppressor works. *J. Natl. Cancer Inst.* (83):158-160, 1991.
46. Werness, B.A., Levine, A.J. and Howley, P.M. Association of human papillomavirus types 16 and 18 E6 proteins with p53. *Science* 248:76-79, 1990.
47. Dyson, N., Howley, P.M., Munger, K. and Harlow, E. The human papillomavirus 16 E7 oncoprotein is able to bind to the retinoblastoma gene product. *Science* 243:934-937, 1989.
48. Hollingworth, R.E. and Lee, W.-H. Tumor suppression genes: New prospects for cancer research. *J. Natl. Cancer Inst.* 83:91-96, 1991.
49. DiPaolo, J.A., Woodworth, C.D., Popescu, N.C., et al. Induction of human cervical squamous cell carcinoma by sequential transfection with human papillomavirus 16 DNA and viral Harvey ras. *Oncogene* 4:395-399, 1989.
50. Riou, G., Barrois, M., Le, M.G., et al. C-myc proto-oncogene expression and prognosis in early carcinoma of the uterine cervix. *Lancet* 1:761-763, 1987.
51. Nuovo, G.J. and Silverstein, S.J. Methods in laboratory investigation: Comparison of formalin, buffered formalin, and Bouin's fixation on the detection of human papillomavirus deoxyribonucleic acid from genital lesions. *Laboratory Investigation* 59(5):720-724, 1988.

CHAPTER 7

LOOP EXCISIONAL PROCEDURES FOR TREATING CERVICAL INTRAEPITHELIAL NEOPLASIA (CIN)

LOOP EXCISIONS FOR EXOCERVICAL CIN

When conservative ablative therapies began being used for treating CIN in the late 1960s and early 1970s, triage rules were developed to insure that a colposcopically missed invasive cancer was not inadvertently ablated. In addition to requiring that the CIN lesion be visualized in its entirety, these rules required that ablation not be performed in cases in which there was a significant discrepancy between the cytologic, colposcopic or biopsy results or in which there was a suggestion of invasion by any of the diagnostic tests. Since the loop technique is excisional rather than ablative, these concerns are less of an issue when loop excision is used. We believe exocervical loop excisions can be performed safely even when there is discordance between the diagnostic tests provided the entire lesion can be visualized colposcopically. A key advantage of loop excisional procedures is that they provide lesional tissue for pathologic analysis. The indications that we use for exocervical loop excision are given in Table 7.1. The clinical indications for exocervical loop excision are different from those for loop excision cone biopsies. The applicability of an individual indication to a particular patient will also depend on a number of factors including the colposcopic expertise of the operator, the quality of the cytology laboratory used and the reliability of the patient.

Table 7.1

Indications for Exocervical Loop Excision

Biopsy-proven CIN lesion of any grade

(or)

Squamous intraepithelial neoplasia (SIL) on Pap smear together with a colposcopically identifiable CIN lesion

(and)

Satisfactory colposcopic exam with no evidence of invasion.

The clearest indication for exocervical loop excision is a patient with a histologically-diagnosed CIN of any grade that is visible in its entirety. These patients can be treated safely with loop excision even if there is discordance between the various diagnostic modalities, i.e., Pap smear, colposcopy and cervical biopsy. In the unlikely event that a patient with an undiagnosed invasive cancer is treated with loop excision, no harm will be done since the procedure can be considered to have been a large diagnostic biopsy. Similarly, it is no longer necessary that patients with CIN lesions undergo pre-treatment endocervical curettage, provided the lesion is colposcopically visible in its entirety. An endocervical curettage can be performed easily once the exocervical excision has been completed. In the unlikely event that a CIN is detected in the endocervical curettage performed at the completion of the exocervical excision, the canal can be re-evaluated 3 months after the procedure and a loop excisional cone biopsy performed if the canal still contains CIN. In patients with CIN lesions fulfilling the criteria listed in Table 7.1, exocervical loop excision should be considered a safe and effective conservative therapeutic approach analogous to cryotherapy or laser ablation.

The use of exocervical loop excision to treat colposcopically-identified CIN in patients with an abnormal Pap smear who have not had a confirmatory cervical biopsy, is a more controversial clinical indication. Certainly in patients with a high-grade squamous intraepithelial lesion (Hi-SIL) on cytology and a fully visualized CIN on colposcopy (i.e., the lesion does not extend into the endocervical canal), there is a clear indication for an exocervical excision. Patients that fulfill these criteria can readily be diagnosed and treated at a single visit (for the so-called "See and Treat" approach, see Chapter 13). Whether patients with a low-grade squamous intraepithelial lesion (Lo-SIL) and an atypical transformation zone that lacks the characteristic colposcopic features of a high-grade CIN should be treated with an exocervical loop excision prior to histopathological documentation of the presence of disease is more controversial due to the potential for overtreating patients with squamous metaplasia. (This is fully discussed in Chapter 13.)

It is important that only cervices with CIN be treated using loop excision procedure. The procedure should not be used to excise transformation zones indiscriminately in patients with either abnormal Pap smears or a positive HPV DNA test in the absence of clear-cut CIN lesions.

There are a number of contraindications to exocervical loop excision. These include a lesion that extends deeply into the endocervical canal, the presence of known microinvasive or invasive cancer and contraindications related to bleeding during and after the procedure. The contraindications are listed in Table 7.2.

A diagnostic/therapeutic conization (either a cold knife, laser or electrosurgical conization) is used in patients with CIN extending deeply into the canal. In patients with clinically apparent invasive cancer, it is simpler to confirm the diagnosis using a standard punch biopsy and proceed to definitive

Table 7.2

Contraindications to Ectocervical Loop Excision

"Positive" endocervical curettage or a lesion in which the endocervical limit cannot be visualized colposcopically.

Clinically apparent invasive carcinoma of the cervix.

A bleeding disorder.

Pregnancy (except in highly experienced hands).

Severe cervicitis.

Less than 3 months postpartum.

DES-exposed patient.

Equivocal cervical abnormality.

---

therapy rather than performing an ectocervical loop excision for diagnostic purposes. For patients with suspected microinvasive carcinoma, the diagnosis can be confirmed by punch biopsy followed by cone biopsy or by loop excision. Because the loop excision procedure can be associated with significant perioperative bleeding in a small proportion of patients (1-2%), the presence of a bleeding disorder is a contraindication. Similarly, patients with severe cervicitis present a significant risk for bleeding and we recommend that loop excision not be performed until the cervicitis is treated. Another group of patients in whom loop excision should not be performed, except by highly experienced clinicians, is pregnant patients or patients less than 3 months postpartum. Finally, despite our limited experience, we feel that electrosurgery should not be used in DES-exposed women due to the high rate of cervical stenosis that has been reported with other treatment techniques.

ELECTROSURGERY FOR HPV-RELATED DISEASES

Exocervical Loop Excision Procedure

Electrosurgical exocervical loop excision is exceptionally fast and technically very simple to perform. In most cases the entire procedure can be completed in less than 5 minutes. The first step is to perform routine colposcopy after inserting a nonconductive speculum adapted for use with a smoke evacuator (Figure 7.1). We routinely use a large Graves speculum since smaller speculums usually do not provide a large enough field of view. Use of a coated, nonconductive, vaginal wall retractor also helps to insure good visualization of the cervix and protects the vaginal side walls.

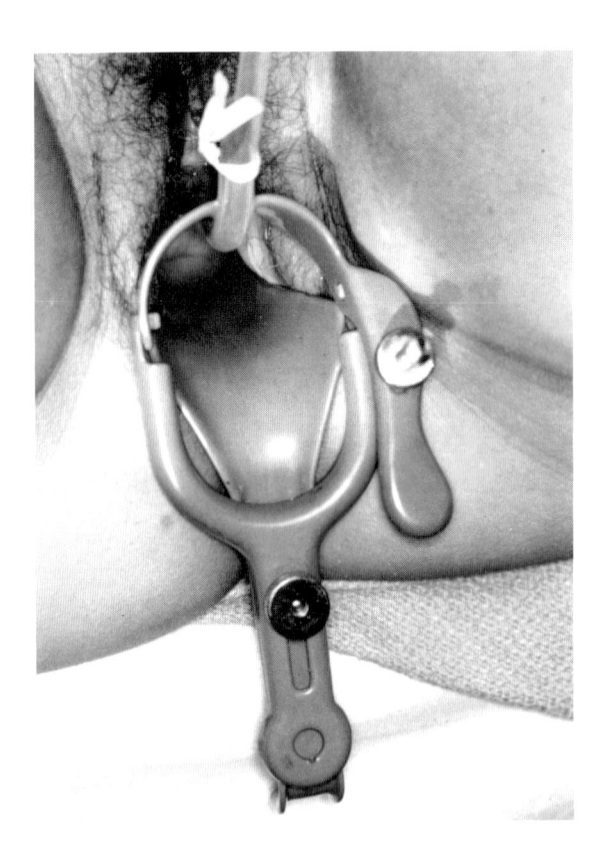

Figure 7.1. A nonconductive speculum equipped with smoke adaptor. This type of speculum is recommended for loop excision procedures.

Once a CIN lesion has been identified and the limits of the lesion delineated, the cervix is painted with full strength aqueous Lugol's Solution (Figure 7.2). This is an important step since it clearly highlights the transformation zone and the staining (or lack thereof) remains intense for a long period of time. In contrast, the effects of 5% acetic acid are transitory and often fade before the procedure is completed. After the cervix has been painted with aqueous Lugol's solution, an intracervical block is applied.

Paracervical blocks can be used for loop excision but they are painful and not necessary. An intracervical block is preferred because it is easier and less painful to perform. The intracervical block is achieved by injecting approximately 0.5-0.9 ml of 2% xylocaine solution with 1:100,000 epinephrine, 2 mm beneath the epithelial surface at the 12:00, 3:00, 6:00 and 9:00 positions (Figure 7.3). The total amount of anesthetic injected is usually 1.8-3.6 ml. Anesthesia sufficient to perform loop excision is achieved within 3 minutes of the injection.

If a woman has an exceptionally large cervix or CIN lesion, it may be advisable to inject an additional 1.8 ml of anesthesia in the spaces between the original injections. For injection it is preferable to use a dental aspirating syringe and a 27 gauge needle (see Chapter 4).

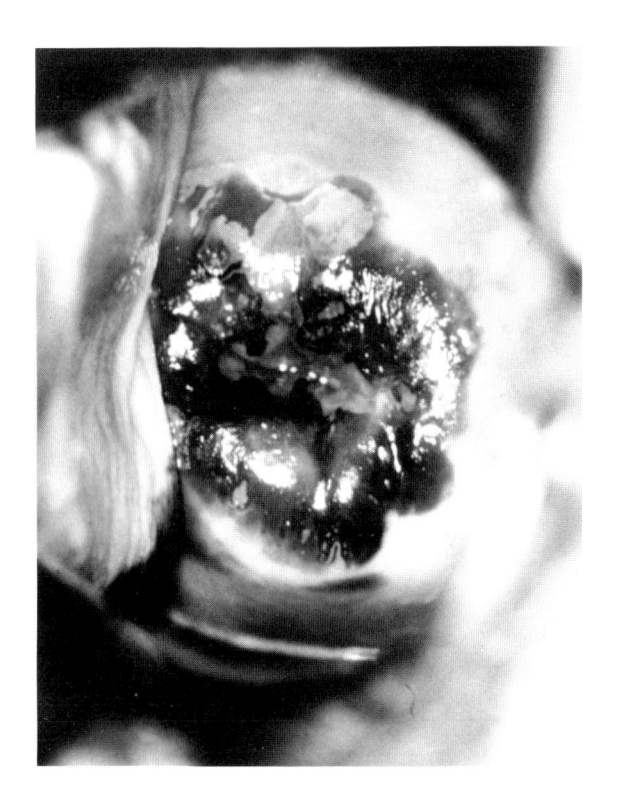

Figure 7.2. The cervix is painted with Lugol's solution. Appearance of a cervix after being painted with Lugol's solution prior to beginning loop excision.

ELECTROSURGERY FOR HPV-RELATED DISEASES

While the anesthetic is taking effect, a patient return ground pad is attached to the patient's thigh (Figure 7.4). A loop of an appropriate size so as to allow the entire CIN lesion to be excised in a single pass (if possible) is selected and attached to a pencil-type electrode handle. A footswitched ESU is preferred to electrode handles with cutting and coagulating switches incorporated into them. For the majority of ectocervical loop excisions, a 2.0 x 0.8 cm electrode is the preferred size loop. These electrodes allow a biopsy with sufficient depth to be taken while protecting against the inadvertent excision of too much tissue. Before performing the excision, make a test pass of the electrode over the region to be excised in order to insure that the path is appropriate.

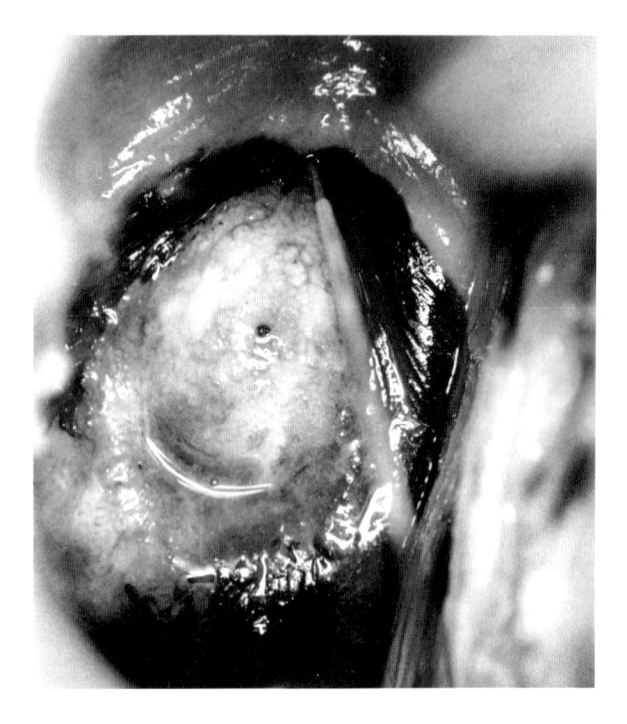

Figure 7.3. Four quadrant injection of 2% xylocaine with 1:100,000 epinephrine intracervically 2 mm beneath the surface using a dental aspirating syringe.

If the vaginal walls prolapse into the field of view or the path of the electrode, a vaginal wall retractor coated with a nonconductive material is inserted before proceeding (Figure 7.5). It is critical that the cervix be perpendicular to the path of the electrode. If the cervix is tilted to one side, an attempt to make it perpendicular to the electrode path is made by packing moistened 2" x 2" gauze pads behind the cervix or by pulling on the anethesized cervix with a skin hook (Figure 7.6).

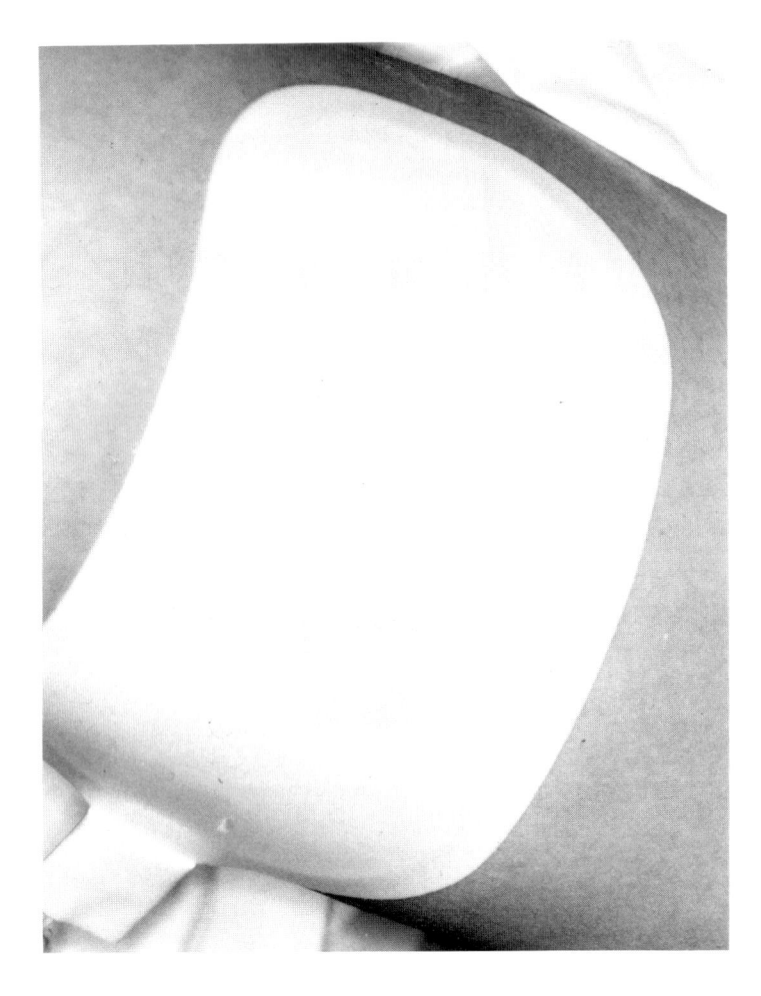

Figure 7.4. Attaching return electrode. A patient return electrode is attached to the patient's thigh.

The ESU is then turned on and adjusted to the appropriate power setting for the wire loop electrode that has been selected. As described in Chapter 4, there are a number of features that we prefer in an ESU which include a digital readout, cord fault alarm, a blended mode, restart capacity, a footswitch and isolated circuitry (Figure 7.7). It is important to keep the unit switched to "Standby" unless actually using the active electrode to prevent inadvertent activation and a patient burn with the active electrode . The size of the loop electrode which is selected, as well as the particular model of ESU, are important variables when selecting the appropriate power setting.

ELECTROSURGERY FOR HPV-RELATED DISEASES

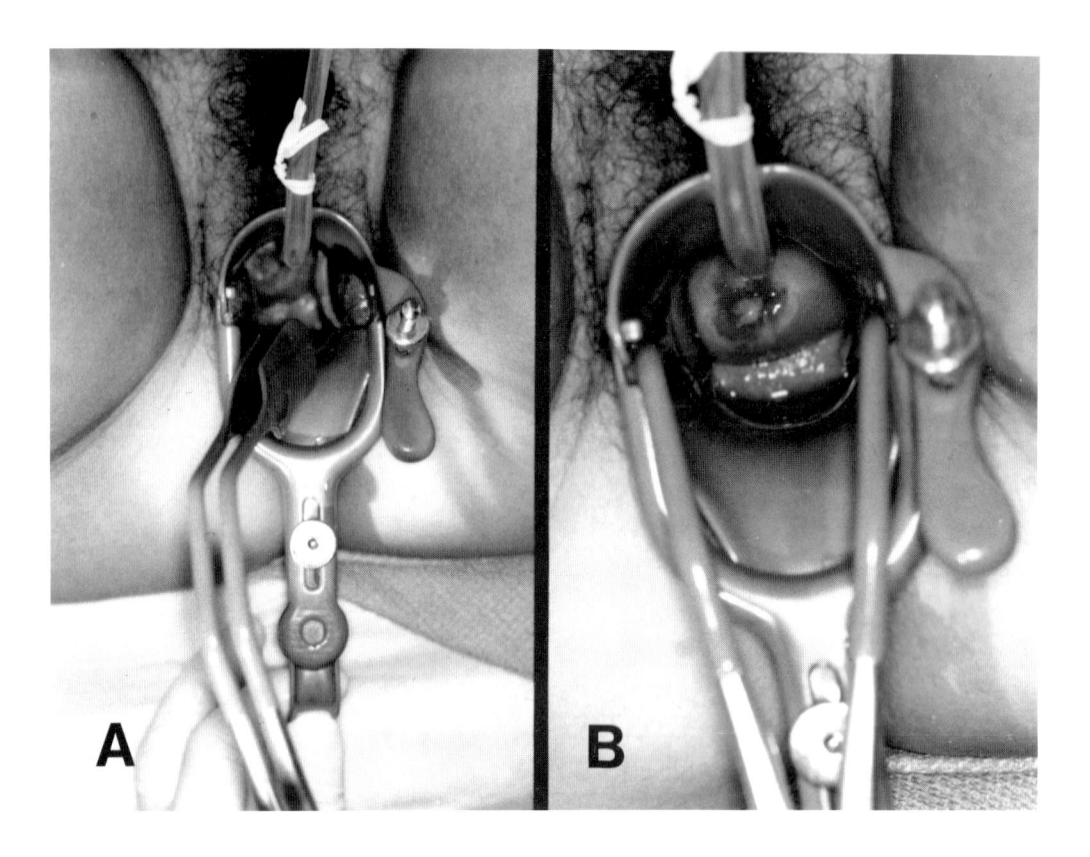

Figure 7.5. A) Coated, nonconductive, vaginal wall retractor. A coated, nonconductive, vaginal wall retractor can be used to exclude the vaginal wall. B) When properly positioned, there is good visualization of the cervix.

Table 7.3 lists the power settings that are recommended for various sized loop electrodes using either the Aspen Excalibur operated in Blend 1 mode or the CooperSurgical LEEP™ System 6000 operated in Blend mode. The appropriate power setting decreases as the size of the loop electrode decreases. If the exact power setting for a particular combination of ESU and loop electrode is not known, the operator must determine the appropriate power setting prior to the procedure. This can be achieved by testing the equipment on either beef tongue or a chicken breast and increasing the power until smooth cutting in the absence of charring is achieved.

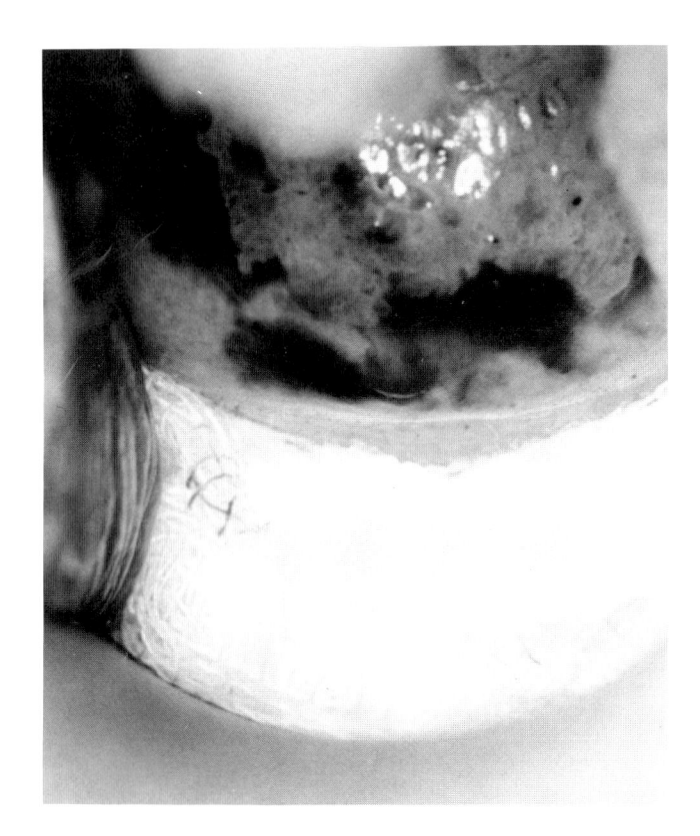

Figure 7.6. Repositioning the cervix. Tilted cervix that has been moved perpendicular to the path of the electrode by packing a moistened 2" x 2" gauze sponge under the posterior lip of the cervix.

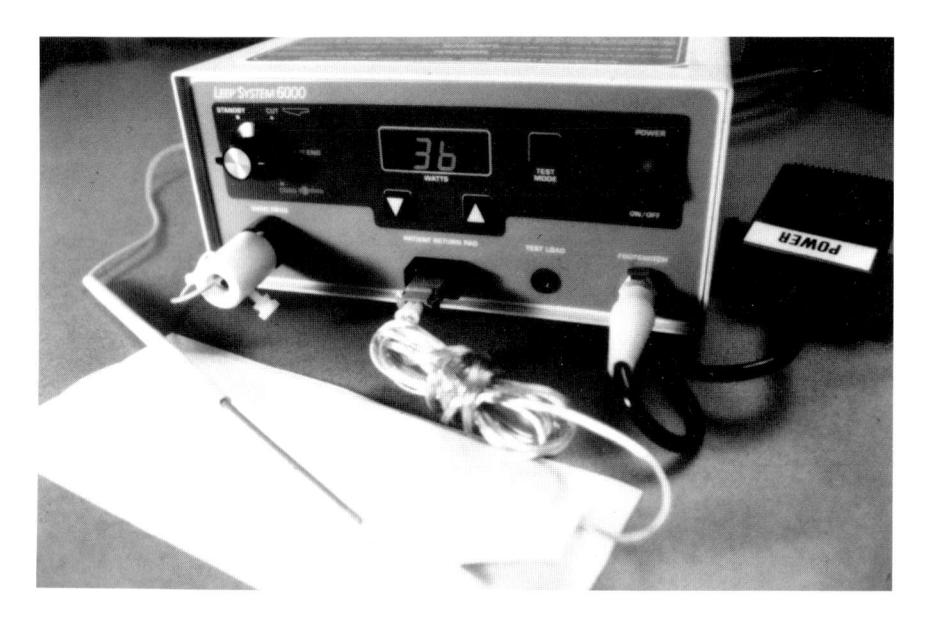

Figure 7.7. ESU that has the recommended features. *(Generator courtesy of CooperSurgical, Inc.)*

Figure 7.8 depicts the approach that is followed for a small central CIN confined to the area around the external os that can be excised in a single pass with the loop electrode. Once everything has been readied for the actual excision, the ESU is switched from "Standby" to "Active", the smoke evacuator is turned on and the electrode is placed 2 - 3 mm lateral to the CIN lesion and several mm from the epithelial surface (Figure 7.8). It is important that the central portion of the CIN lesion be excised in the first pass if more than one pass is to be made. This is because the most likely location of an invasive cancer will be in the central portion of the lesion adjacent to the squamocolumnar junction. It is important not to cut through this area with the loop electrode if it can be avoided. The electrode is then activated by depressing the footpedal, and is pushed perpendicularly into the cervical stroma to a depth of approximately 5 mm. The electrode is then drawn across the cervix parallel

Table 7.3

Power Settings for Different Sizes of Electrode

Size of Electrode	CooperSurgical LEEP™ System 6000	Aspen Excalibur
1 x 1 cm loop	26 watts	25 watts
1.5 x 0.5 cm loop	32 watts	32 watts
2 x 0.8 cm loop	36 watts	35 watts
2 x 1.0 cm loop	36 watts	35 watts
2 x 1.5 cm loop	not recommended	35 watts
2 x 2 cm loop	not recommended	40 watts
3 mm ball electrode	30 watts	30 watts
5 mm ball electrode	50 watts	50 watts

to the surface and sunk progressively deeper into the stroma until a depth of 7 - 8 mm is reached in the region of the endocervical canal. Once the electrode has passed through the region of the endocervical canal, it is progressively

LOOP EXCISIONAL PROCEDURES FOR TREATING CIN

withdrawn to a more shallow depth so that by the time it has cleared the transformation zone on the side of the cervix opposite the starting point it is only 5 mm deep. The electrode is then removed perpendicularly.

When excising lesional tissue it is important to have a stable hand; this can be achieved by resting the shaft of the loop electrode on the posterior blade of the speculum (Figure 7.10). This position will give support to the operator's hand, reduce hand tremor and help to control the depth of excision.

Sometimes the procedure must be stopped midway through an excision or, for some reason, the electrode may stop cutting. Should this occur, we recommend removal of the electrode and excising from the opposite side, meeting the original line of excision (Figure 7.11).

The depth of excision that should be achieved when excising a CIN lesion confined to the ectocervix is identical to the amount of tissue that should be destroyed when performing a CO_2 laser ablation or cryotherapeutic ablation of a similar lesion. Several studies have documented the depth of extension of CIN into endocervical glands. Perhaps the most extensive of these is that of Anderson and Hartley who found that the maximum depth of extension of CIN into the endocervical glands was 5.2 mm but that the mean $\pm$ three standard deviations depth of extension, was only 3.8 mm (Table 7.4).[1]

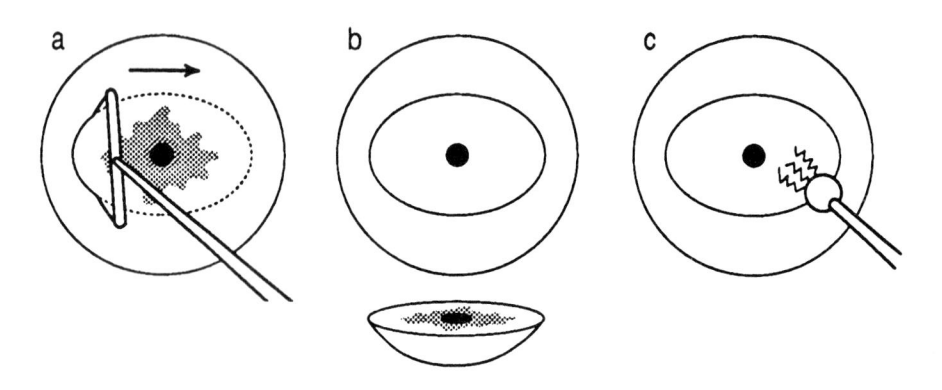

Figure 7.8. Sequence of steps for small CIN lesion confined to the exocervix.

ELECTROSURGERY FOR HPV-RELATED DISEASES

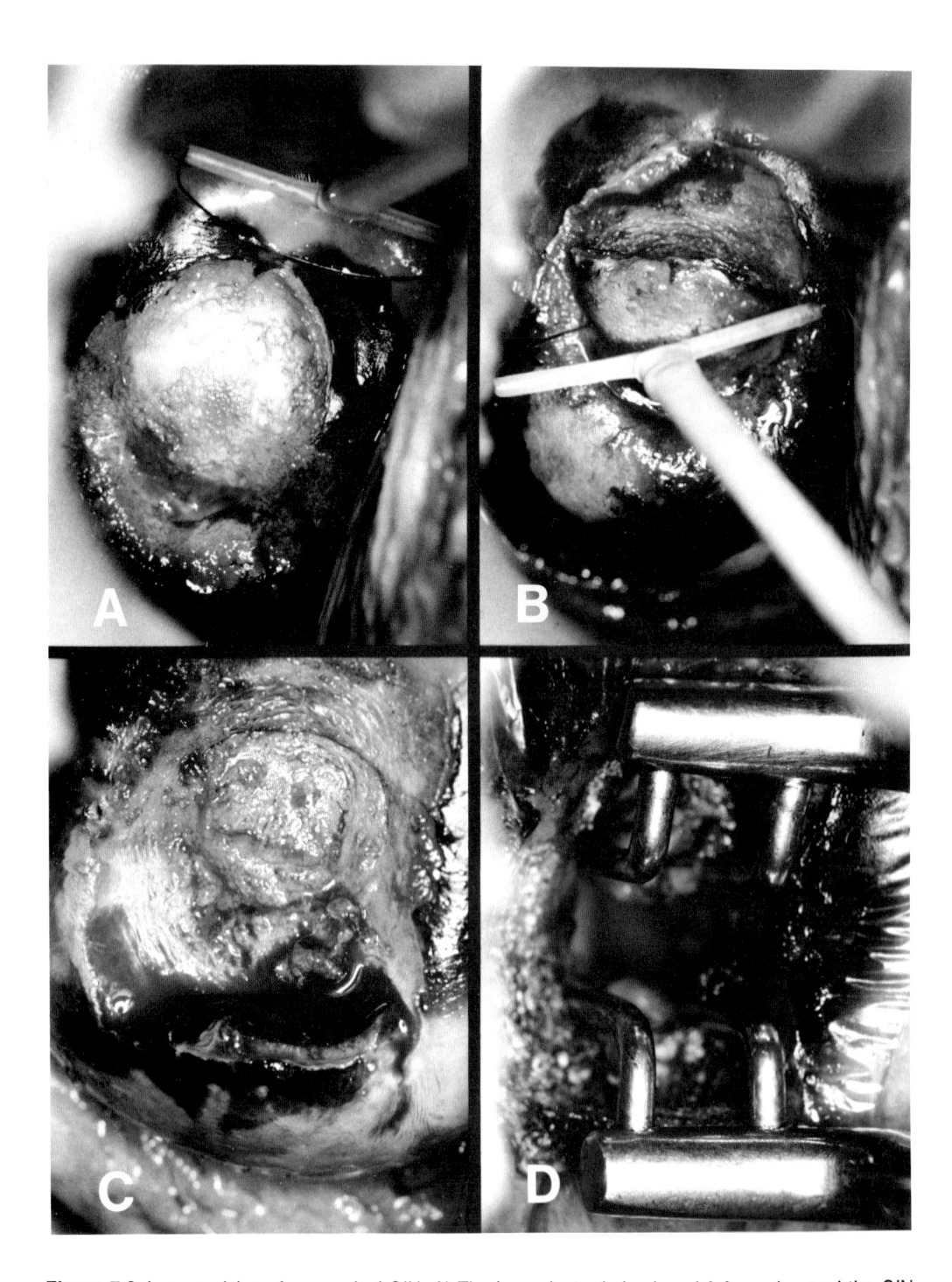

Figure 7.9. Loop excision of exocervical CIN. A) The loop electrode is placed 2-3 mm beyond the CIN lesion and activated. B) Partway through. C) The crater base which has little charring. D) Inspecting the endocervical canal to insure the lesion is completely excised.

LOOP EXCISIONAL PROCEDURES FOR TREATING CIN

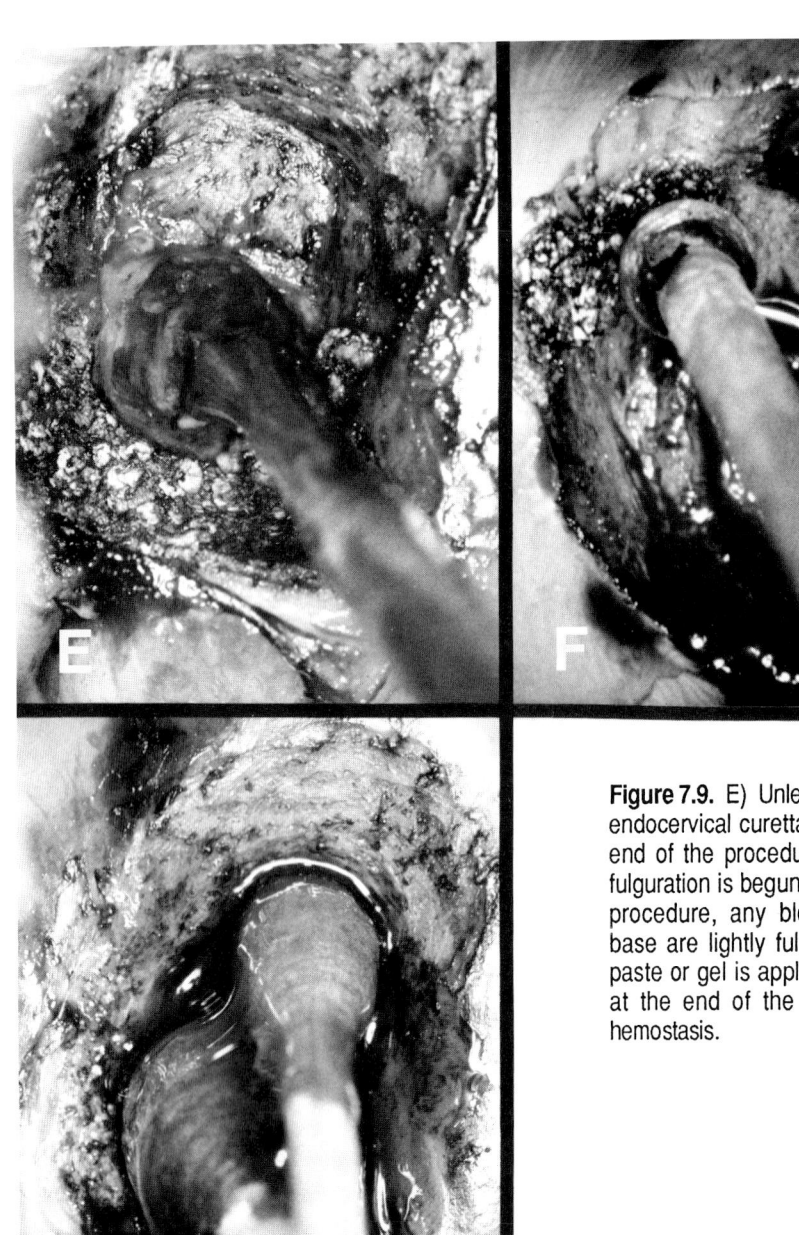

Figure 7.9. E) Unless previously done, an endocervical curettage is obtained at the end of the procedure, preferably before fulguration is begun. F) At the end of the procedure, any bleeders in the crater base are lightly fulgurated. G) Monsel's paste or gel is applied to the crater base at the end of the procedure to insure hemostasis.

ELECTROSURGERY FOR HPV-RELATED DISEASES

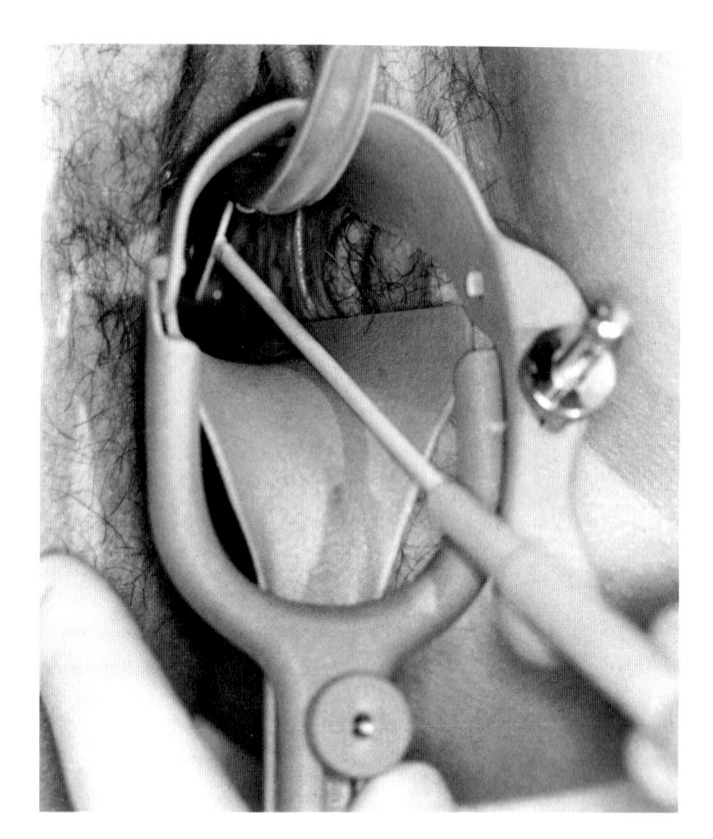

Figure 7.10. Stabilizing the electrode. The loop electrode can be stabilized by resting the electrode on the posterior blade of the speculum.

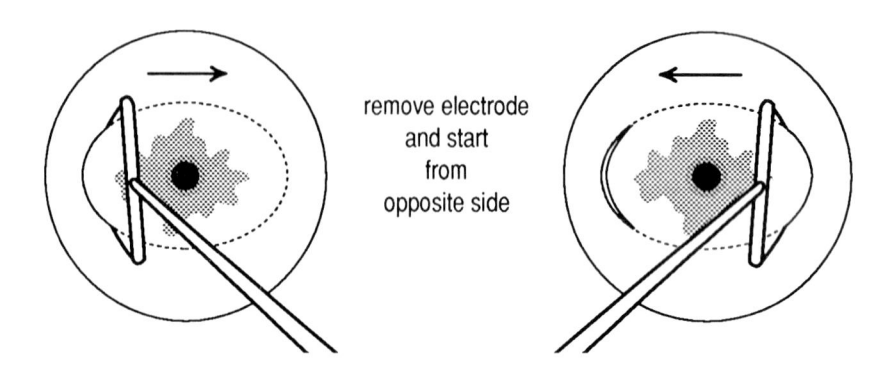

remove electrode and start from opposite side

Figure 7.11. What to do if a "stall" occurs.

LOOP EXCISIONAL PROCEDURES FOR TREATING CIN

A typical specimen excised from the cervix during a loop excision procedure has a minimal amount of charring and carbonization at the edges (Figure 7.12).

Table 7.4

Extension of CIN Into Endocervical Glands

	Depth of Extension (mm)		
	Mean	Max	Mean (+) 3 S.D.
Depth of uninvolved gland	3.4	7.8	6.3
Depth to which CIN extends into glands	1.2	5.2	3.8

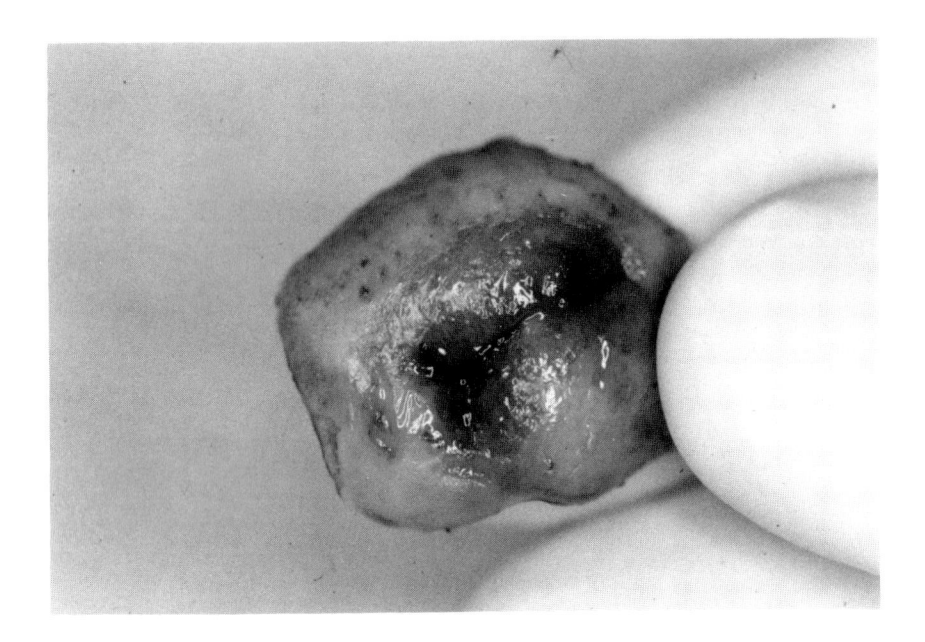

Figure 7.12. Cervical tissue specimen excised using a 0.8 cm x 2.0 cm loop electrode.

Based on these (and other) morphological studies, it is now generally recommended that CIN confined to the exocervix be ablated using the CO_2 laser to a depth of 6 - 8 mm at the lateral margins and to a depth of 8 - 10 mm in the region of the endocervical canal (Figure 7.13).[2] Such an ablation approach produces a "dome-shaped" crater in the cervix with rounded edges. Similarly, using loop excision, the excised tissue should contain the cervical os in the center and should measure 5 - 6 mm deep at the margins and 8 - 10 mm deep in the center. It is important that the excised tissue not have the appearance of a "quonset hut" with blunt ends. Since the cervical branches of the uterine artery are at the 3:00 and 9:00 positions, inserting the electrode deeper than 5 mm can cause significant bleeding. In order to control the depth of the electrode at various points along its path it is important to perform the procedure under direct colposcopic control. A colposcope equipped with low magnification (4-7.5x) is best for loop excision. If the colposcope that is available does not have variable magnification, a lower magnification than is usually used can be obtained economically by equipping the colposcope with 5x oculars.

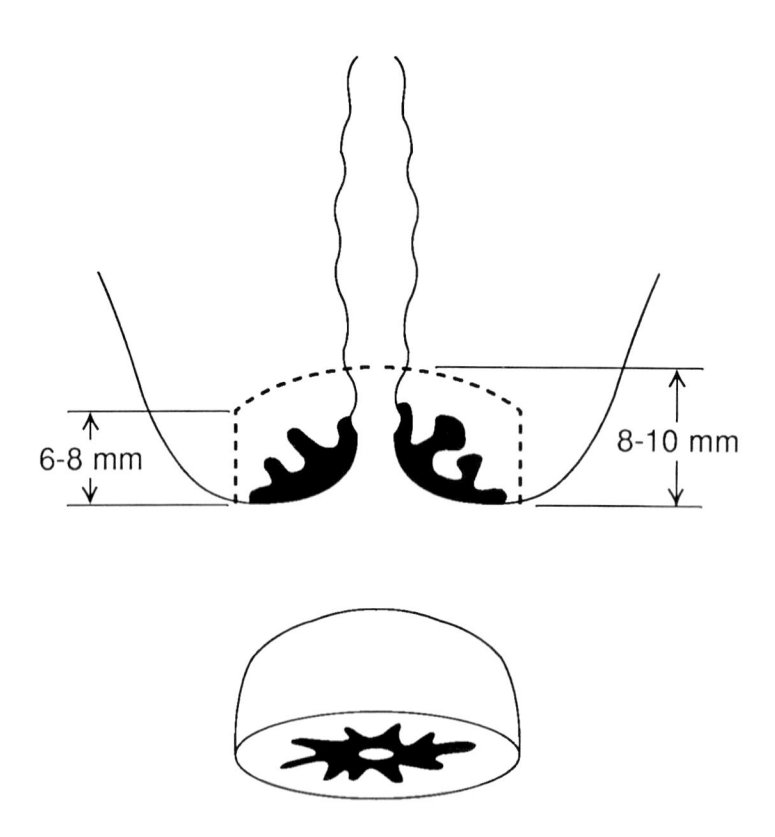

Figure 7.13. Recommended dimensions of tissue defect using CO_2 laser. Dome-shaped ablation is suggested for laser ablation of CIN by others. Tissue excised using the loop electrodes should be of similar dimensions and shape. If a 0.8 X 2.0 cm loop is used, the maximum depth of excision will be limited to 0.8 cm.

The approach described above is used for relatively small, central lesions that can be excised in a single pass with the loop electrode. Larger lesions may require more than a single pass. When this occurs, the central portion of the lesion is excised in the first pass. Then additional passes are made with the electrode to remove any remaining CIN tissue (Figure 7.14).

In some cases it is advantageous to combine wire loop excision of the central portion of the CIN with electrosurgical fulguration ablation of more peripheral portions of the CIN lesion using "Coagulation" current and the 5 mm ball electrode (Figure 7.15). A combined excisional and ablational approach is particularly useful for large CIN lesions that extend onto the vaginal fornices (Figure 7.16). Additional anesthesia may be required when large lesions are treated, especially if they extend on to the vagina. When performing electrosurgical fulguration of CIN, it is important to keep the cervix moist to increase arcing from the ball electrode to the tissue. It is also important to remove the charred tissue from the ball electrode tip frequently and to keep the ball electrode in place until a full cautery effect is achieved (Table 7.5).

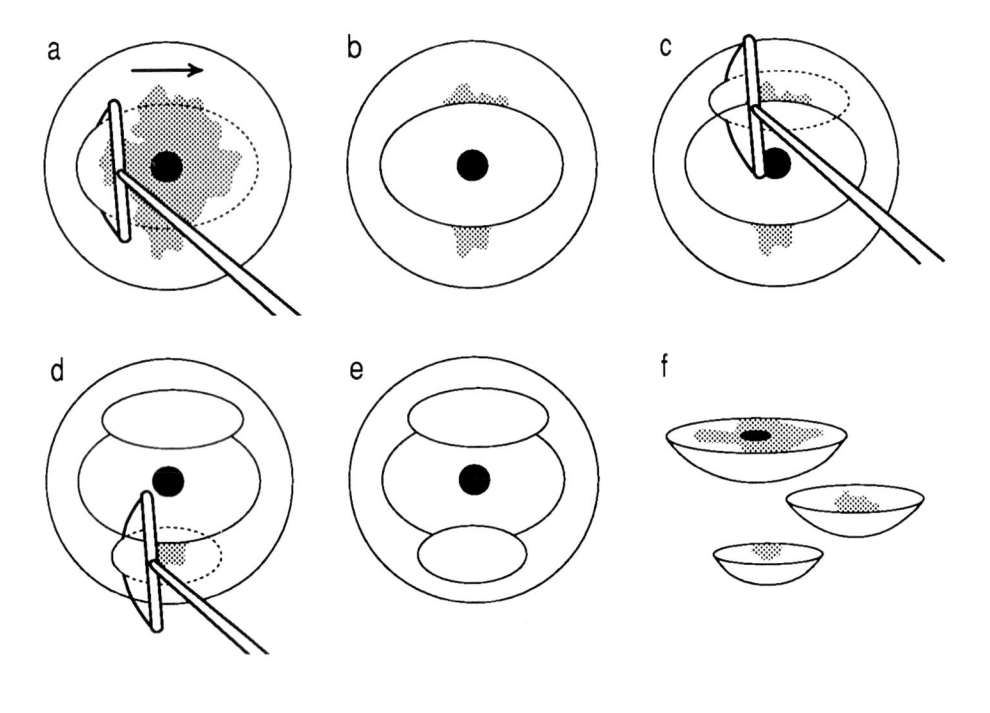

Figure 7.14. Excision of large CIN lesions confined to exocervix. After the central portion is excised, additional passes with the loop electrodes are made to excise the peripheral portions of the lesion.

ELECTROSURGERY FOR HPV-RELATED DISEASES

Once the CIN has been excised, the crater base and the endocervical canal must be examined with the colposcope. This allows the operator to insure that the entire lesion has been excised and that no endocervical glands are still present in the crater base. The endocervical canal should also be examined for residual CIN by placing a cotton-tipped applicator stick soaked with 5% acetic acid in the canal once the excised tissue has been removed, and then examining the canal using an endocervical speculum. The normal endocervical mucosa will appear salmon pink whereas residual CIN will appear bright white. Be careful to distinguish between the thin, 1 mm zone of white thermal artifact, which is almost invariably present at the resection margin, and residual CIN, which will be present deeper in the canal.

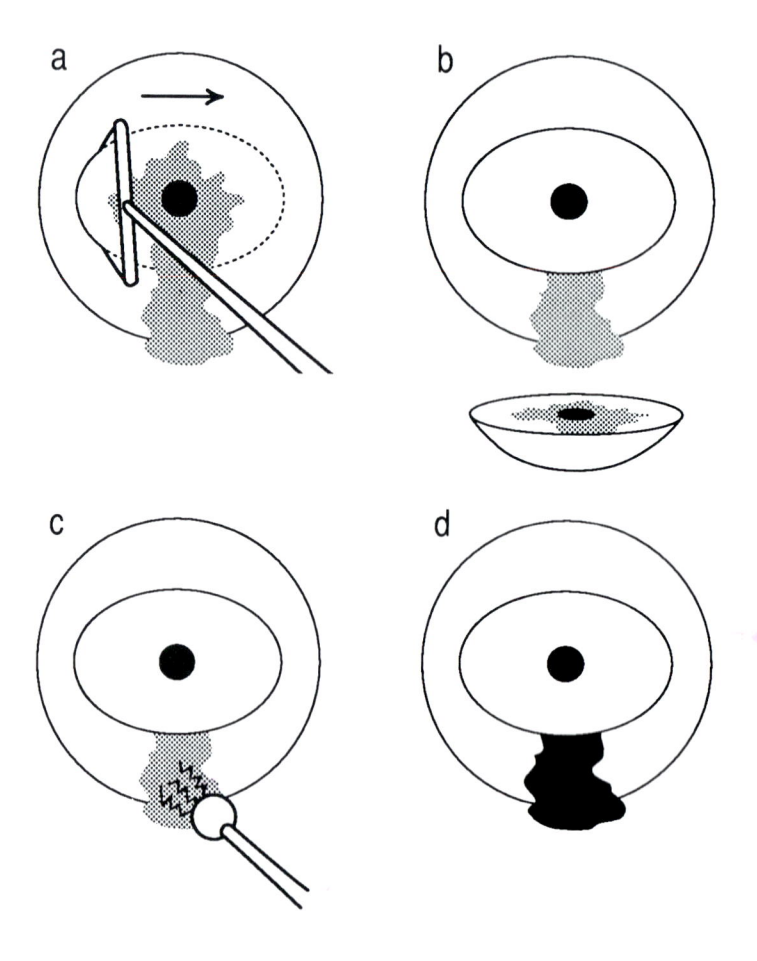

Figure 7.15. Combined excision/fulguration. This approach to treating CIN is used for large lesions and combines wire loop excision of the central portion of CIN with electrosurgical ablation of peripheral portions of the CIN using coagulation current and a ball electrode.

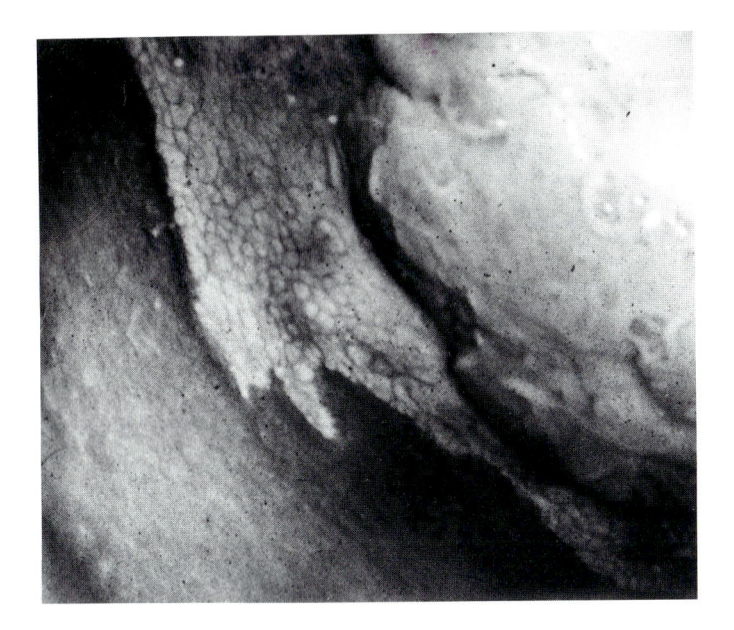

Figure 7.16. Large lesion with extension of CIN on to the vagina. This lesion cannot be excised in its entirety but a combination of loop excision and electrosurgical fulguration can be used to treat it.

Table 7.5

Tips for Good Electrosurgical Fulguration

Keep cervix moist to increase arcing.
Frequently remove char from electrode.
Fulgurate until mucus stops bubbling.
Fulgurate in overlapping circles.

When examining the crater base colposcopically, it is also important that residual endocervical glands be identified as they may contain CIN. Residual endocervical glands have a green-white mucinous appearance against a background of yellow denatured collagen. If either residual CIN in the endocervical canal or residual endocervical glands in the excisional crater are detected, it is important that additional tissue be removed in order to prevent recurrence.

At the end of the excision, an endocervical curettage should be performed (provided one was not previously performed and the endocervical canal was found to be free of disease) and the crater base should be fulgurated lightly using a 5 mm ball electrode and pure coagulation current if there is active bleeding. Fulguration is intended to stop active bleeding from the crater base and to coagulate the tissue lightly. In cases in which bleeding is severe, we fulgurate active bleeders using a macroneedle electrode before performing the ECC. This prevents the curettings from becoming lost in the blood. The base of the crater should not be heavily charred since this produces a large amount of devitalized tissue which may become infected and subsequently produce postoperative bleeding. In all cases, including those in which active bleeding is not encountered, we place either Monsel's paste or gel in the crater base. This acts as a long-acting astringent and prevents subsequent bleeding.

In our early experience with the loop excision procedure, the incidence of postoperative bleeding was greatly reduced by packing the crater base with Monsel's paste. Of the first 40 patients treated before using Monsel's paste routinely, six returned to the clinic 4 - 6 days after the procedure complaining of persistent bleeding.[3] In all these patients the amount of bleeding was minimal but sufficient to be of concern to the patient. In some patients a blood clot was found in the crater base that appeared to be inhibiting healing. Since bleeding in these 6 cases was readily controlled by removing the blood clot and applying Monsel's paste to the oozing crater base, the protocol was modified to apply Monsel's paste routinely at the end of the procedure. Once this was done, the incidence of postoperative bleeding was greatly reduced.[3]

LOOP EXCISION CONE BIOPSY FOR ENDOCERVICAL EXTENSION OF CIN

The development of techniques for electrosurgical cone biopsy allows many patients with CIN extending into the endocervical canal to be safely and effectively managed electrosurgically. As originally described by Mor-Yosef and co-workers[4], loop excision cone biopsies (loop diathermy cone biopsies) were usually performed in the operating room under general anesthesia using the large loop electrodes. The major difference between the Prendiville technique for treating ectocervical disease and Mor-Yosef's technique for cone biopsy was that the electrode was inserted much deeper into the cervix for the cone biopsy. Because of the significant amount of tissue removed (the average length of the loop excision cone biopsy was 20.2 mm) there was a 2% incidence of perioperative bleeding and a 6% incidence of postoperative bleeding.[4]

Cone biopsies can be performed on some patients electrosurgically (loop excisional cone biopsy) on an outpatient basis using local anesthesia. The recommended outpatient procedure is modeled on methods used to treat CIN extending into the endocervical canal with laser ablation and combines excision with the shallow large loop electrodes used for ectocervical loop excision with excision of endocervical CIN using a 1 x 1 cm loop or rectangular electrode.

Results with this method have been excellent with no significant perioperative bleeding and only a single case of significant postoperative bleeding.

Indications for Loop Excision Cone Biopsy

Loop excision cone biopsy is a useful diagnostic and therapeutic procedure for patients that have CIN extending a limited distance into the endocervical canal (Table 7.6). The typical patient treated with this approach on an outpatient basis is one in whom CIN extends into the endocervical canal but in whom the upper limit of the lesion can be identified (although often incompletely visualized) by careful inspection with an endocervical speculum. This approach is limited to lesions whose canal extension can be excised with a single pass of a 1 x 1 cm loop electrode. It should be emphasized that this approach should not be used for CIN lesions that extend so deeply into the canal that the upper limits of the lesion cannot be seen and the entire lesion can not be excised using a 1 x 1 cm electrode. In these cases either a cold knife conization or an electrosurgical needle electrode conization is performed.

Table 7.6

Indications/Contraindications for Loop Excision Cone Biopsy

Indications

CIN extending into the endocervical canal to a depth that can be excised with a 1 x 1 cm loop electrode.

Contraindications

CIN extending deeper into the endocervical canal than can be excised with a single pass of a 1 x 1 cm loop electrode.

Loop Excision Cone Biopsy Procedure

Patients are initially evaluated colposcopically and prepared for a loop excisional biopsy in a manner similar to that described above for ectocervical CIN with the exception that, in addition to the four quadrant intracervical block, 0.25 - 0.5 ml of 2% xylocaine with 1:100,000 epinephrine is directly injected into the anterior and posterior endocervical canal.

Two approaches for performing outpatient electrosurgical cones can be used. We recommend the use of a 1.0 x 1.0 cm square or loop style electrode

ELECTROSURGERY FOR HPV-RELATED DISEASES

to excise first a 0.8 - 1.0 cm deep cylinder of endocervical tissue. After the first pass with the electrode, any CIN extending onto the portio can be excised with the 2.0 x 0.8 cm loop electrode (Figures 7.17A, 7.18A). This approach is preferred and will usually excise any lesion extending up to 7 mm into the endocervical canal. A typical loop excision cone biopsy sequence is shown in Figure 7.19. The specimens obtained are illustrated in Figure 7.20. Another method of performing loop excision cone biopsies is to excise first the exocervical portion of the lesion using a 2.0 x 0.8 cm loop electrode and then using a 1.0 x 1.0 cm loop or rectangular electrode to excise any residual disease extending into the canal (Figures 7.17B, 7.18B). There are two problems with

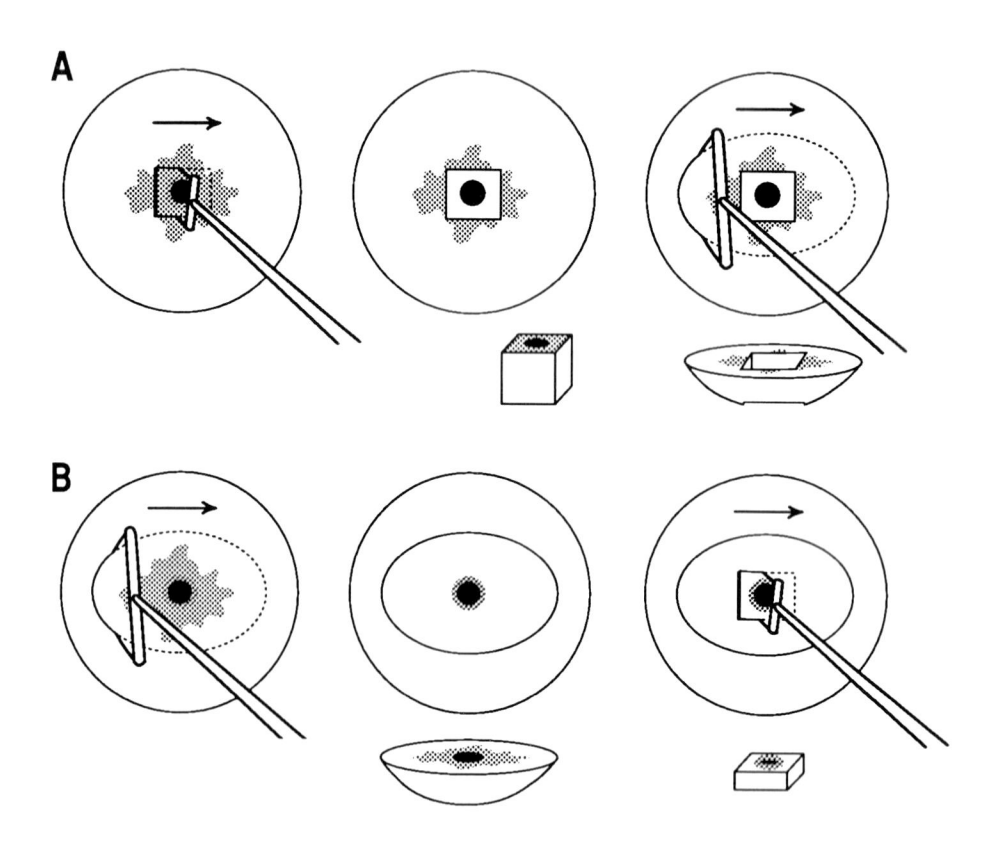

Figure 7.17. Loop excision cone biopsy. Two different approaches for performing outpatient loop excisional cones using wire loop electrodes. A) The recommended method excises the canal first. B) Alternate method recommended for selected cases.

the latter approach. First, there is the potential for cutting across disease within the endocervical canal if the first pass is too shallow. This may present

142

problems for histopathologic interpretation. Second, there is a tendency to excise deeply into the canal. As shown in Figure 7.18C, it is easy to excise to a depth of 1.6 cm using this approach but it is advisable not to perform loop excision cone biopsies to this depth on an outpatient basis. Although there are

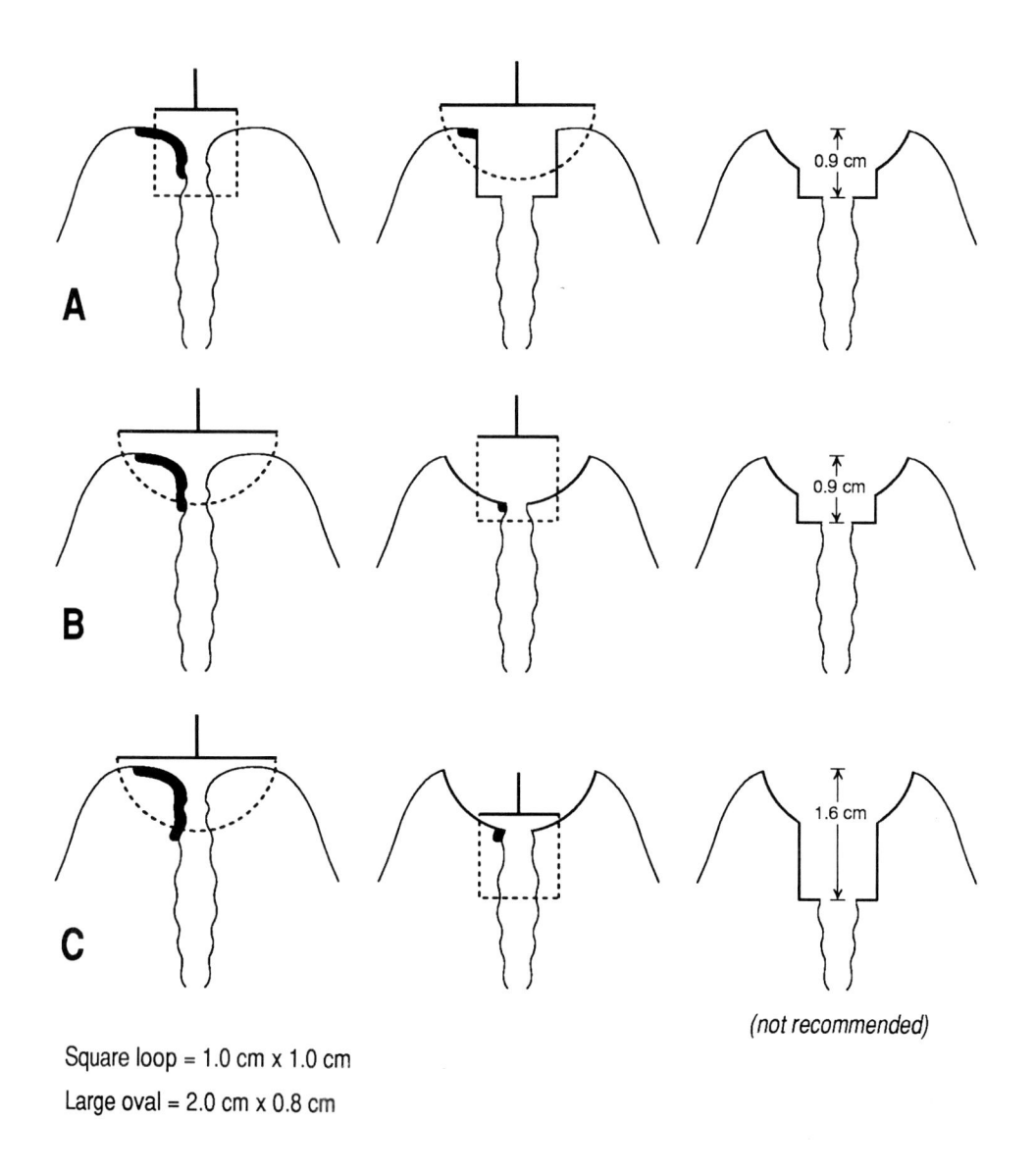

Square loop = 1.0 cm x 1.0 cm
Large oval = 2.0 cm x 0.8 cm

Figure 7.18. Loop excision cone biopsies. A) The recommended approach involves excising the endocervical canal first. B) A second approach that is useful in some cases. C) Excessively deep excision of the canal for an outpatient setting can occur if the endocervical canal is excised after the exocervical portion.

ELECTROSURGERY FOR HPV-RELATED DISEASES

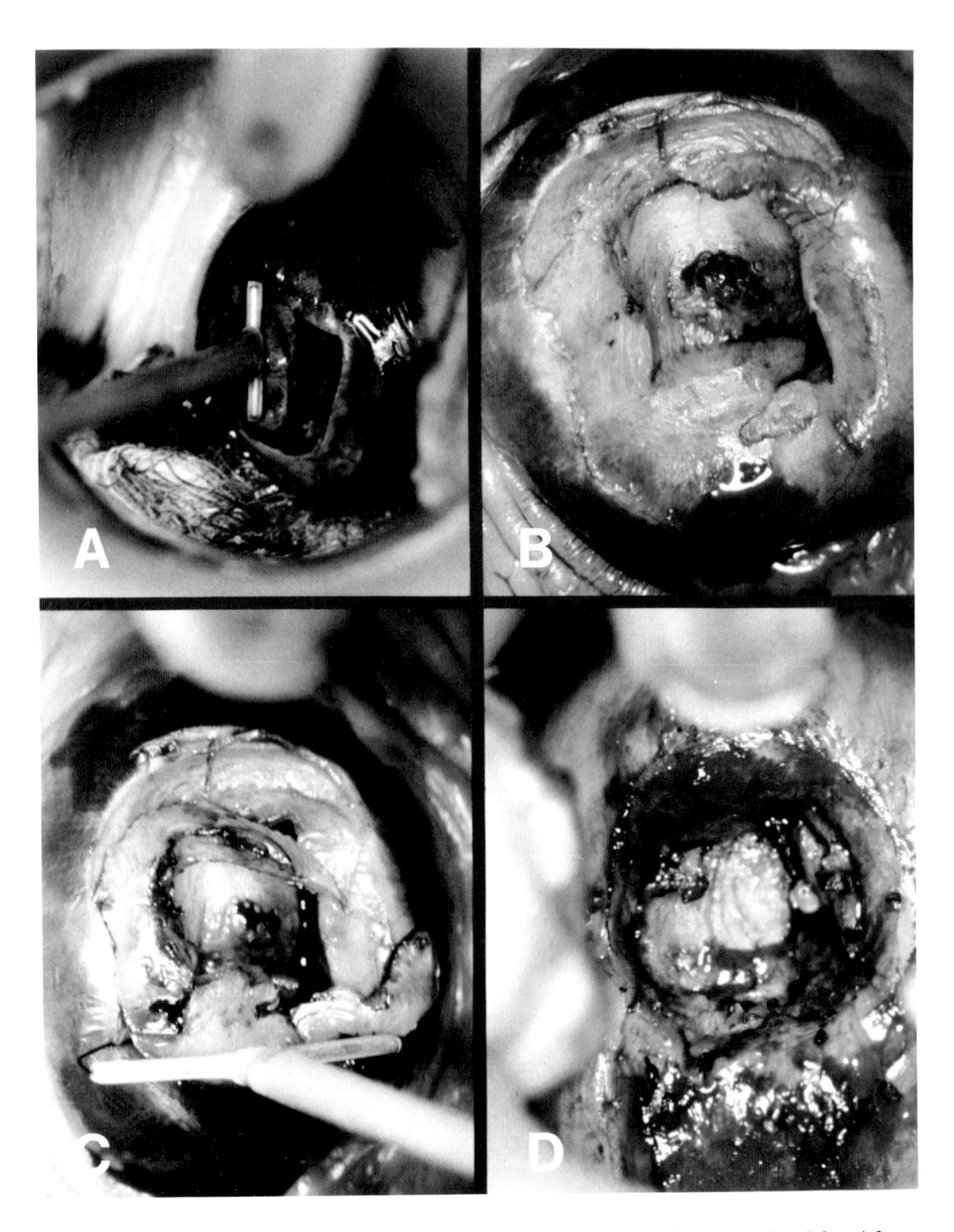

Figure 7.19. Loop excision cone biopsy. A) Removal of endocervical disease using 1.0 x 1.0 cm rectangular loop. B) Crater base after removal of endocervical portion. C) Excision of exocervical disease using a 0.8 x 2.0 cm loop. D) Crater base at end of procedure.

LOOP EXCISIONAL PROCEDURES FOR TREATING CIN

potential problems with this method, excising the exocervical portion first can be useful in selected cases such as patients with irregular cervices in whom it is difficult to approach the endocervical canal with a 1.0 x 1.0 cm rectangular electrode.

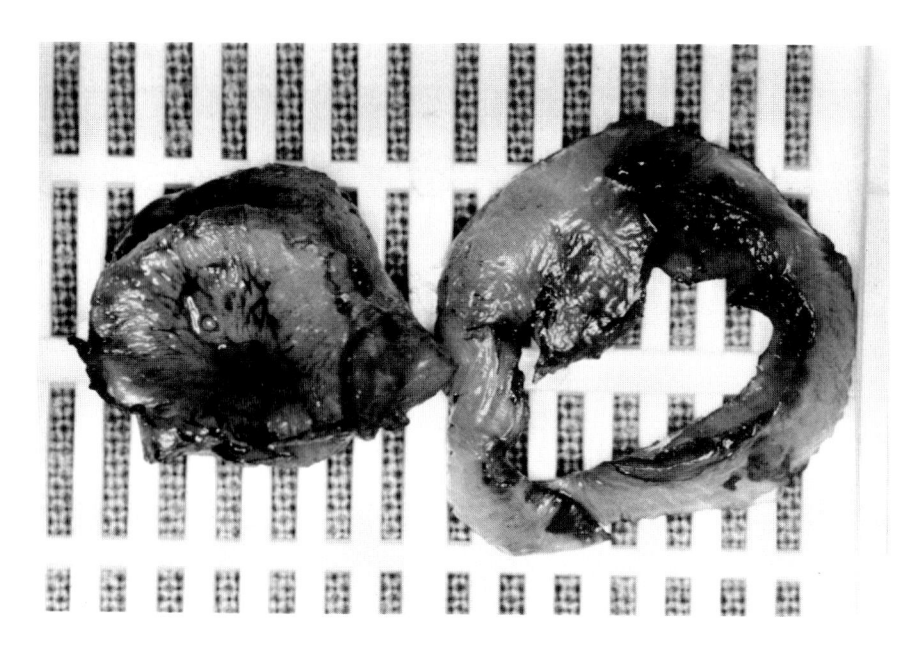

Figure 7.20. Specimens from loop excision cone biopsy. The one on left contains endocervical portion of excision and the specimen on right is exocervical portion.

Always check the endocervical canal colposcopically for residual CIN by placing a cotton-tipped applicator stick soaked with 5% acetic acid into the endocervical canal and examining the canal with an endocervical speculum. As described previously, the normal endocervical mucosa will appear salmon pink, whereas residual CIN will appear bright white. Again, it should be noted that there will usually be a 1 mm zone of white thermal artifact at the resection margin and that this does not represent residual CIN. If CIN remains in the canal, excise another piece of tissue using the 1 x 1 cm loop or rectangular electrode. After the excisions are completed, endocervical curettage may be performed. If there is active bleeding, both the endocervical and the ectocervical portions of the crater base are fulgurated using a ball electrode. As with ectocervical electrosurgical loop excision, if bleeding is absent or negligible, the crater base is packed with Monsel's paste or gel, instead of being fulgurated, and the patient is discharged.

ELECTROSURGICAL NEEDLE CONIZATIONS

Patients with endocervical canal involvement whose lesions extend too deeply into the canal to be excised with a single pass with a 1 cm deep loop can still be treated with electrosurgery. In these cases, a microneedle electrode, rather than a cold knife, can be used to perform a conization. The criteria for determining which patients are appropriate for microneedle conization are given in Table 7.7.

Table 7.7

Indications for Electrosurgical Needle Cone Biopsy

Biopsy-proven CIN lesion of any grade that extends far enough into the endocervical canal that the endocervical extension cannot be excised with a single pass of a 1 x 1 cm loop electrode.

A needle conization sequence is presented in Figure 7.21. Patients can be operated on either under general or local anesthesia. Prior to conization, the cervix and endocervical canal is infiltrated with dilute vasopressin. Ten units of vasopressin (1/2 ampule) is mixed with 30 ml of normal saline if the procedure is performed under general anesthesia or 30 ml of 1% xylocaine if the procedure is performed under local anesthesia. Ten ml of the mixture is injected into the cervical stroma around the area to be excised. The microneedle is used to excise down to the appropriate depth in the endocervical canal. A skin hook is useful to provide traction on the specimen during the excision. At the end of the excision, the apex of the cone is severed using a tonsillar snare or curved scissors in order to avoid thermal artifact at the endocervical margin. The crater base is fulgurated with a ball electrode and coagulation current.

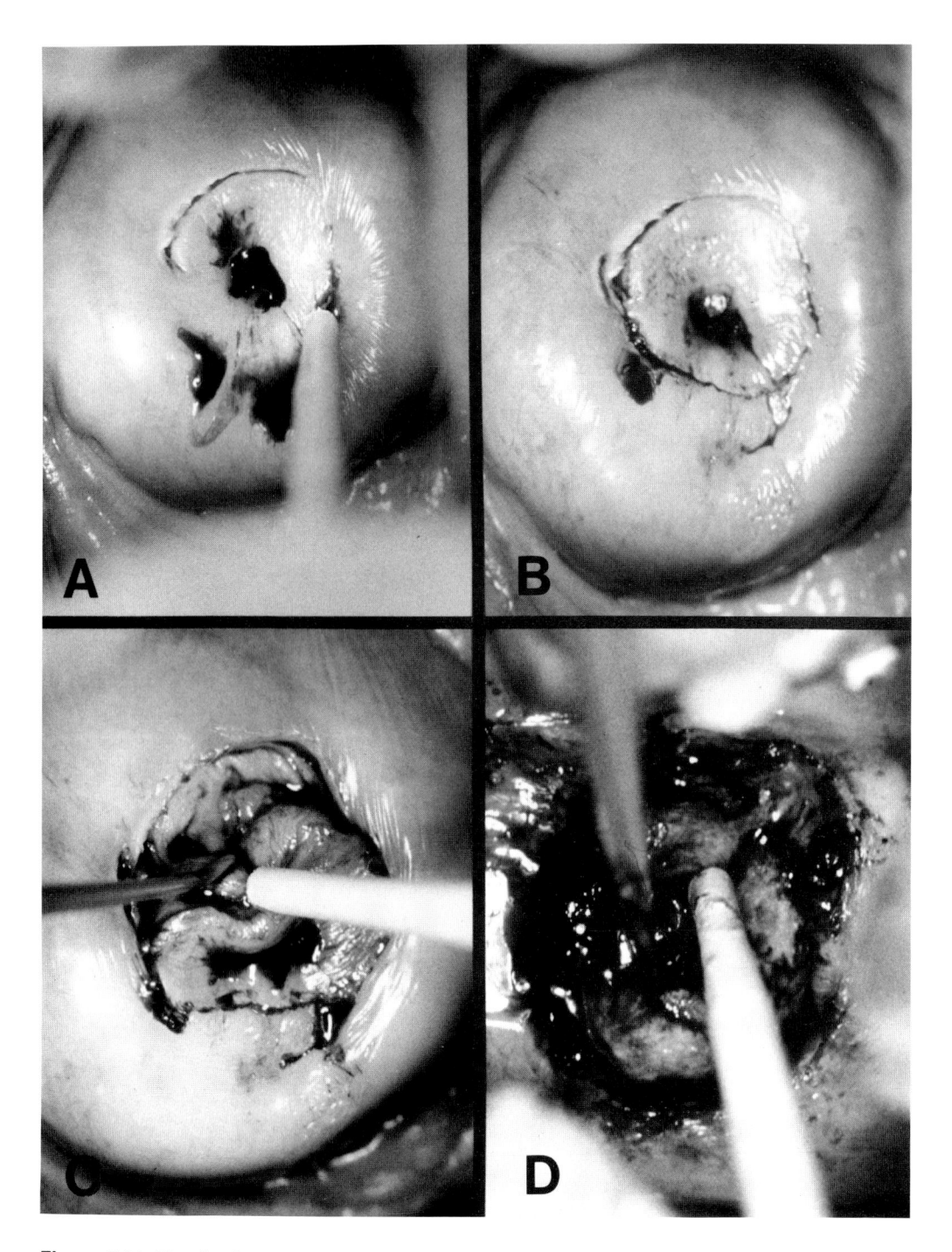

Figure 7.21. Needle Cone Biopsy. A, B) The region to be excised is encircled using a microneedle electrode. C, D) Using a skin hook to retract the tissue, the incision is continued to the desired depth *(figure continues on page 148).*

ELECTROSURGERY FOR HPV-RELATED DISEASES

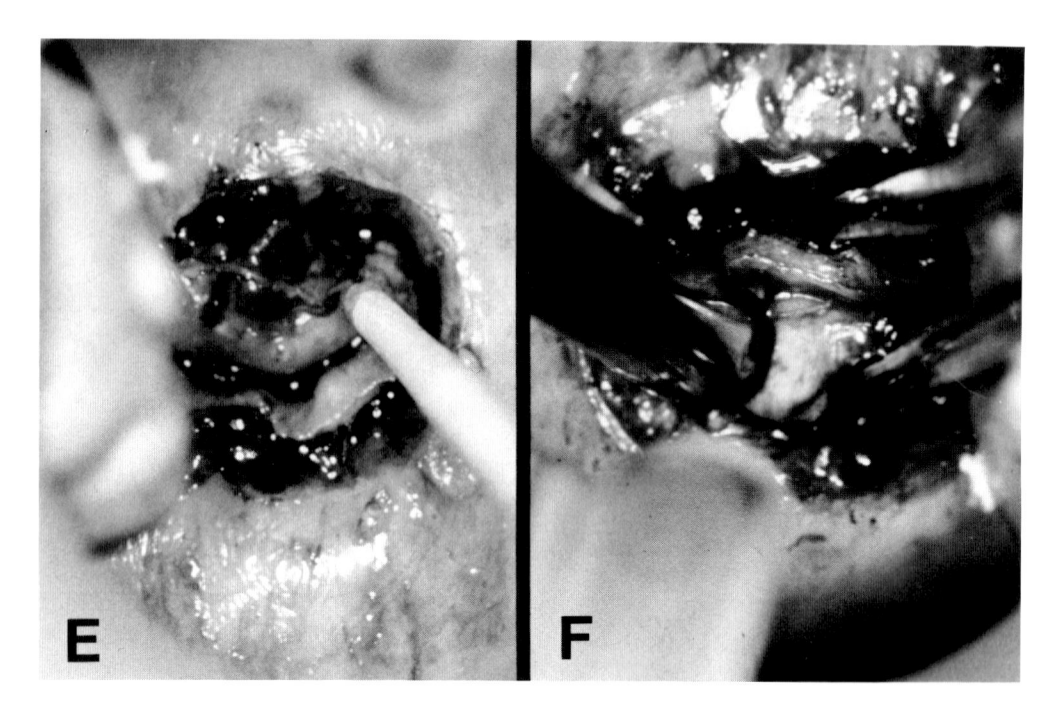

E) Using a skin hook to retract the tissue, the incision is continued to the desired depth *(continued from page 147)*. F) A tonsillar snare is used to excise the base of the cone.

Postoperative Instructions After Electrosurgery

We give all patients who have received ectocervical electrosurgical excision the same set of printed postoperative instructions that we give to patients who have had laser ablations. These instructions are designed to prevent behaviors which might produce postoperative bleeding, to allay the patients fears about the discharge that usually occurs after the procedure and to prevent unnecessary telephone calls while, at the same time, clearly alerting the patient to the warning signs of a significant postoperative complication. A reproduction of our standard printed instructions is given in Chapter 8.

All patients are advised to forego sexual intercourse or the use of vaginal tampons and douching for a period of three weeks in order to prevent newly developing scar tissue from being dislodged and traumatized. We also advise patients to reduce the amount of strenuous exercise that they perform, especially lifting heavy objects over their head.

Many patients will have a moderate amount of reddish-black discharge for a period of one to two weeks after electrosurgery. The amount of this discharge is similar to that which occurs after laser ablation and is much less than is generally encountered after cryosurgery. If loop excision is performed during the early proliferative phase of the menstrual cycle it will prevent the patient from misconstruing menstrual blood flow as significant postoperative hemorrhage. If bleeding becomes as heavy as a normal menstrual period during the first postoperative week, the patient is instructed to call. Similarly, if bleeding persists for more than one week or if the vaginal discharge becomes malodorous the patient is asked to call. Many patients have noted that their first menstrual period after electrosurgical excision is especially heavy but this does not seem to be associated with later problems.

COMPLICATIONS OF ELECTROSURGERY

The major complications of electrosurgery are listed in Table 7.8 and the incidence of these complications in the large published series of patients treated with loop excision that list complications are given in Table 7.9.

Table 7.8

Potential Complications of Electrosurgery

Perioperative bleeding
Postoperative bleeding
Cervical infection
Cervical stenosis
Effects on fertility/pregnancy

Perioperative Bleeding

Perioperative and postoperative bleeding are the major complications of loop excision, whether ectocervical or cone biopsy, and have occurred in all the major published series. Significant perioperative bleeding appears to be much more common in patients with acute cervicitis and this condition should be considered to be a contraindication to loop excision. The bleeding that occurs in patients with acute cervicitis appears to be a diffuse (non-arterial type) bleeding from the crater base that is often very difficult to stop using fulguration. If such bleeding does occur, placing liberal amounts of Monsel's paste in the crater base and then packing the vagina with iodoform gauze has been used successfully. The patients are asked to rest in the waiting room for several hours after which the pack is removed. In all our cases to date this has been highly effective. None of the patients have required further treatment or returned to the office with postoperative bleeding.

Table 7.9

Complications of Electrosurgery for CIN

Author	Recessed SCJ	Stenosis	Severe Periop. Bleed	Severe Postop. Bleed	Moderate Postop. Bleed
Prendiville	7%	0%	2%	2%	9%
Whiteley	9%	0%	0%	1%	3%
Luesley	10%	1%	1%	4%	N.D.
Wright	2%	1%	0%	0%	4%

Another type of perioperative bleeding, that rarely occurs, is significant arterial-type bleeding. In the majority of instances this appears to have developed when the operator inadvertently inserted the wire loop electrode too deeply at the 3:00 or 9:00 position and cut a branch of the uterine artery. Although this complication has been quite uncommon in our experience, when it does occur it can produce significant hemorrhage and the operator must be equipped to handle it. A mattress suture may be required to stop arterial bleeding and a 12 inch long needle driver and 00 Vicryl suture material should be available in the colposcopy suite should the necessity of placing a suture arise.

Significant perioperative bleeding appears to be a relatively uncommon event during exocervical loop excision. In our experience, and in the large published series, it occurs in about 1% of cases.[3-8] The one large series with a higher rate is that of Murdoch *et al.*[8] In that study a large number of patients actually underwent "loop diathermy cone biopsies" as opposed to simple exocervical loop excisions. Therefore, the incidence of severe perioperative bleeding of 5% is not surprising. Even in the women undergoing loop excision cone biopsy, all of the perioperative hemorrhages responded to cauterization and vaginal tampons.

Obviously the patient population (e.g., a high incidence of acute cervicitis) and the experience of the operator will influence the incidence of significant perioperative bleeding. As one would anticipate, significant perioperative bleeding is a much more frequent complication when loop excision cone biopsies (as opposed to ectocervical loop excisions) are performed.

Postoperative Bleeding

Significant postoperative bleeding requiring hospital admission, transfusion, or suturing, also appears to be an uncommon complication of ectocervical electrosurgical excision. In our series of over 800 cases of ectocervical electrosurgical excision we have not had a single instance in which a patient required hospitalization, transfusion or suturing for postoperative bleeding. We have had, however, a number of patients return either to the colposcopy suite or to the emergency room for postoperative bleeding. The majority of these patients have presented 4 to 6 days after the procedure with either persistent or increased vaginal bleeding. Colposcopic examination usually reveals necrotic debris and granulation tissue in the crater base from which slight oozing can be demonstrated by asking the patient to "bear down". Rarely a blood clot will be present in the crater (Figure 7.22).

In patients with mild degrees of postoperative bleeding, the crater base can be re-cauterized using the ball electrode or, preferably, Monsel's paste can be applied to the crater. If a blood clot is present it can be removed using a ring forceps and then Monsel's applied to the crater base. If it appears that a cervical infection is contributing to the persistent bleeding, antibiotics should be prescribed.

The United Kingdom studies have reported higher rates of serious postoperative bleeds than we have experienced. In the series of patients reported by Luesley *et al.* the incidence of severe postoperative bleeding requiring either transfusion, vaginal packs or sutures was 4%.[7] This incidence is similar to that of Murdoch *et al.* who reported a 2% incidence of severe postoperative bleeding requiring either transfusion, sutures or vaginal packs and a 2% incidence of moderate postoperative bleeding which responded to tampons and/or antibiotics.[8] The somewhat higher incidence of complications in the United Kingdom series compared to our experience may be related to the fact that the Europeans tend to excise more deeply than we do. We attempt to excise to a depth of 7 - 8 mm in the center of the lesion whereas in the United Kingdom there is a tendency to excise to a greater depth.

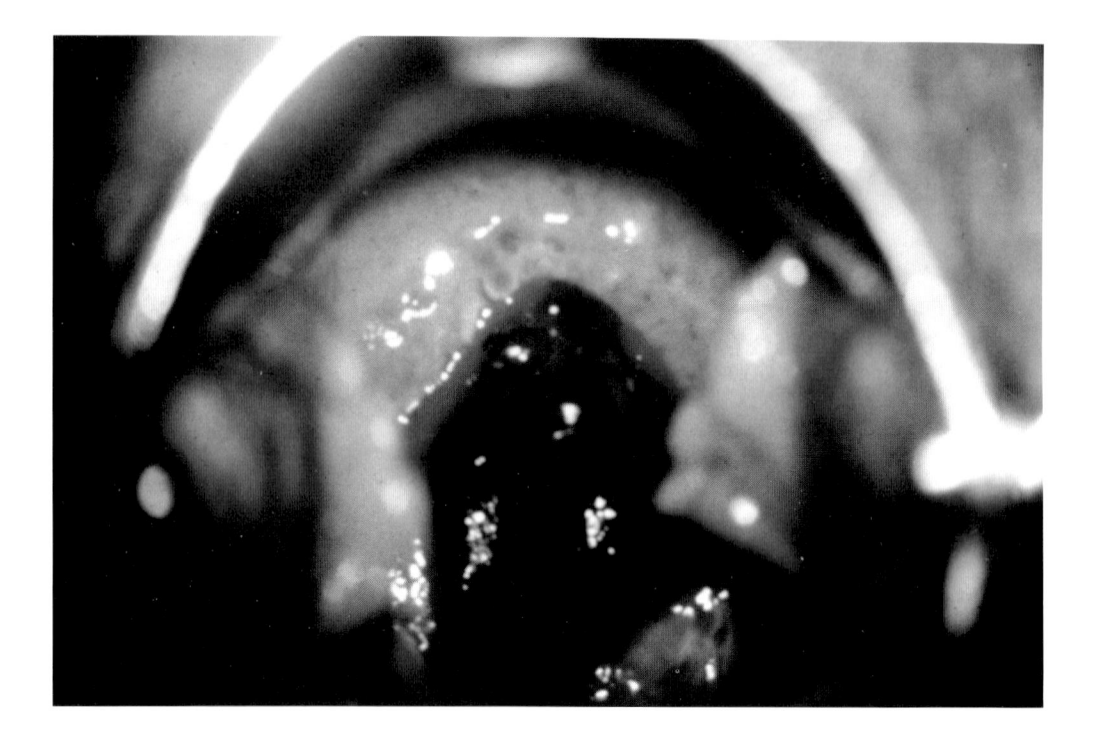

Figure 7.22. Postoperative bleeding. Blood clot that formed in the crater base 5 days after an electrosurgical excision.

Recessed Squamocolumnar Junction and Cervical Stenosis

The frequency of recessed squamocolumnar junctions after loop excision varies greatly in the different published series. A primary cause of this variation may be in how a particular cervix is interpreted and the depth of excision. In our experience, truly recessed squamocolumnar junctions have occurred in 2% of patients after electrosurgical excision. Although many cervices will have the squamocolumnar junction at the external os, in most of these cases a satisfactory colposcopic examination can be obtained provided the examiner is patient and uses an endocervical speculum. In contrast to our experience, in the large study of Luesley *et al.*, an incidence of recessed SCJ of 10% was reported after electrosurgical excision.[7] Figure 7.23 illustrates a typical post-excision cervix one month after the procedure and 7.24 is a treated cervix at 3 months.

True cervical stenosis is also an infrequent complication of loop excision. In all of the reported series the incidence of cervical stenosis has been either 1% or less.

LOOP EXCISIONAL PROCEDURES FOR TREATING CIN

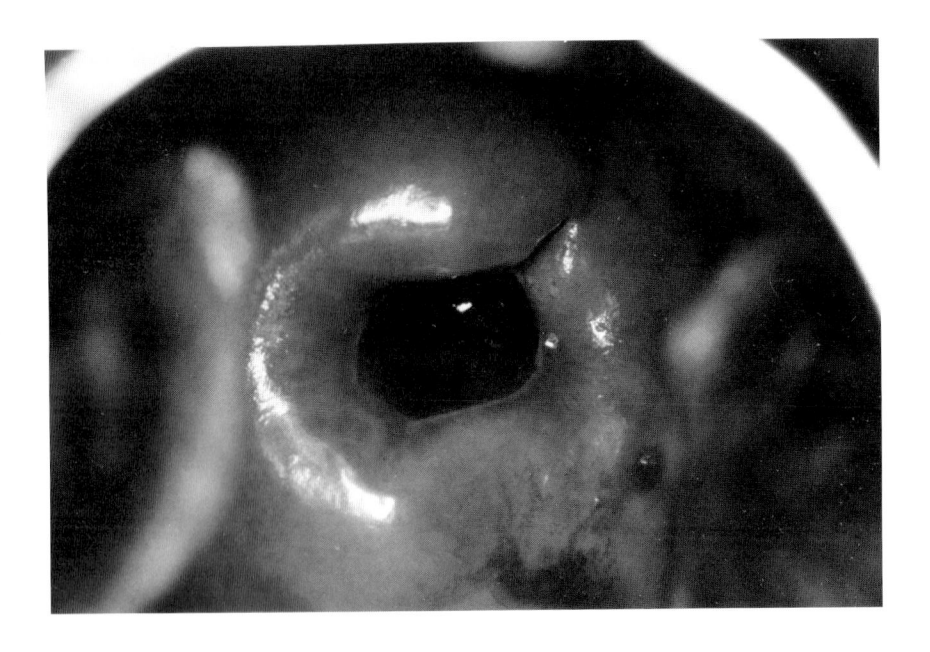

Figure 7.23. Typical appearance of cervix four weeks after loop excision.

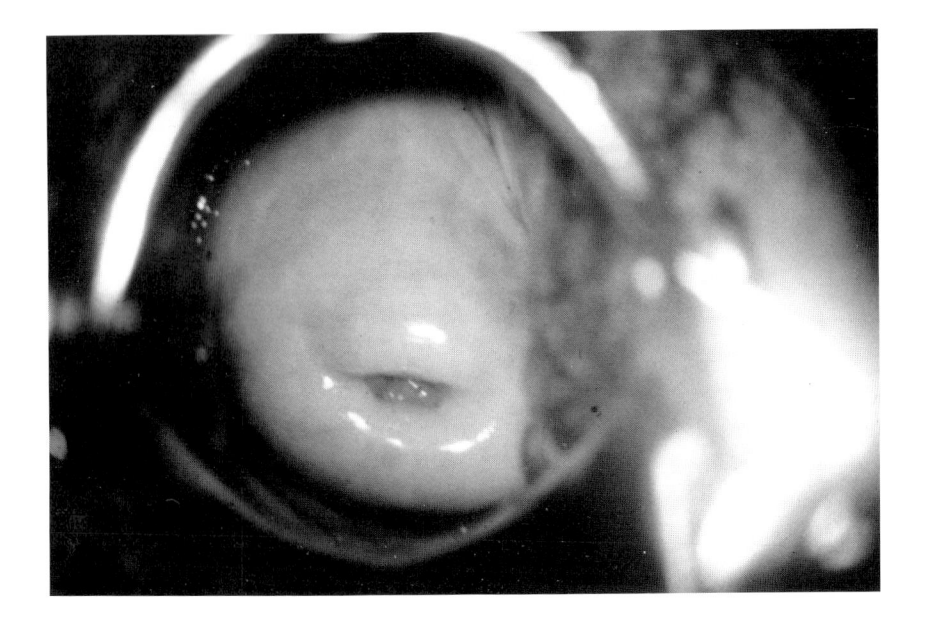

Figure 7.24. Typical cervix 3 months after a loop excision.

Postoperative Follow-up

Patients are requested to return to the office 3 months after cervical loop excision. At this first follow-up visit, a Pap smear is obtained, colposcopy is performed and an endocervical curettage is performed when indicated. Colposcopically-directed biopsies are taken from any abnormal areas. Provided all tests are negative, the patient is seen again at 6 and 12 months after treatment. At these visits only a Pap smear is obtained and colposcopy is not performed. Once there have been three consecutive negative smears the patient is discharged from postoperative follow-up and returned to routine screening.

REFERENCES

1. Anderson, M.C. and Hartley, R.B. Cervical crypt involvement by intraepithelial neoplasia. *Obstet. Gynecol.* 55:546-550, 1980.
2. Wright, V.C. Carbon dioxide laser surgery for cervical intraepithelial neoplasia. *Lasers in Surgery and Medicine* 4:145-152, 1984.
3. Wright, T.C., Gagnon, M.D., Richart, R.M. and Ferenczy, A. Treatment of cervical intraepithelial neoplasia using the loop electrosurgical excision procedure. *Obstet. Gynecol.* 79:173-178, 1992.
4. Mor-Yosef, S., Lopes, A., Pearson, S. and Monaghan, J. Loop diathermy cone biopsy. *Obstet. Gynecol.* 75:884-886, 1990.
5. Prendiville, W., Cullimore, J. and Norman, S. Large loop excision of the transformation zone (LLETZ). A new method of management for women with cervical intraepithelial neoplasia. *Br. J. Obstet. Gynecol.* 96:1054-1060, 1989.
6. Whiteley, P.F. and Olah, K.S. Treatment of cervical intraepithelial neoplasia: Experience with the low-voltage diathermy loop. *Am. J. Obstet. Gynecol.* 162:1272-1277, 1990.
7. Luesley, D.M., Cullimore, J., Redman, C.W.E., *et al*. Loop diathermy excision of the cervical transformation zone in patients with abnormal cervical smears. *B.M.J.* 300:1690-1693, 1990.
8. Murdoch, J.B., Grimshaw, R.N. and Monaghan, J.M. Loop diathermy excision of the abnormal cervical transformation zone. *Int. J. Gynecol. Cancer* 1:105-111, 1991.

CHAPTER 8

ELECTROSURGERY OF THE CERVIX: A STEP-BY-STEP GUIDE

ELECTROSURGICAL LOOP EXCISION FOR EXOCERVICAL DISEASE
Indications and Contraindications

The indications for loop excision of exocervical CIN are identical to those used to identify CIN lesions that can be treated with ablative therapy.

Table 8.1

Indications for Exocervical Loop Excision

Biopsy-proven CIN lesion of any grade

(or)

Squamous intraepithelial neoplasia (SIL) on Pap smear together with a colposcopically identifiable CIN lesion

(and)

Satisfactory colposcopic exam and no evidence for invasion.

Table 8.2

Contraindications to Exocervical Loop Excision

"Positive" endocervical curettage or a lesion in which the endocervical limit cannot be visualized colposcopically.

Clinically apparent invasive carcinoma of the cervix.

A bleeding disorder.

Pregnancy (except in highly experienced hands).

Severe cervicitis.

Less than 3 months post-partum.

DES-exposed patient.

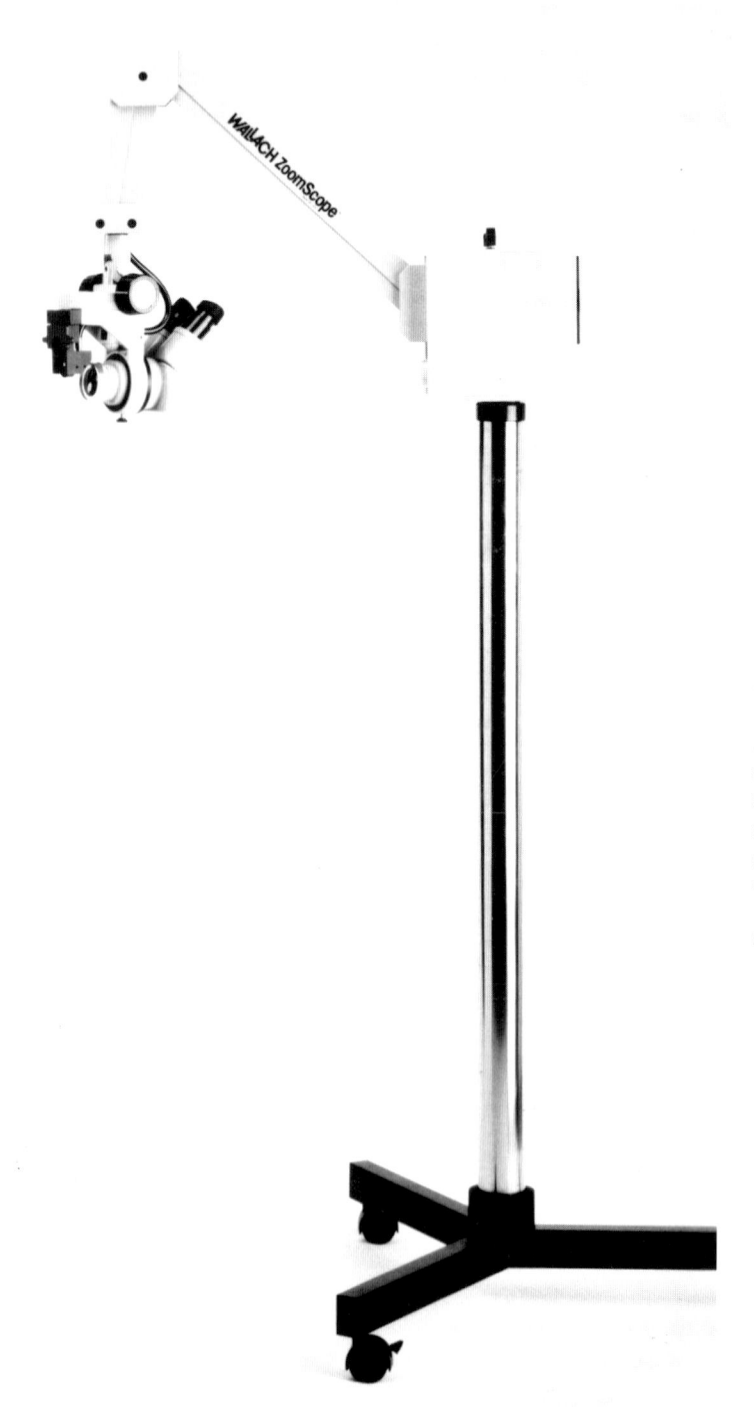

Figure 8.1. Colposcope that can be used at low (4 to 7.5x) magnification. Patients are always treated under colposcopic guidance at 4 to 7.5x magnification. This requires a colposcope that is equipped for low magnification work. *(Photograph of Zoom Scope courtesy of Wallach Surgical Devices, Inc.)*

ELECTROSURGERY OF THE CERVIX: A STEP-BY-STEP GUIDE

Treatment Procedure

Step 1 Explain the procedure to the patient and obtain informed consent.

CONSENT FORM FOR ELECTROSURGERY

It was explained to me by Dr. _____or assistants, and I understand that my precancerous areas of the cervix or anogenital area (vulva, vagina, anus, penis) or genital warts will be removed using thin wire loop and small ball-like electrodes and electric power. I understand furthermore, that this procedure requires iodine application to the cervix and local anesthesia of the areas being treated. To my knowledge, I am not allergic to either xylocaine or iodine.

Also, it was explained to me that severe bleeding can rarely occur during the procedure necessitating additional treatment or hospitalization. Bleeding and/or infection occasionally may develop a few days to a week after electrosurgery of my cervix or anogenital areas and, in such case, I will have to return immediately to the Colposcopy Clinic or, if the Clinic is closed, the Emergency Room of the _____ Hospital.

I was also told that, occasionally, when the genital skin containing warts is treated by electrosurgery, the newly formed skin may appear either lighter or darker than the untreated normal skin. Scars may also form after electrosurgery. This, however, is a rare event.

It was also explained to me that in some women this treatment, when applied to the cervix, can cause cervical stenosis (obstruction of the pathway between the vagina and the uterus). If this should occur, additional surgery may be required. It was also explained to me that long-term effects of this treatment on fertility are unknown.

I accept treatment by electrosurgery using thin wire and other electrodes as seen fit by Dr._____ or colleagues qualified in electrosurgical procedures.

_____   _____
Witness   Patient

ELECTROSURGERY FOR HPV-RELATED DISEASES

Step 2 Have patient undress from the waist down and lie on gynecological examining table in lithotomy position with feet in stirrups. Select and set-up the equipment required for the procedure (listed in Chapters 4 and 7). Disposable set-up trays containing the necessary disposable items are available (Figure 8.2).

Step 3 Attach a return electrode to the inner thigh. Insert a nonconductive, insulated speculum and connect the speculum's smoke evacuator tube to the vacuum system. (It is important that the speculum be large enough to allow complete, unobstructed visualization of the cervix. If the vaginal side walls remain in the way, a nonconductive, insulated vaginal spreader should be used.)

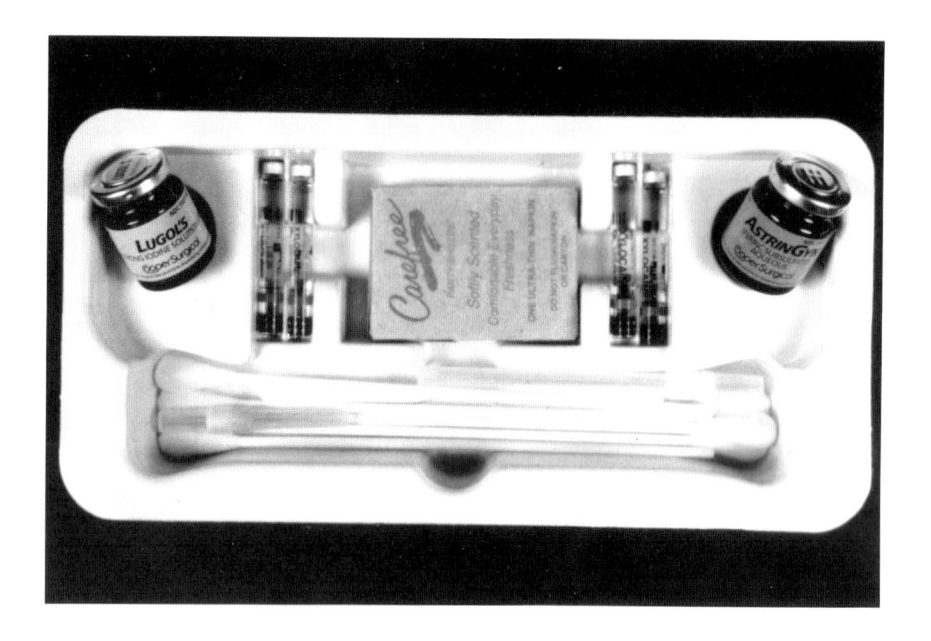

Figure 8.2. Disposable set-up tray designed for cervical loop excisions. This set-up tray contains many of the items required for the procedure including an extended, 4 inch needle. *(Tray courtesy of CooperSurgical, Inc.)*

Step 4 Apply 5% acetic acid to the cervix and examine the cervix with the colposcope to identify the presence and distribution of CIN.

Step 5 Apply strong, aqueous iodine solution to outline the margins of the lesional tissues (Figure 8.3).

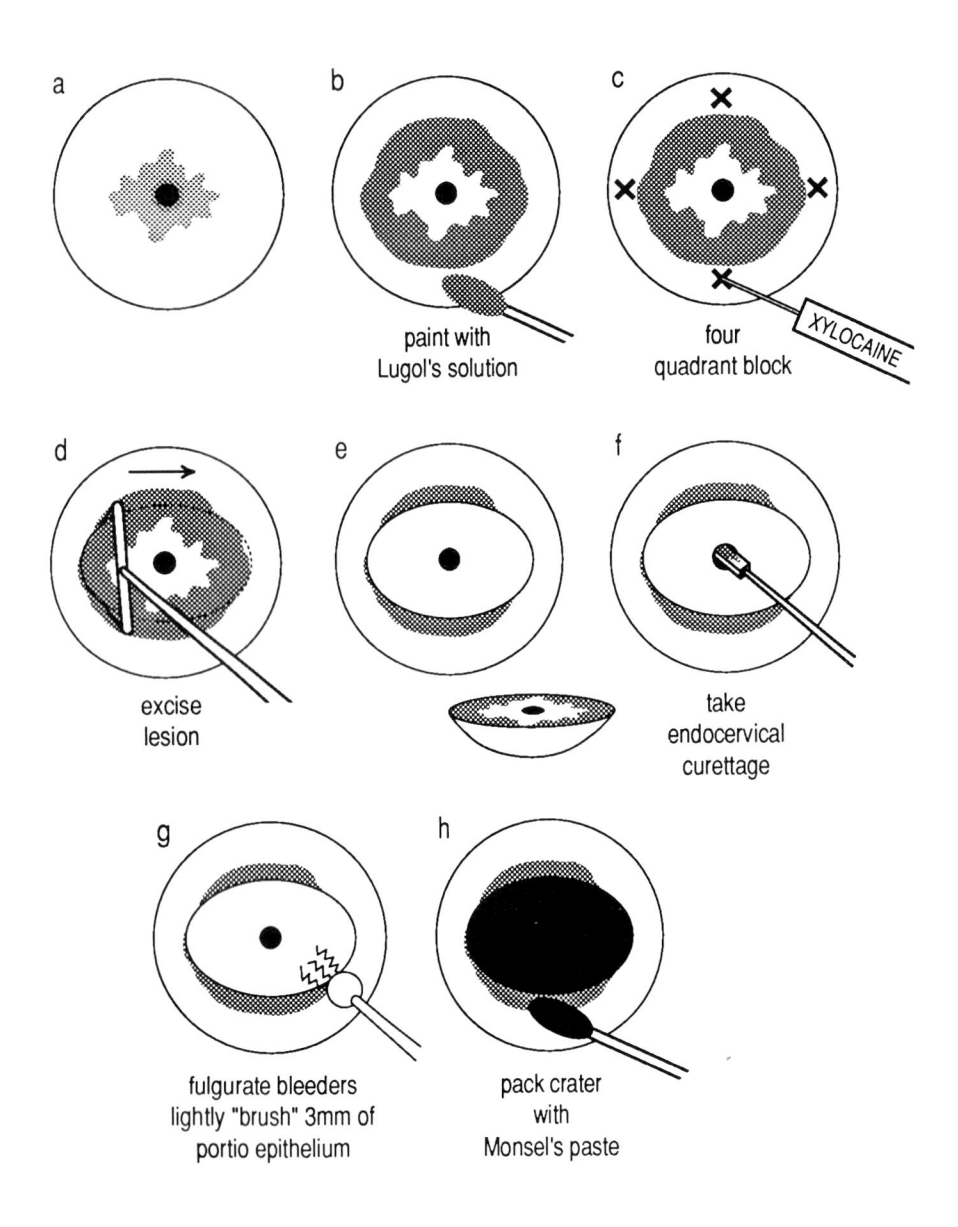

ELECTROSURGERY OF THE CERVIX: A STEP-BY-STEP GUIDE

Figure 8.3. Sequence of steps for loop excision of CIN confined to exocervix.

ELECTROSURGERY FOR HPV-RELATED DISEASES

Step 6   Provide anesthesia using an intracervical block. This is obtained by injecting 2% xylocaine with 1:100,000 epinephrine just beneath the cervical epithelium at the 12 o'clock, 3 o'clock, 6 o'clock and 9 o'clock positions. A dental syringe equipped with a 27 gauge needle is best for injecting the cervix. A total of 1.8-3.6 ml of anesthetic is generally used (up to 1 ml per quadrant). More anesthetic is rarely needed. Wait three minutes to obtain the desired anesthesia effect.

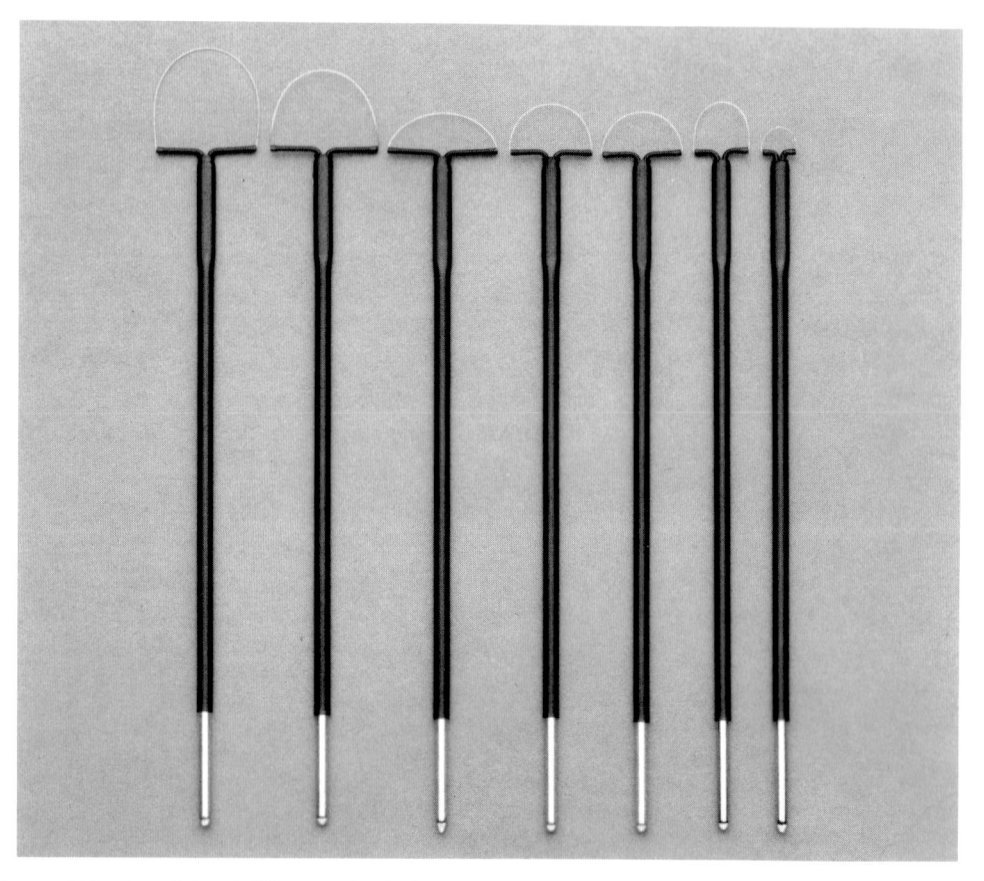

Figure 8.4. A variety of different sized electrodes are available for cervical loop excisions. We recommend that only "shallow-style" electrodes, such as the third loop from the left, be used for the routine treatment of exocervical CIN. That electrode measures 0.8 x 2.0 cm. *(Photograph courtesy of Cabot Medical Corp.)*

Step 7   Select appropriate electrode for the electrosurgery which will allow the entire CIN lesion or atypical transformation zone to be excised in a single pass, if possible (Figure 8.4). Small, low-grade CIN lesions in nulliparous women with small cervices are best excised

ELECTROSURGERY OF THE CERVIX: A STEP-BY-STEP GUIDE

using a 1.5 cm wide by 0.5 cm deep loop electrode. Larger lesions or lesions in multiparous women are best excised using a 2.0 cm wide by 0.8 cm deep loop electrode. We recommend that large loop electrodes that measure more than 1 cm in depth rarely, if ever, be used for excision of CIN that is confined to the exocervix.

Step 8 Select the appropriate power settings. The power settings that will be used for a particular application will depend on the size, design and composition of the electrode, whether fulguration or cutting is desired, as well as the electrosurgical generator used (Figure 8.5). Table 8.3 lists the appropriate settings for one of the generators that is commonly used. Always be certain that the ESU is maintained in "Standby Mode" until the actual procedure is begun.

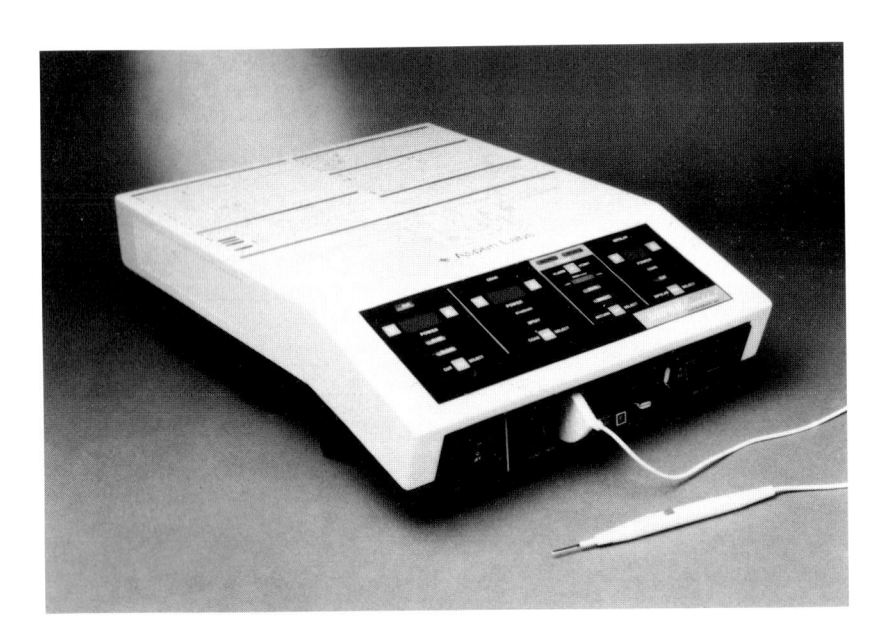

Figure 8.5. An electrosurgical generator that incorporates the recommended safety features. *(Photograph courtesy of Aspen Labs.)*

Step 9 Make a test pass with the electrode to insure that the path of the electrode is unobstructed.

ELECTROSURGERY FOR HPV-RELATED DISEASES

Step 10   Turn vacuum suction "on".

Step 11   Activate ESU and excise the CIN lesion.

Hints for Loop Excision

When excising lesional tissue, it is important to have a stable hand; this can be achieved by resting the shaft of the loop electrode on the posterior blade of the speculum. Performing the procedure under colposcopic guidance also helps the operator control the depth of excision.

It is critical that the cervix be well visualized and approximately perpendicular to the path of the electrode. If the cervix is not perpendicular place saline-soaked 2" x 2" gauze pads behind the cervix to align it correctly or use a hook.

The lesion should be excised with a continuous motion without stopping, whenever possible. Stopping the excision or stalling the electrode may produce excessive thermal damage and prevent accurate interpretation by the pathologist. If the procedure must be stopped or the electrode "stalls", the electrode should be removed from the tissue and the operator should begin from the opposite side, meeting the original line of excision. We usually move from left to right or right to left since the cervical os is usually oriented in this direction. However, if an anterior to posterior excision is better suited to remove the most suspicious areas of the lesion in the first pass, this is the direction that should be used.

We begin the excision 2 - 4 mm lateral to lesional tissue. The ESU is activated with the electrode not yet touching the tissue. Once the ESU is activated, the electrode is pushed perpendicularly into the tissue to a depth of 4-5 mm and then drawn laterally across and through the cervix and pulled to the other side. As the electrode is drawn through the endocervical canal it is pushed to a depth of 8 mm. This produces a dome-shaped circle of tissue with the endocervical canal in the center. Do not insert the electrode deeper than 5 mm at the 3 o'clock and 9 o'clock positions since deeper insertion can result in significant bleeding from the cervical branches of the uterine artery.

Step 12   After the central portion of tissue has been excised, additional passes with the loop electrode can be made to excise residual tissue. All excised tissues are picked up with a ring forceps and submitted for histological diagnosis.

ELECTROSURGERY OF THE CERVIX: A STEP-BY-STEP GUIDE

Table 8.3

Power Settings for Electrodes Used for Cervical Lesions*

Electrodes	Power Setting
Loop Style	**Blend**
1.0 x 1.0 cm	26 watts
1.5 x 0.5 cm	32 watts
2.0 x 0.8 cm	36 watts
Ball Style	**Coagulation**
3 mm	30 watts
5 mm	50 watts

*Values used with the CooperSurgical LEEP™ System 6000

Step 13 After all lesional tissue has been excised, the crater base is inspected to insure that all endocervical glands have been excised. An endocervical curettage is then performed.

Table 8.4

Postoperative Instructions for Patients after Electrosurgery of Cervical Lesions

You may develop a brown-black vaginal discharge which may last from a few days to 2 weeks. This is normal. **If discharge persists longer than 2 weeks, if profuse bleeding develops, if discharge becomes malodorous and/or is associated with pelvic pain, please call the office.**

Do not douche or use vaginal tampons for 3 weeks.

Refrain from intercourse for 3 weeks.

Avoid lifting heavy weights over the head for 2 weeks.

Return to the office in 3 months.

Step 14 Any bleeders in the crater base are lightly fulgurated using a ball electrode and "coagulation" current (Figure 8.3). Monsel's paste or gel is then applied to the crater base to maintain hemostasis. Printed postoperative instructions are given to the patient (Table 8.4) and the patient is instructed to return to the office in 3 months for a follow-up visit.

Problems That Can Develop During and After the Procedure

Intraoperative Bleeding

Significant intraoperative bleeding, including arterial-type bleeding, can occasionally develop during the loop excision. Diffuse bleeding from the crater bed is best managed through a combination of pressure and "coagulation" using either a ball type or a macroneedle electrode. Arterial bleeding can usually be controlled by placing the ball electrode in firm contact with the bleeding source and then "desiccating" the bleeder using coagulation current. Rarely, arterial bleeding will require the placement of a mattress-style chromic suture.

Postoperative Bleeding

Any blood clot is removed under colposcopic guidance and the bleeding area(s) is/are identified, cleaned with 5% acetic acid, and anesthetized with 2% xylocaine with epinephrine. Hemostasis is achieved by fulgurating the area using either the 5 mm ball or a macroneedle electrode and "coag" power outputs or by placing Monsel's paste or gel on the bleeder.

Postoperative Infection

Clean cervix with 5% acetic acid. Prescribe oral metronidazole, 2 gms as a single dose, and have the patient begin vaginal douches with peroxide solution (1 tbsp. in 3 cups of warm water), once a day for 7 days. If discharge is associated with abdominal pain and fever, prescribe antibiotics.

ELECTROSURGICAL CONE BIOPSIES FOR CIN INVOLVING ENDOCERVICAL CANAL

Electrosurgical cone biopsies may be performed in many patients on an outpatient basis under local anesthesia Two different types of electrosurgical cone biopsies can be performed. In one type, a thin wire loop electrode (loop excision cone biopsy) is used. This procedure can be performed on an outpatient basis under local anesthesia. In the other type (needle cone biopsy), a thin tungsten needle electrode (microneedle) is used to excise the tissue much like a scalpel is used for a cold knife cone biopsy. A tonsillar snare or curved scissors can be used for excising the base of the excised cone. The needle cone biopsy is usually performed in the operating room. Although the indications for loop excision cone biopsies and needle cone biopsies are still being defined, in general these two procedures are being performed on patients who are considered to be at relatively low and high risk, respectively, for having invasive cervical cancer.

Indications and Contraindications

The indications for loop excision cone biopsies and needle cone biopsies are different. Loop excision cone biopsies are contraindicated in patients requiring needle cone biopsies.

Table 8.5

Indications for Loop Excisional Cone Biopsy

Biopsy-proven CIN lesion of any grade

(or)

Squamous intraepithelial neoplasia (SIL) on Pap smear together with a colposcopically identifiable CIN lesion

(and)

The lesion extends 7 mm into the endocervical canal to a limited extent and can be excised in its entirety in a single pass with a 1 x 1 cm loop electrode.

Table 8.6

Contraindications to Loop Excisional Cone Biopsy

Clinically apparent invasive cancer.

CIN extending so far into the canal it cannot be excised with a single pass with a 1 x 1 cm loop electrode.

A bleeding disorder.

Pregnancy (except in highly experience hands).

Severe cervicitis.

Less than 3 months post-partum.

Table 8.7

Indications for Electrosurgical Needle Cone Biopsy

Biopsy-proven CIN lesion of any grade that extends far enough into the endocervical canal that it cannot be excised with a single pass with a 1 x 1 cm loop electrode.

LOOP EXCISION CONE BIOPSY

Treatment Procedure

The treatment procedure for loop excision cone biopsy (Figure 8.6) is almost identical to that used for loop excision of exocervical disease.

ELECTROSURGERY OF THE CERVIX: A STEP-BY-STEP GUIDE

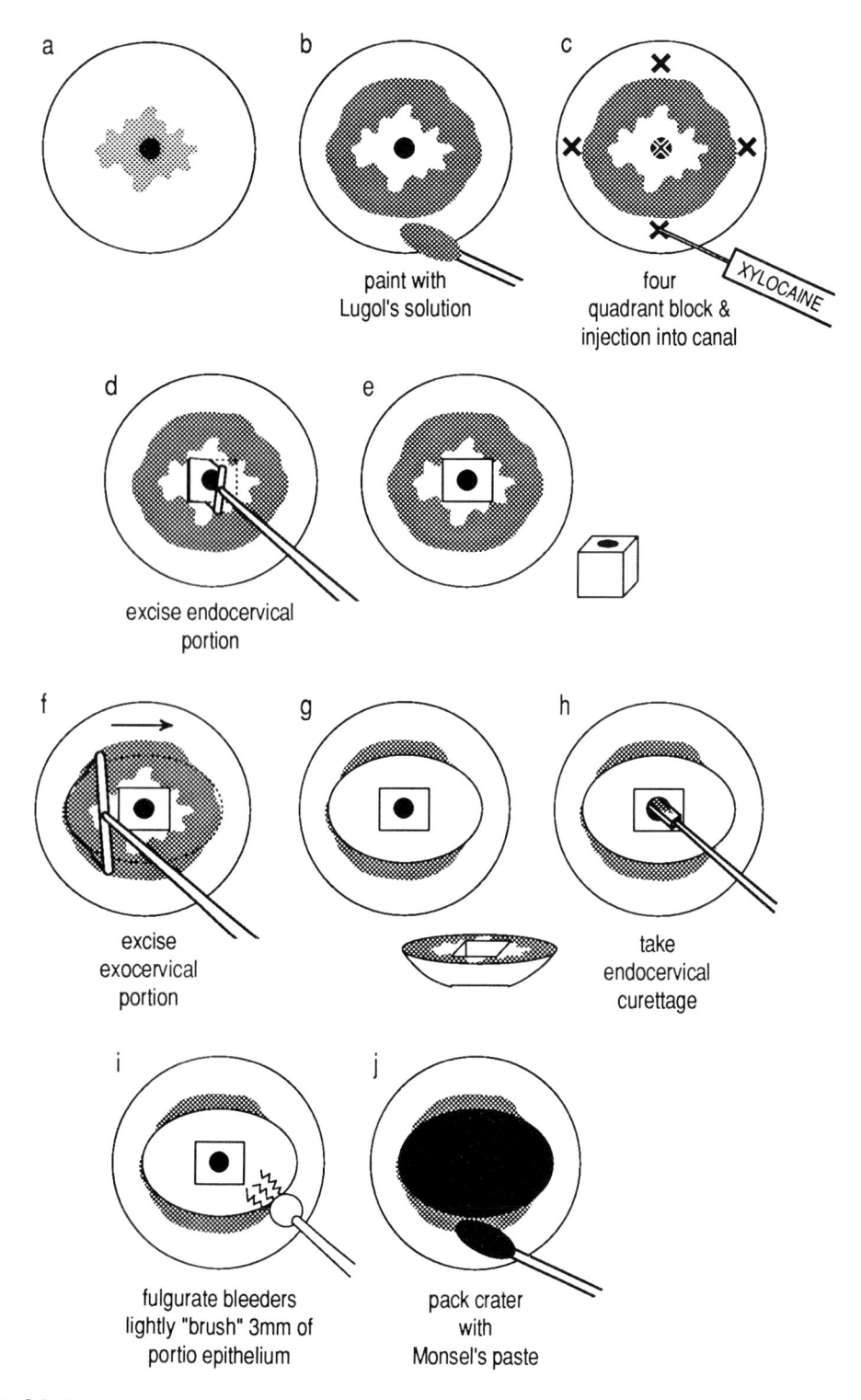

Figure 8.6. Sequence of steps for performing loop excisional cone biopsy.

ELECTROSURGERY FOR HPV-RELATED DISEASES

Step 1   Explain the procedure to the patient and obtain informed consent.

Step 2   Have patient undress from the waist down and lie on gynecological examining table in lithotomy position with feet in stirrups. Select and set-up the equipment required for the procedure (listed in Chapters 4 and 7). Disposable set-up trays containing the necessary disposable items are available (Figure 8.2).

Step 3   Attach a return electrode to the inner thigh. Insert a nonconductive, insulated speculum and connect the speculum's smoke evacuator tube to the vacuum system. (It is important that the speculum be large enough to allow complete, unobstructed visualization of the cervix. If the vaginal side walls remain in the way, a nonconductive, insulated vaginal spreader should be used.)

Step 4   Apply 5% acetic acid to the cervix and examine the cervix with the colposcope to identify the presence and distribution of CIN.

Step 5   Apply strong, aqueous iodine solution to outline the margins of the lesional tissues.

Step 6   Obtain anesthesia with an intracervical block as used for exocervical disease. The one difference between the two procedures is that for cone biopsies an additional 0.5 ml of anesthesia is injected into both the anterior and posterior aspects of the endocervical canal after having injected the exocervix.

Step 7   Select appropriate electrode or combination of electrodes. (Generally loop excisional cone biopsies are performed using both a 1.0 by 1.0 cm loop or rectangular electrode for excising the endocervical portion of the lesion and a 2.0 cm wide by 0.8 cm deep loop style electrode for excising the exocervical portion of the lesion.)

Step 8   Select the appropriate power settings. The power settings that will be used for a particular application will depend on the size, design and composition of the electrode, whether fulguration or cutting is desired, as well as the electrosurgical generator used (Figure 8.5). Table 8.3 lists the appropriate settings for one of the generators that is commonly used. Always be certain that the ESU is maintained in "Standby Mode" until the actual procedure is begun.

Step 9 Make a test pass with the electrode to insure that the path of the electrode is unobstructed.

Step 10 Turn vacuum suction "on".

Step 11 Activate ESU and excise the CIN lesion.

Hints for Loop Excision Cone Biopsies

Two different approaches can be used for performing outpatient electrosurgical cones. We recommend the approach of excising the central portion of the lesion using a 1.0 x 1.0 cm rectangular electrode and subsequently excising any residual disease on the portio using a 2.0 x 0.8 cm loop electrode (Figure 8.7).

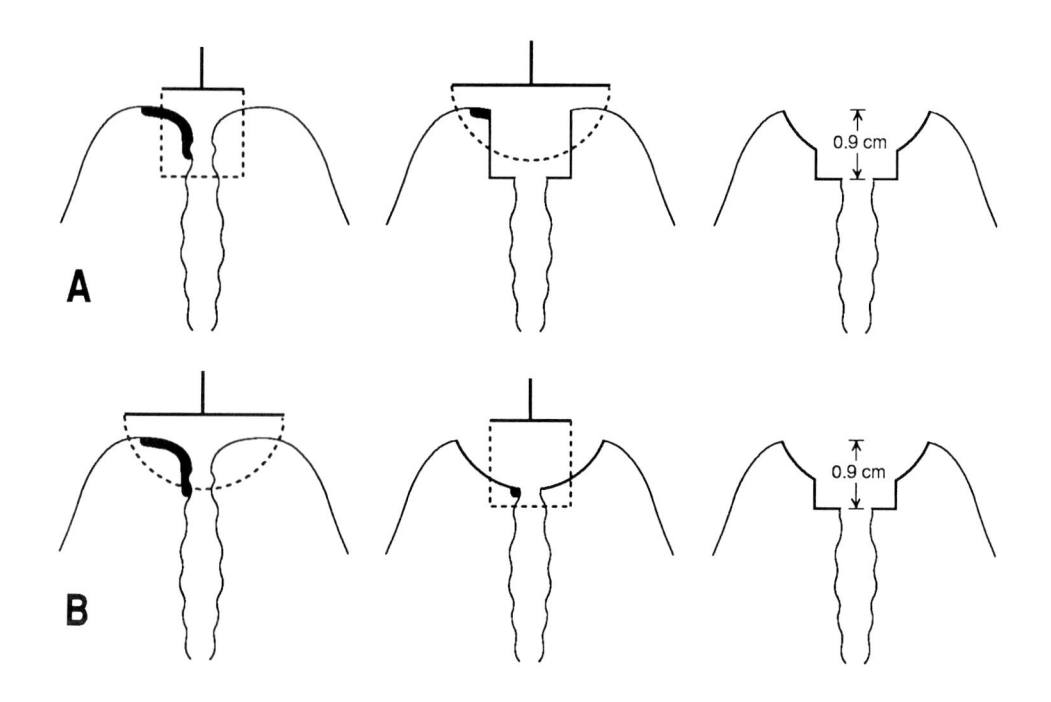

Figure 8.7. Two approaches to loop excisional cone biopsies. A) Recommended approach. B) Approach used in selected cases.

ELECTROSURGERY FOR HPV-RELATED DISEASES

Step 12 Place a vinegar soaked cotton-tipped applicator into the canal and use an endocervical speculum to check that all lesional tissue in the canal has been removed. (Residual disease will appear as white rather than salmon pink.) If acetowhite epithelium remains in the canal, make an additional pass with the 1.0 x 1.0 cm electrode. When all lesional tissue has been excised, an endocervical curettage is performed.

Step 13 After all lesional tissue has been excised, the crater base is inspected to insure that all endocervical glands have been excised. An endocervical curettage is performed.

Step 14 Any bleeders in the crater base are lightly fulgurated using a ball electrode and "coagulation" current (Figure 8.6). Monsel's paste or gel is applied to the crater base to maintain hemostasis. Printed postoperative instructions are given to the patient.

Step 15 After loop excisional cone biopsy, use the ball electrode and coagulation current to lightly "brush" about 5 mm of portio squamous epithelium. (This serves to retard ingrowth of the squamous epithelium slightly and helps position the healed squamocolumnar junction at the external os.)

Step 16 Postoperative instructions, follow-up and management of complications are identical to those used after loop excision of exocervical disease. Patients are asked to return to the office 3 months after loop cone biopsy for colposcopy, endocervical curettage (if indicated), Pap smear and biopsy of any abnormal areas.

CHAPTER 9

DIAGNOSIS AND MANAGEMENT OF VAGINAL AND EXTERNAL ANOGENITAL HPV-RELATED DISEASES

HPV infections of the lower anogenital tract epithelium are common in both men and women and are considered to be sexually transmitted diseases. Curative therapy reduces the risk of HPV-related neoplasia and the transmission of the virus to sex partners and infants.

DEFINITIONS

Lower genital tract infection with human papillomaviruses may result in three types of disease: Clinical, subclinical and latent[1] (Table 9.1). Clinical

Table 9.1

Types of HPV Infections of the Lower Genital Tract
Clinical
Subclinical
Latent

disease is defined as being grossly evident and includes condylomata acuminata and their variants such as papular condylomata. Acuminate warts are most commonly seen in the vagina and on keratinizing epithelia. Subclinical disease is defined as disease that can only be seen using magnification after the application of 5% acetic acid. These lesions are usually slightly raised. Subclinical disease is particularly prevalent on the cervix. In latent infections, HPV DNA can be detected using molecular techniques (hybridization or polymerase chain reaction) in patients without clinical, colposcopic or morphologic evidence of disease. These patients appear to "carry" HPV DNA in their lower anogenital squamous epithelium in the absence of clinical disease.

Both clinically and subclinically infected epithelia contain morphologic alterations consistent with either benign disease (condylomatous infections) or intraepithelial neoplasia. The vast majority of acuminate condylomata of the vagina and external anogenital skin are morphologically and clinically benign and contain HPV types 6/11, whereas papular, pigmented or white, hyperkeratotic lesions, cancer precursors and acetowhite subclinical lesions may contain HPV 16 and related oncogenic virus types[2,3] (Table 9.2).

Table 9.2

Distinctive Characteristics of HPV Infections of Vaginal and External Anogenital Skin by Viral Type

Clinical Finding	6/11	HPV 16 and related oncogenic viruses*
Acuminate condylomata	mostly	rarely
Papular or flat acetowhite, intraepithelial neoplasia (VAIN, VIN, PAIN, PIN)	rarely	usually
Subclinical acetowhite lesions	often	rarely
Spontaneous regression	about 30%	rarely
Persisting lesions	often	usually
Progress to invasion if untreated	rarely or never	frequently

*18, 30s, 50s, 60s groups
VAIN: vaginal intraepithelial neoplasia; **VIN**: vulvar intraepithelial neoplasia; **PAIN**: perianal intraepithelial neoplasia; **PIN**: penile intraepithelial neoplasia

Regardless of its anatomical site in the lower genital tract, intraepithelial neoplasia contains nuclear atypia characterized by pleomorphism, hyperchromasia and coarsely clumped chromatin, as well as abnormal mitotic figures, altered cell cohesion, and altered maturation.[3] Other external anogenital skin lesions such as epithelial hyperplasia (previously called hyperplastic dystrophy) and diffuse condylomatosis may be mistaken for intraepithelial neoplasia clinically. The distinctive morphologic features that allow discrimination between intraepithelial neoplasia and epithelial hyperplasia or condyloma are presented in Table 9.3.

Table 9.3

Distinctive Histologic Features of Epithelial Hyperplasia, Condyloma and Intraepithelial Neoplasia*

Histology	EH	Condyloma	IN
Surface asperities	no	yes	yes
Cell cohesion	yes	yes	disturbed
Nuclear pleomorphism	absent	in koilocytes	yes
Nuclear aneuploidy	no	no	yes
Abnormal mitotic figures	no	no	yes
Koilocytes	no	yes	few/none
Mitoses	in basal/parabasal cells	lower 1/3	full thickness

*External anogenital skin. **EH** = epithelial hyperplasia; **IN** = intraepithelial neoplasia

DIAGNOSING VAGINAL AND EXTERNAL ANOGENITAL LESIONS

Although typical condylomata acuminata are easily recognized without the use of magnification, histologic verification is recommended prior to beginning therapy. The primary rationale for this is that occasionally even an experienced clinician can be fooled since seborrheic keratosis, molluscum contagiosum, or other conditions may sometimes appear clinically to be classical condylomata. Many of these HPV mimics require excisional treatment rather than topical therapy with cytolytic/cytotoxic agents. A second reason is that it is best to have histologic proof of the disease which is going to be treated, particularly if cytodestructive methods under general anesthesia are to be used. Histological proof of disease is very helpful in cases in which complications develop. Histology is also useful for those physicians who are less familiar with the clinical diagnosis of acuminate condylomata and wish to obtain clinical/pathologic correlations of disease. **Histologic sampling of lesions which are not classical acuminate condylomata is mandatory.**

Routine histologic evaluation should be obtained in the following conditions: Papular, pigmented lesions with a granular or shiny surface that might be vulvar intraepithelial neoplasia (VIN); junctional nevi or melanoma; white, hyperkeratotic lesions, either diffuse or multi-focal, to rule out the

ELECTROSURGERY FOR HPV-RELATED DISEASES

presence of VIN, epithelial hyperplasia or lichen sclerosis; red, erosion-like or exophytic, ulcerated lesions to rule out VIN, invasive squamous cell carcinoma, Paget's disease or syphilitic chancre; and all rapidly growing or long-standing, large papillary lesions to rule out squamous cell carcinoma or the rare verrucous carcinoma (giant condyloma of Buschke-Lowenstein).

Slightly raised, subclinical, acetowhite lesions in the vagina or the external anogenital skin may contain neoplasia and should be sampled. Areas of white epithelium with abnormal vessels or very coarse mosaic patterns suggestive of early stromal invasion should diligently be searched for, and, if present, generously sampled for histologic examination. A number of subclinical, acetowhite lesions of the external anogenital skin may not contain HPV-related changes. In the absence of features which are diagnostic of other conditions, HPV DNA *in situ* hybridization may usefully be applied to determine whether HPV is present (see Chapter 6).

Techniques for Histologic Sampling

Specimens for histology may be obtained using a small cervical type punch biopsy, a Keyes' punch, a scalpel or loop/needle electrodes. The first two devices provide specimens primarily for diagnosis, whereas the latter two

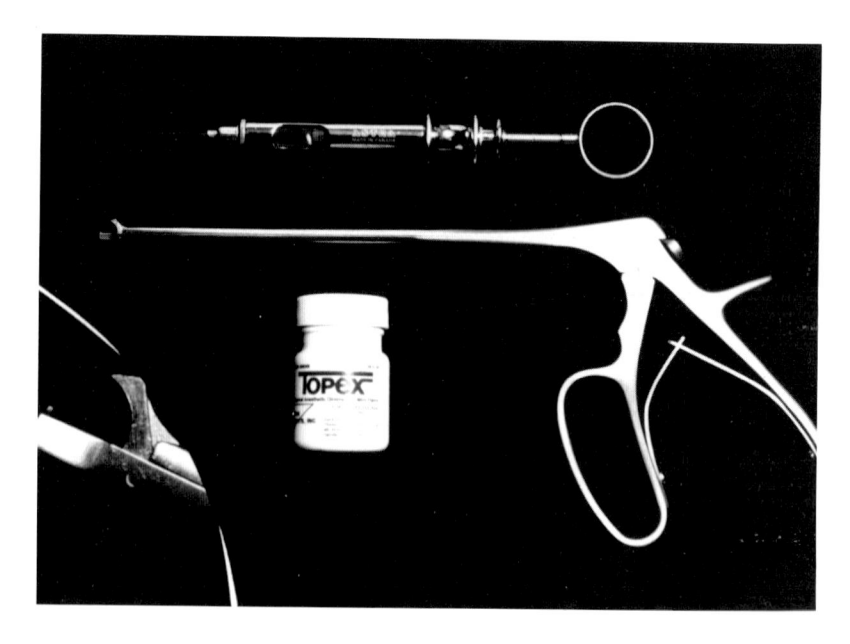

Figure 9.1. Biopsy punches. Small-jawed forceps designed for obtaining shallow biopsies of the vagina and the non-hairy skin. The local anesthetic kit consists of a metal syringe, 27-30 gauge disposable needles, 2% xylocaine solution and 20% benzocaine ointment. The latter is applied on the area to be anesthetized 5 minutes prior to needle insertion.

provide excisional-type specimens which are often both diagnostic and therapeutic. Small biopsy punches and Keyes' punches are available from a number of medical instrument makers. We prefer to use biopsy punches rather than Keyes' punches. They are more versatile for the gynecologist who does not specialize in vulvar disease since they can also be used for taking vaginal and cervical biopsies (Figure 9.1). Another advantage of the small-jawed biopsy forceps is that the vast majority of lesional tissues in the lower genital tract are intraepithelial and sampling the deep dermis and subcutaneous tissue (better performed with the Keyes' punch rather than gynecologic punch) is seldom necessary.

In order to obtain well oriented histologic sections, large specimens should be placed in a plastic cassette (provided by the pathology laboratory) or on a cardboard or paraffin plate and pinned out while being fixed in 10% neutral buffered formalin.

Table 9.4

Techniques for Performing Punch Biopsies

1. Examine area to be sampled after applying 5% acetic acid.
2. Infiltrate area to be excised with 2% xylocaine with 1:100,000 epinephrine (except for penis).
3. Using a 27 gauge dental needle inject anesthetic just beneath the lesional tissue so as to "separate" the latter from the deeper reticular dermis.
4. Wait 3 minutes for anesthesia to take effect.
5. Grasp the apex of the lesion with the front half of the biopsy forceps and excise. Try to limit the amount of tissue excised to 1/2 the bite of the forceps.
6. Recover the specimen from the biopsy forceps with fine-toothed forceps or a toothpick and place it on a piece of paper towel or lens paper. (A drop of lubricating jelly on the towel helps hold the biopsy in place.)
7. Treat the excised area with Monsel's paste or gel to insure hemostasis.
8. Wipe off the excess Monsel's paste or gel to prevent scarring of the biopsied area once hemostasis has been obtained.
9. Place antibiotic cream on the biopsied area and retain using a 2" x 2" gauze.

Table 9.5

Techniques for Performing Electrosurgical Excisional Biopsy

1. Depending on the size and location of disease, either local or general anesthesia may be used.
2. If invasion is suspected, excise the area in question with a microneedle electrode that is approximately 0.01 inches in thickness.
3. Excisional procedures can also be performed using a number 11 scalpel blade.
4. Most excisions are carried out along the second or third surgical plane, or about 1 to 3 mm from the surface epithelium.
5. Bleeding vessels may be fulgurated using a macroneedle electrode and coagulation current.
6. If the wound is relatively small, excisions may be left to granulate by second intention, but larger excised areas are best closed by 3-0 sutures.

CLINICAL FEATURES OF HPV INFECTIONS
Condylomata Acuminata

There are two principal types of acuminate condylomata (Table 9.6).

Table 9.6

Clinical Features of Condylomata Acuminata

Site	Appearance
Nonkeratinizing squamous epithelium	Soft and fleshy
Hairy skin	Firm, hyperkeratotic, sessile wart

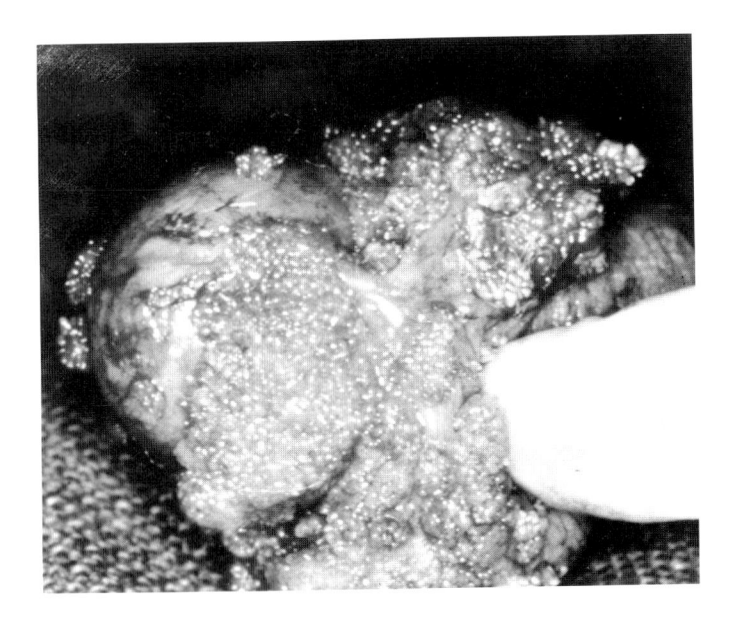

DIAGNOSIS AND MANAGEMENT OF HPV-RELATED DISEASES

Figure 9.2. Condylomata acuminata of penis. The glans and foreskin are extensively involved by confluent cauliflower-like masses.

The soft, fleshy, acuminate condylomata often grow and spread rapidly. This type arises from the non-keratinized squamous epithelium of the vagina, labia, vestibule, meatus, anal canal, glans penis, and the inner lining of the prepuce (Figure 9.2). The second type is the sessile wart. This generally firm, hyperkeratotic lesion arises on the hairy, external, anogenital skin (Figure 9.3).

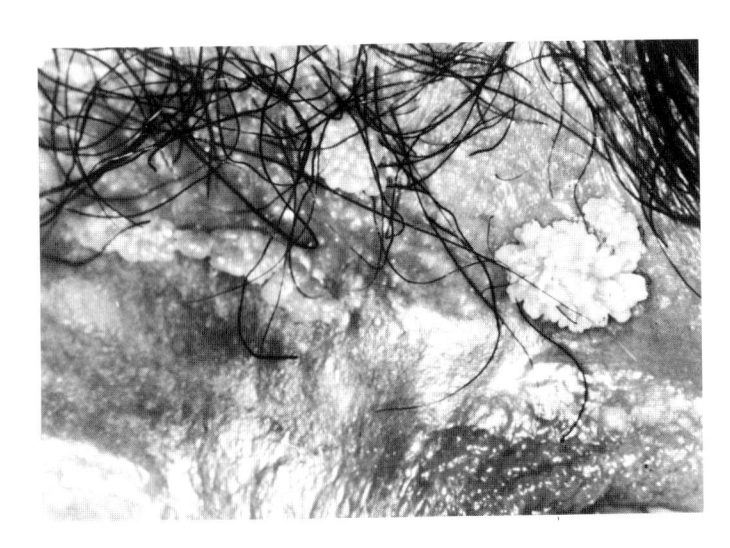

Figure 9.3. Acuminate condylomata of the vulva. Sessile condylomata of the hairy skin.

The distal portion of the penis is the area most often involved with HPV infection (over 70% of the cases). Squamous cell carcinoma of the penis has a

ELECTROSURGERY FOR HPV-RELATED DISEASES

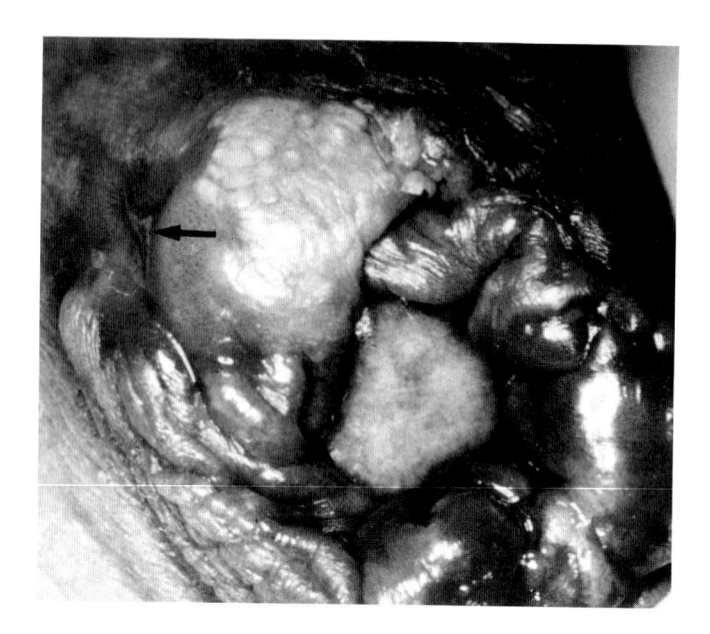

Figure 9.4. Invasive squamous cell carcinoma of the penis. Early ulcerative lesion (arrow) arising in fields of acetowhite intraepithelial neoplasia with irregular mosaic pattern.

anatomical distribution (Figure 9.4). In 30% of the cases, the perianal skin, the base of the penile shaft, scrotum or terminal urethra is infected. The proximal urethra, near the urinary bladder, is only rarely infected by HPV.[4] In women, the introitus and the labia minora are the most frequent sites of external anogenital warts. About 15% of men with penile warts and 40% of women with vulvar condylomata have perianal involvement. The incidence of intra-anal condylomata is greatly increased in homosexual men. Condylomata located past the external anal sphincter are usually associated with a history of anal intercourse. Approximately 15% of heterosexual patients and 90% of homosexuals with perianal condylomata have intra-anal lesions as well. All patients with perianal condylomata should be anuscoped for possible internal lesions.

Intraepithelial Neoplasia

Extracervical intraepithelial neoplasia most often involves the upper third of the vagina and the non-hairy areas of the external anogenital skin. Its clinical appearance is variable (Table 9.7). The most frequent form occurs on the non-hairy skin of the vulva, and is raised, broad-based, papular, pigmented/ greyish with hyperkeratotic areas (Figure 9.5). This type of VIN is often associated

DIAGNOSIS AND MANAGEMENT OF HPV-RELATED DISEASES

Table 9.7

Clinical Appearance of Intraepithelial Neoplasia

Most commonly raised, pigmented, papular lesion.

Less commonly white, hyperkeratotic lesions with papillary surface that are often confused with condyloma.

Occasionally pink, flat, multifocal lesions that appear as ulcers.

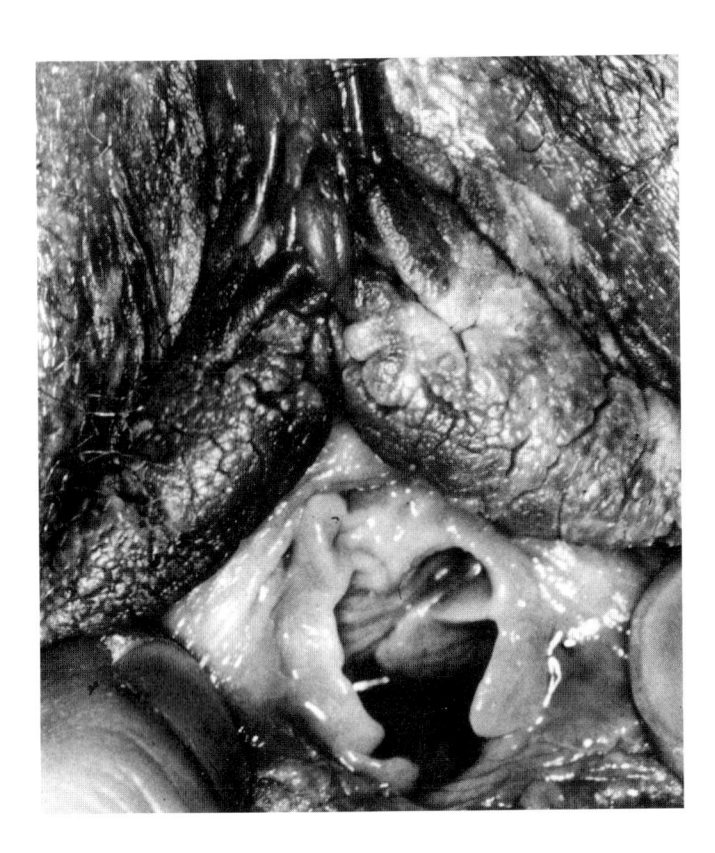

Figure 9.5. Vulvar intraepithelial neoplasia (VIN). Thickened, pigmented epithelium with white areas and verrucoid surface involving both labia minora.

with CIN. Less frequently, intraepithelial neoplasia presents either as white, papular (Figure 9.6) or confluent, hyperkeratotic lesions with papillary surfaces that masquerade as condylomata (Figure 9.7), or as pink/dull red (ulcer-like), flat, multifocal lesions (Figure 9.8).

ELECTROSURGERY FOR HPV-RELATED DISEASES

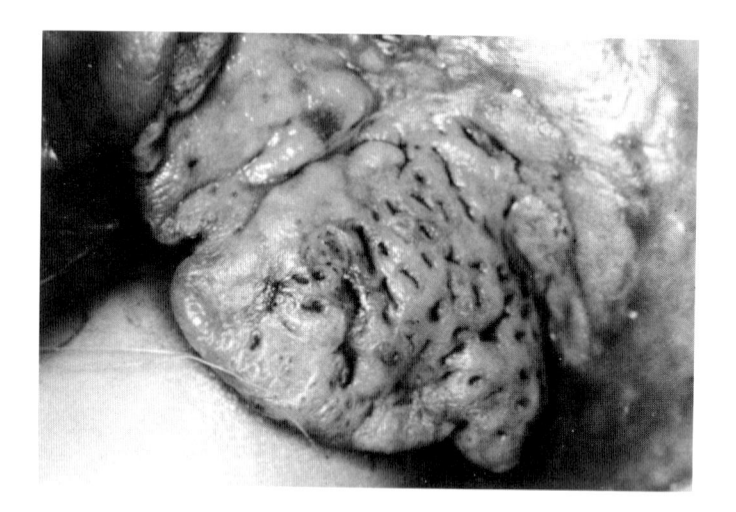

Figure 9.6. Vulvar intraepithelial neoplasia (VIN). Thickened, papular, sharply demarcated, acetowhite epithelium. Such lesions require tissue destruction to the second surgical plane (reticular dermis).

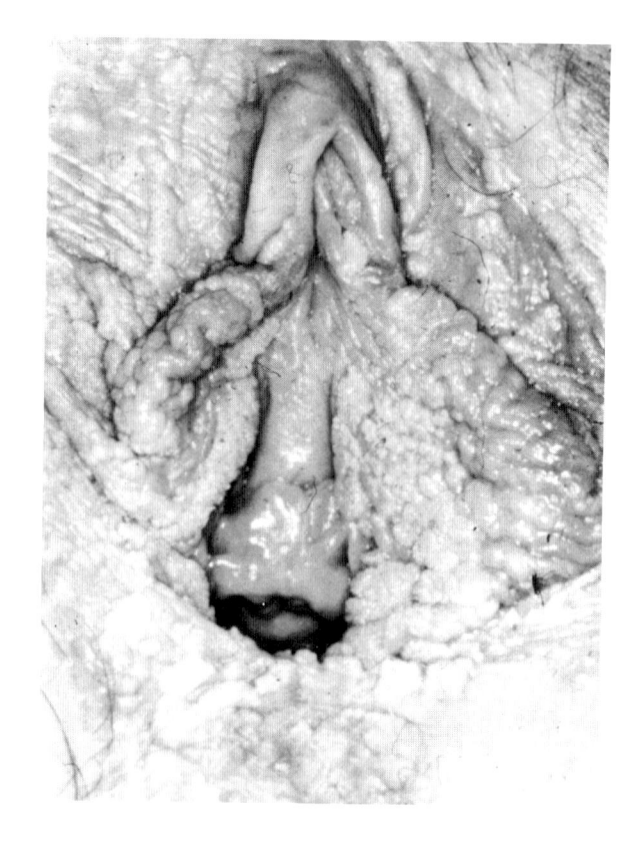

Figure 9.7. Vulvar intraepithelial neoplasia (VIN). Raised, confluent masses with verrucous surface resembling condylomata acuminata of the non-hairy skin of the vulva. This patient had been treated with podophyllin for 4 years without histologic assessment prior to the diagnosis of VIN being made.

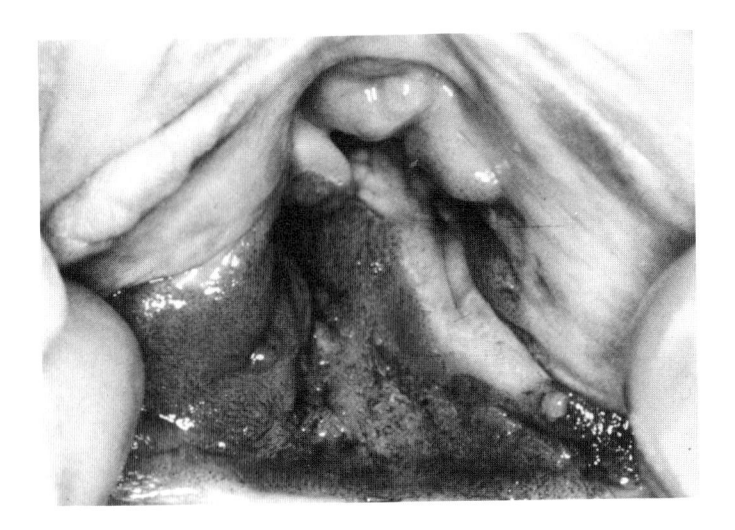

Figure 9.8. Vulvar intraepithelial neoplasia (VIN). A red lesion resembling a vulvar ulcer. Note coarse mosaic and punctation patterns. The lesion has extended into the lower 1/3 of the vagina.

SUBCLINICAL HPV INFECTIONS

Subclinical, acetowhite lesions of the external anogenital tract have a distribution similar to their clinically visible counterparts, but are often much more extensive (Figures 9.9, 9.10).

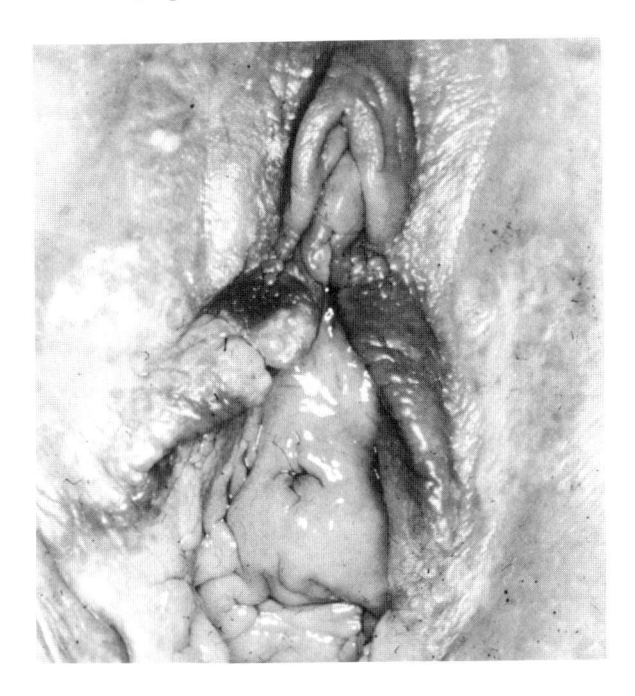

Figure 9.9. Subclinical HPV infection of vulva. Acetowhite, confluent, asymptomatic lesions of the non-hairy skin of the vulva. The patient has been followed for 7 years without a change in the lesions' characteristics. Histologically there was koilocytosis in the upper layers of the epithelium.

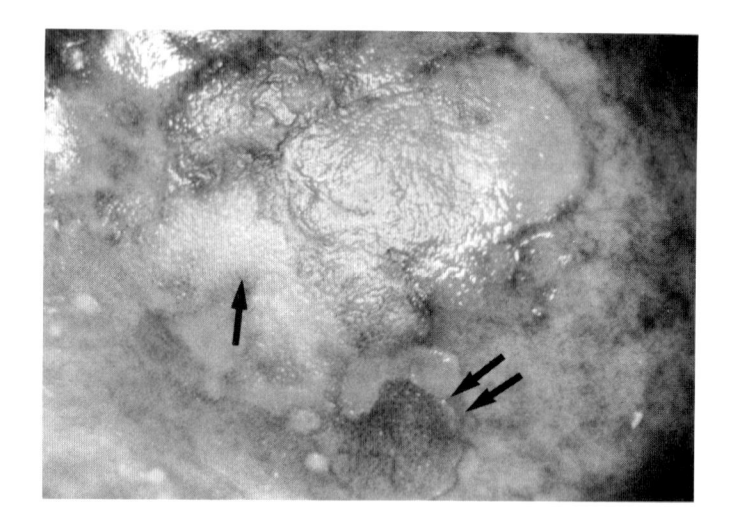

Figure 9.10. Subclinical HPV infection of the penis. Multiple, confluent, acetowhite lesions of the glans with finely granular (arrow) and punctation surface pattern (double arrow). Histologically, the lesion was an intraepithelial neoplasm.

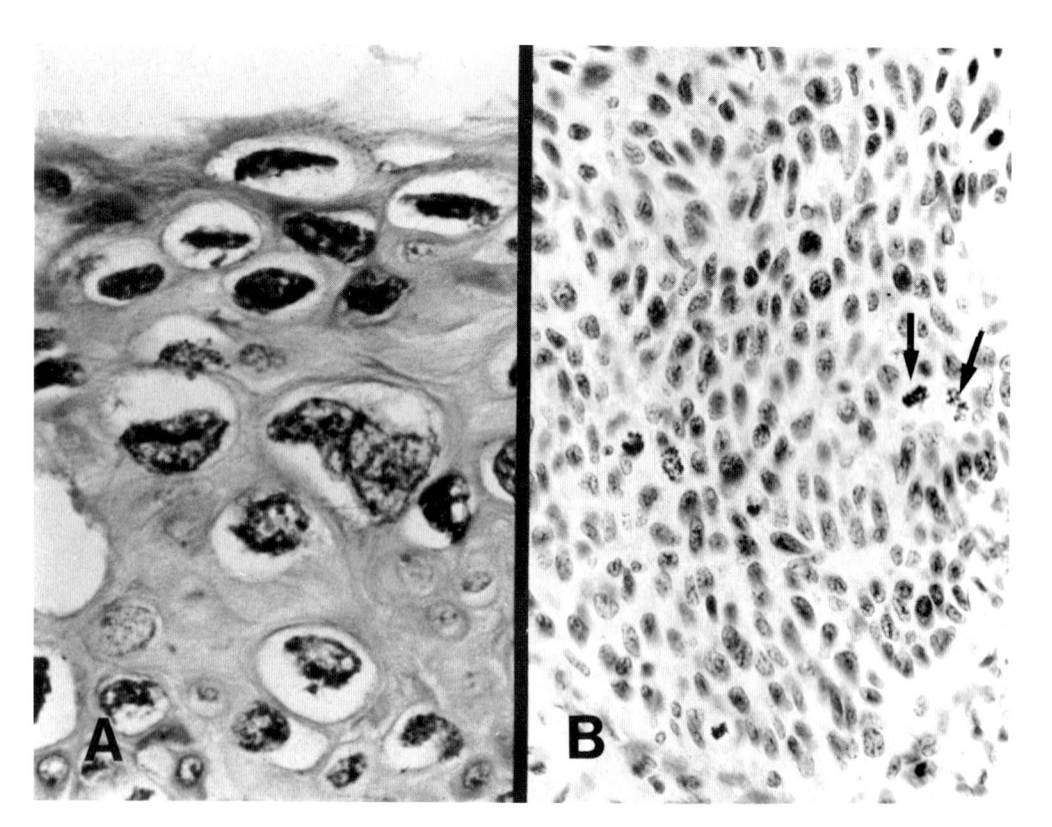

Figure 9.11. Histology of subclinical HPV infections of the genital skin. A) Flat condyloma/low-grade intraepithelial neoplasm with koilocytosis. B) Intraepithelial neoplasia with several abnormal mitotic figures (arrows).

DIAGNOSIS AND MANAGEMENT OF HPV-RELATED DISEASES

Subclinical lesions are usually multifocal, flat to slightly raised, and may have irregular punctation and mosaic patterns. In the vagina they are iodine-negative and are prevalent in the upper 1/3. Their surface may be smooth or finely granular and covered by tiny papillae or asperities. The histology of subclinical white lesions ranges from the typical flat condyloma with koilocytosis (Figure 9.11A) to intraepithelial neoplasia with aneuploid nuclear DNA content and abnormal mitotic figures (Figure 9.11B). Others contain

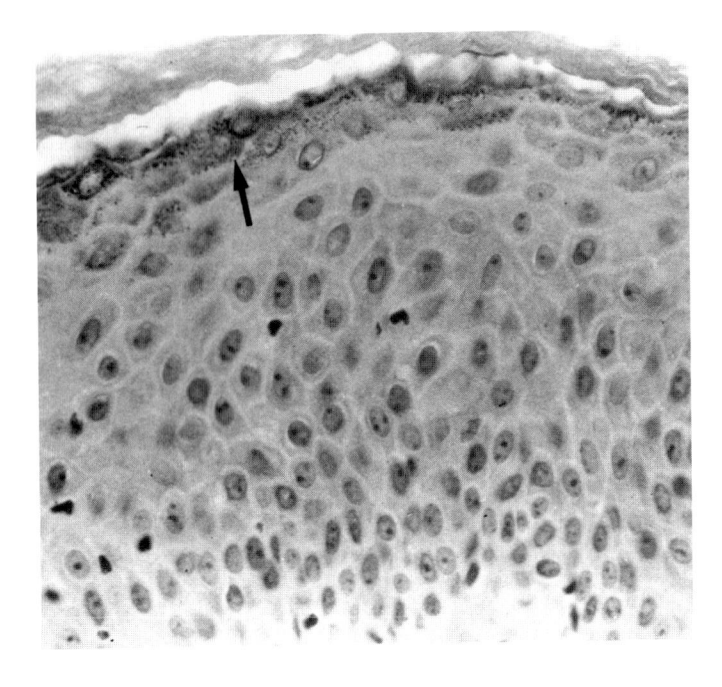

Figure 9.12. Histology of subclinical acetowhite area of the genital skin. There is acanthosis and a prominent granular cell layer (arrow). Koilocytosis, binucleation and dyskeratosis are absent. However, *in situ* hybridization with a HPV 6/11 RNA probe was positive in occasional cells of the upper epithelial strata.

nonspecific changes including acanthosis and surface para-/hyperkeratosis (Figure 9.12) most of which are not associated with HPV. Histologically equivocal lesions are found chiefly on the external anogenital skin (penis). About 50% of such cases contain HPV DNA by *in situ* hybridization (see Chapter 6).

Table 9.8

Condyloma and Intraepithelial Neoplasia Mimics

Micropapillomatosis labialis
Pearly penile papules
Molluscum contagosium
Epithelial hyperplasia (hyperplastic dystrophy)
Contact dermatitis
Epidermal inclusion cysts
Vaginal atrophy
Immature squamous metaplasia
Nevi, seborrheic keratosis
Condyloma lata (syphilis)
Acanthosis nigricans

MIMICS OF HPV-RELATED DISEASES

It is important to distinguish clinical and subclinical HPV infections from their mimics. These are presented in Table 9.8.

In most instances, an accurate diagnosis can be made either through clinical and/or colposcopic examination or by histology. Because of the relatively high false-negative rates of the viral tests that are currently available, only an unequivocally positive test is meaningful.[3] In women, the most frequent clinically visible condyloma mimic is micropapillomatosis labialis (Figure 9.13) and in men, pearly penile papules (Figure 9.14). Diffuse and, less frequently, focal vulvar and anal epithelial hyperplasia (hyperplastic dystrophy) is often confused with intraepithelial neoplasia of the external anogenital tract. Acetowhite, absolutely flat, focal lesions are not specific for HPV infections. They may be produced by acute and chronic irritations due to candida albicans and to allergic reactions to endogenous or exogenous agents including foreign material, heat and other irritants.

DIAGNOSIS AND MANAGEMENT OF HPV-RELATED DISEASES

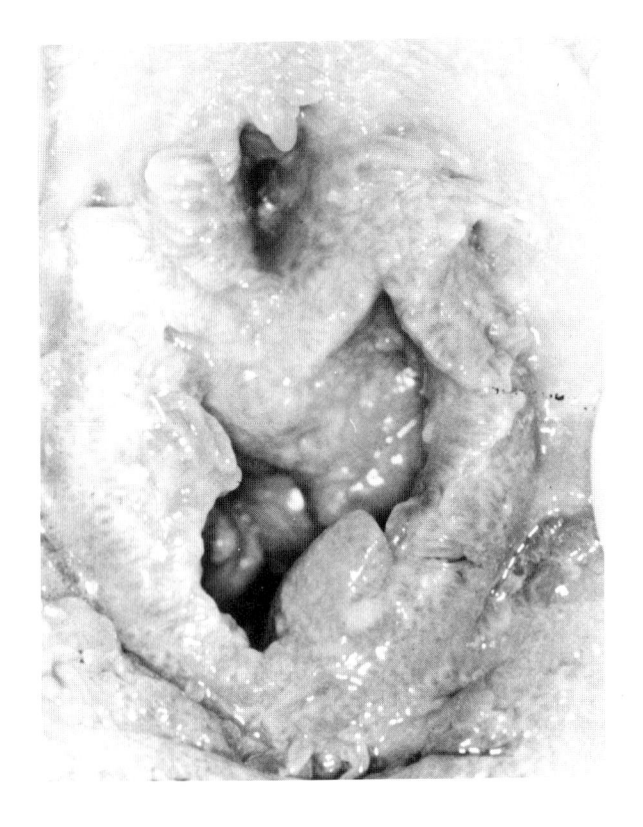

Figure 9.13. Micropapillomatosis labialis (MPL). Each labial papilla has its own base (stalk). In contrast, the papillary fronds in condyloma often share a base. The patient had a history of past and current vulvovaginal candidiasis.[6]

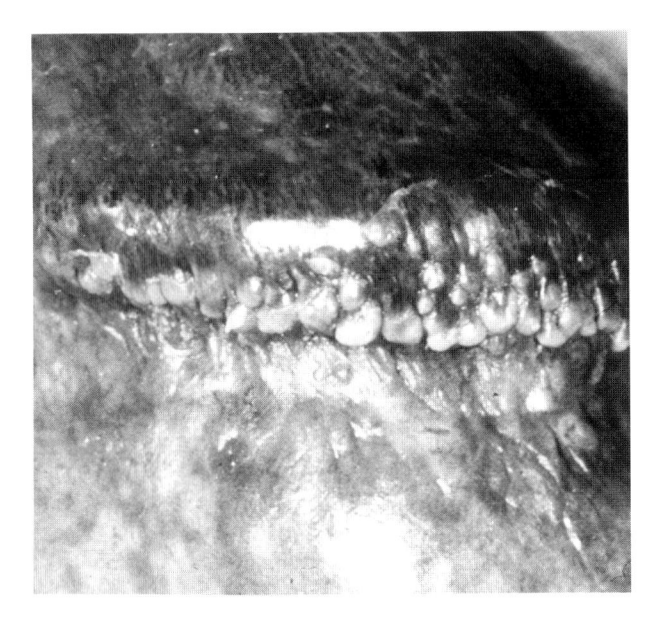

Figure 9.14. Pearly penile papules (PPP). The corona glandis contains rows of blunt ended papules with hyperkeratotic surfaces. This condition should not be confused with condylomata acuminata.[7]

The diagnosis of HPV-related diseases is particularly difficult in elderly women since atrophic changes detected on vaginal cytology are frequently difficult to distinguish from VAIN (Table 9.9). In postmenopausal women

Table 9.9

Approach to Postmenopausal Patients with Mildly Abnormal Cytology

Atrophy is difficult to distinguish cytologically from mild atypia.

Treat with Premarin (1 gm intravaginal cream h.s. for 4-6 wks) and repeat smear.

If repeat Pap is abnormal, perform colposcopy and stain vagina with iodine.

Biopsy all unstained areas.

Have biopsies reviewed by expert prior to definitive therapy.

---

with abnormal Pap tests suggestive of either condyloma or low-grade intraepithelial neoplasia, the use of Premarin vaginal cream, 1 gm. h.s. for four to six weeks is recommended. The rationale for using estrogen in such cases is to mature the atrophic squamous epithelium of the vagina. Atrophy may masquerade as condyloma or VAIN (Figure 9.15A, B) and lead to a Pap smear being interpreted as being abnormal. If the repeat Pap test contains persistent abnormalities, the vagina should be colposcoped and iodine stained. Unstained areas should be biopsied to confirm the presence of intraepithelial neoplasia or condyloma (Figure 9.16). DES-exposed offspring also often present diagnostic problems. Colposcopically, a large number of DES-exposed women have abnormal colposcopic patterns including white focal lesions with or without mosaic and punctation. In the vagina these changes represent immature squamous metaplasia involving vaginal adenosis and should not be confused with VAIN (Figure 9.17). Review of all cytologic and histologic material suggestive of VAIN in the DES patient by cytopathologists with expertise in the field is recommended prior to any form of treatment.[3,8]

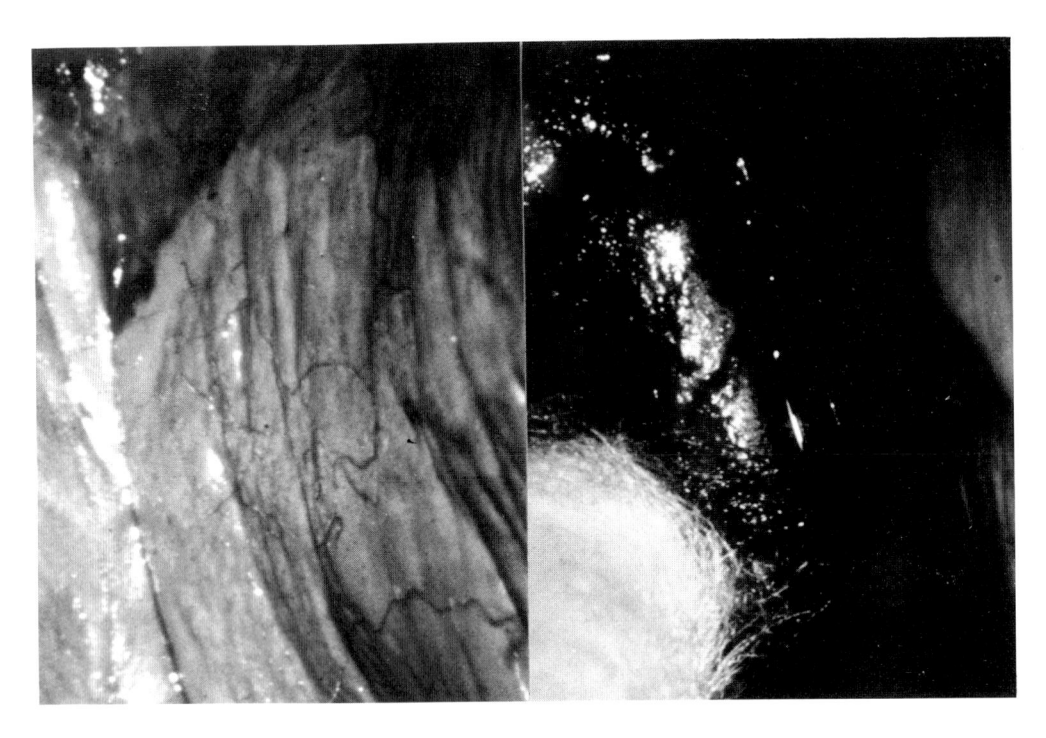

Figure 9.15. Atrophic epithelium of vagina. A) In this 61 year old woman with an abnormal Pap smear suggestive of VAIN, there is total lack of iodine staining of the vaginal epithelium. B) Eight weeks after Premarin vaginal cream therapy, iodine staining is retained throughout. The white spots above the cotton-tipped applicator are due to light reflection. A repeat Pap smear was normal.

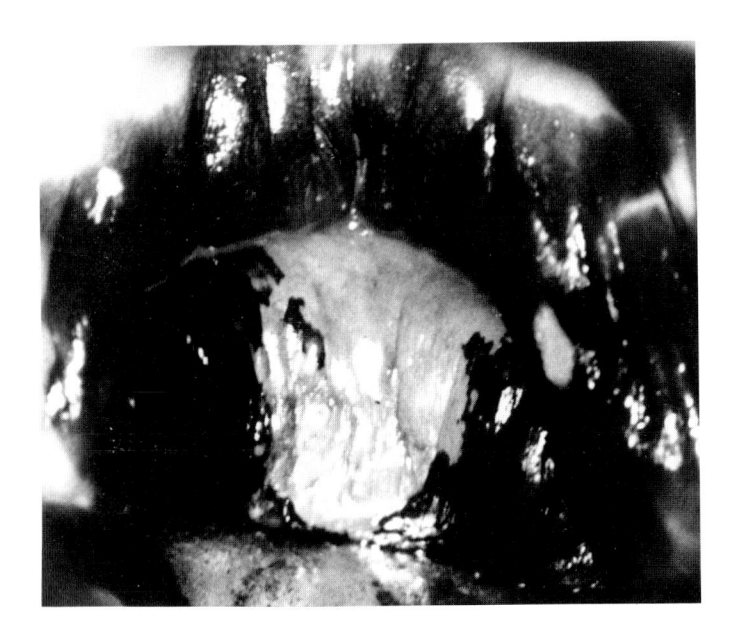

Figure 9.16. Vaginal intraepithelial neoplasia (VAIN). Extensive iodine-negative, sharply demarcated, lesional tissue in the vaginal vault of a 40 year old patient who had a hysterectomy for CIN grade 3 two years previously. Biopsy contained VAIN grade 3.

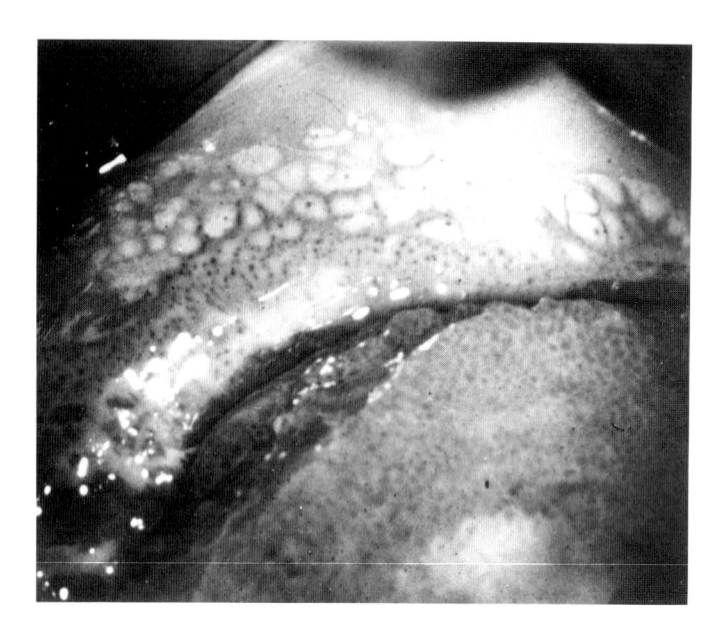

Figure 9.17. Diethylstilbestrol (DES) cervix. This 21 year old woman was exposed in utero to DES. She has an abnormal transformation zone with irregular, coarse mosaic and punctation patterns adjacent to a cervical collar and a pseudopolyp (right). Biopsy of the abnormal area at 3 o'clock contained immature squamous metaplasia.

TREATMENT OPTIONS

A vast range of chemotherapeutic, surgical and immuno-modulating treatment modalities are available for anogenital HPV infections in both men and women. These include topical cytotoxic agents such as 20% podophyllin, 0.5% podofilox, various concentrations of bi- and trichloroacetic acid solutions (BCA, TCA), 5% 5-fluorouracil (5-FU) in the form of a cream, and cryotherapy with liquid nitrogen or nitrous oxide[11,12]. Unfortunately, the efficacy of the different modalities are difficult to compare since many of the published series are uncontrolled clinical trials. In placebo-controlled studies, the treatment results, particularly with podophyllin, have not been significantly superior to those obtained with placebo[10], unless the regimen was carried out for long periods. Lesions that are difficult for the patient to reach (e.g., anus) are inappropriate for home therapy. Among the topical cytotoxic agents, 0.5% podofilox (Condylox™ in the USA and Condyline™ in Canada) (Figure 9.18) and TCA have been the most successful for treating external anogenital condylomata.[9,13] The advantage of 0.5% podofilox over TCA is that the former is approved for home use and, in addition, is associated with comparatively fewer and less severe side effects, including discomfort, erosions and ulcerations, than the latter.

DIAGNOSIS AND MANAGEMENT OF HPV-RELATED DISEASES

For acuminate condylomata of the vagina, topical 5-FU cream has been associated with complete response rates of approximately 75%.[14] However, 5-FU cream therapy for intraepithelial neoplasia of the vagina and the external anogenital skin has not met therapeutic expectations and complications such as corrosive denudation and scarring of the treated areas have been significant.[3] In addition, 5-FU is a teratogen and there is concern about its use in women of reproductive age. Among the various types of interferon therapy given to patients with refractory or recurrent genital warts, the multi-subspecies α–interferons (Figure 9.19) provide the most favorable response rates, i.e., three times higher rates of complete regression than are observed with placebo.[15] Interferon therapy requires repeated administrations by a physician (2 times a week for up to 8 weeks) and side effects are relatively frequent but of a transitory nature.[16] The majority of recurrences with any treatment modality are observed six weeks after the last treatment; they are relatively uncommon after a six month disease-free period in patients with condylomata but are frequent in patients with intraepithelial neoplasia.

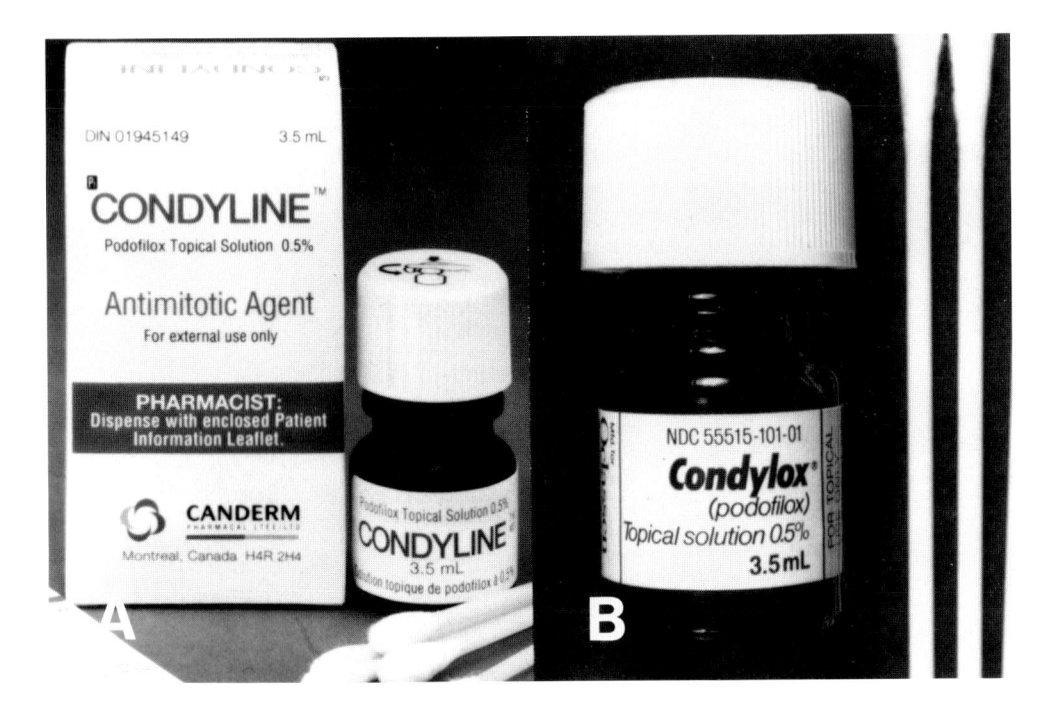

Figure 9.18. 0.5% purified podophyllotoxin (podofilox) is approved and recommended for home therapy because of its low concentration of podophyllotoxin. In Canada, 0.5% podofilox is sold as Condyline™ and in the U.S. as Condylox™. *(Photographs courtesy of Canderm Pharmacal Ltd., and Oclassen Pharmaceuticals, Inc.)*

Recently, laser technology has been applied to the treatment of extensive anogenital flat and acuminate condylomata and intraepithelial neoplasia as well as to persistent or recurrent disease after traditional, conservative therapy.[14,17-20] CO_2 laser vaporization has the advantage of being precise and rapid, and the cosmetic results are highly acceptable; the disadvantage of CO_2 laser therapy is that the equipment is expensive. In addition, therapy may have to be repeated several times to offset frequent recurrences.[19,20] The therapeutic effectiveness of combining CO_2 laser ablation or electrosurgery with interferon therapy is being evaluated in several medical centers.

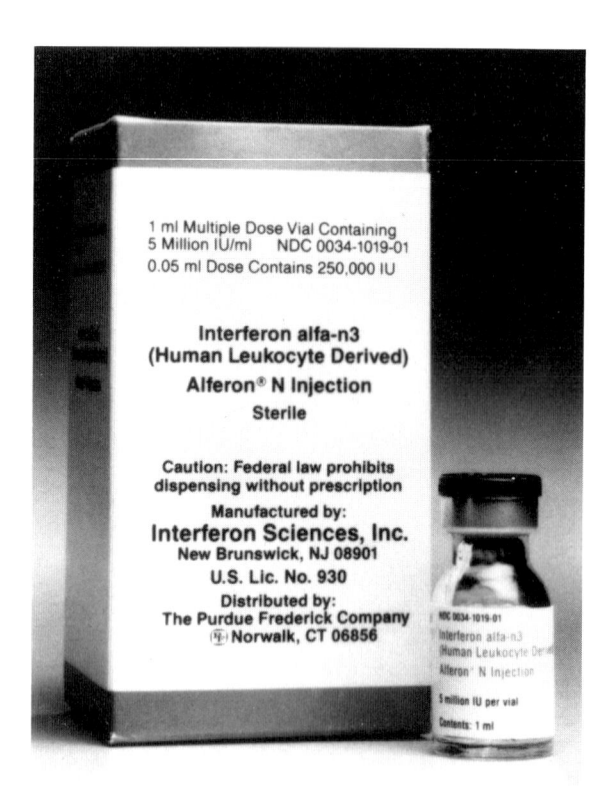

Figure 9.19. Multi-subspecies Alferon(R) N injections contain as many as 14 α-interferon subtypes and is administered intralesionally twice a week at a dose of 0.05 ml per wart. It is recommended for refractory or recurrent external anogenital condylomata. *(Photograph courtesy of the Purdue Frederick Co.)*

REFERENCES

1. Wright, T.C. and Richart, R.M. Role of human papillomavirus in the pathogenesis of genital tract warts and cancer. *Gynecol. Oncol.* 37:151-164, 1990.
2. Crum, P.C., Fu, Y.S., Levine, R.V., *et al.* Intraepithelial squamous lesions of the vulva: Biologic and histologic criteria for the distinction of condylomas from vulvar intraepithelial neoplasia. *Amer. J. Obstet. Gynecol.* 144:77-83, 1982.
3. Ferenczy, A. Intraepithelial neoplasia of the vulva. In *Gynecological Oncology, Fundamental Principles and Clinical Practice.* 1, 3rd ed. M. Coppleson, ed. Churchill Livingstone, London, 1992.
4. Oriel, J.D. Natural history of genital warts. *Br. J. Vener. Dis.* 47:1-13, 1971.
5. Barrasso, R., de Brux, J., Croissant, O., *et al.* High prevalence of papillomavirus-associated penile intraepithelial neoplasia in sexual partners of women with cervical intraepithelial neoplasia. *N. Engl. J. Med.* 317:916-923, 1987.
6. Bergeron, C., Ferenczy, A., Richart, R.M. and Guralnick, M. Micropapillomatosis labialis appears unrelated to human papillomavirus. *Obstet. Gynecol.* 76:281-286, 1990.
7. Ferenczy, A., Richart, R.M. and Wright, T.C. Pearly penile papules: Absence of human papillomavirus DNA by the polymerase chain reaction. *Obstet. Gynecol.* 78:118-122, 1991.
8. Malus, M. and Ferenczy, A. Screening and management of diethylstilbestrol-exposed offspring. *Can. Family Physician* 30:1679-1685, 1984.
9. Beutner, K.R. Podophyllin in the treatment of genital human papillomavirus infection: A review. *Sem. Dermatol.* 6:10-18, 1987.
10. Jensen, S.L. Comparison of podophyllin application with simple surgical excision in clearance and recurrence of perianal condylomata acuminata. *Lancet* ii:1146-1148, 1985.
11. Gosh, A.K. Cryosurgery of genital warts in cases in which podophyllin treatment failed or was contraindicated. *Br. J. Vener. Dis.* 53:49-53, 1977.
12. Simmons, P.D., Langlet, F. and Thin, R.N.T. Cryotherapy versus electrocautery in the treatment of genital warts. *Br. J. Vener. Dis.* 57:273-274, 1981.
13. Greenberg, M., Rutledge, L.H., Reid, R., *et al.* A double-blind, randomized trial of 0.5% podofilox and placebo for the treatment of genital warts in women. *Obstet. Gynecol.* 77:735-739, 1991.
14. Ferenczy, A. Comparison of 5-fluorouracil and CO_2 laser for the treatment of vaginal condylomata. *Obstet. Gynecol.* 64:773-778, 1984.
15. Freidman-Klein, A.E., Eron, L.J., Conant, M., *et al.* Natural interferon alpha for treatment of condylomata acuminata. *J.A.M.A.* 259:533-538, 1988.
16. Condylomata International Collaborative Study Group. Recurrent condylomata acuminata treated with recombinant interferon alpha-2a. A multicenter double-blind placebo-controlled clinical trial. *J.A.M.A.* 265:2684-2687, 1991.
17. Baggish, M.S. Improved laser technnique for the elimination of genital warts. *Amer. J. Obstet. Gynecol.* 153:545-550, 1985.
18. Wright, C.E. and Davies, E. Laser surgery for vulvar intraepithelial neoplasia: Principles and results. *Amer. J. Obstet. Gynecol.* 156:374-378, 1987.
19. Ferenczy, A. Laser treatment of patients with condylomata and squamous carcinoma precursors of the lower female genital tract. *Ca-A Cancer J. for Clinic.* 37:334-347, 1987.
20. Ferenczy, A. Laser treatment of genital human papillomavirus infections in the male patient. In *Lasers in Gynecology.* J. Dorsey, ed. *Obstet. Gynecol. Clin. North Amer.* 18:525-535, 1991.

CHAPTER 10

ELECTROSURGERY FOR VAGINAL AND EXTERNAL ANOGENITAL LESIONS

As described in Chapter 7, electrosurgery using low-voltage, high-frequency alternating current and either thin wire loop or ball electrodes for diagnosing and treating cervical disease has recently become an attractive alternative to traditional diagnostic triage and ablative therapies such as cryocoagulation and laser vaporization. Electrosurgery, in the form of electrodesiccation, has been used for decades by dermatologists and surgeons for treating external anogenital condylomata.[1-3] Although the equipment needed for electrodesiccation is considerably less expensive than the CO_2 laser and the treatment results are good (50%-75% cure rates), gynecologists have generally not used electrosurgery as a method of treating condylomata and intraepithelial neoplasia of the vagina and the external anogenital skin. In this chapter, electrosurgical techniques for treating vaginal and external anogenital lesions are described.

Indications for Electrosurgery for Vaginal and External Anogenital Lesions

Excision with loop and needle electrodes and fulguration with ball and needle electrodes can be used to manage vaginal and external anogenital condylomata[4] and intraepithelial neoplasia[5] as well as for a myriad of other intraepithelial lesions (Table 10.1). Excision and fulguration are highly effective and safe techniques and produce results similar to those obtained by CO_2 laser excision/vaporization, but at a significantly lower equipment cost.

Lesional tissues in the vagina and external anogenital region are usually excised using thin wire loop electrodes or microneedle electrodes or are fulgurated using ball and macroneedle electrodes. In general, electrosurgical excision is faster than fulguration. Therefore, extensive and large condylomata are usually excised ("mini-debulking"), whereas smaller ones are fulgurated. In cases of intraepithelial neoplasia in which early invasion is suspected, the area in question can be excised with a microneedle electrode providing a tissue specimen suitable for histologic diagnosis.

Electrosurgery is also useful for the removal of a wide variety of benign conditions such as molluscum contagiosum, polypoid granulation tissue, polyps, seborrheic keratoses and Bartholin's duct cyst (Table 10.1).

Table 10.1

> **Indications for Electrosurgery**
>
> Condylomata acuminata
>
> Intraepithelial neoplasia
>
> Subclinical, flat condylomata (plana)*
>
> Miscellaneous
>
> *with intractable pruritus and/or burning

Management of Asymptomatic Subclinical Infections

Treating asymptomatic patients with diffuse, acetowhite, vulvar lesions is not recommended. The relatively high cost and possible complications associated with therapy of such areas, particularly those with extensive involvement of the anogenital skin, do not seem to be justified on the basis of their clinical significance. In one recent study, the results of treating condylomata acuminata with subcutaneous injections of α-2-interferon were not affected if the patient had coexisting (untreated) acetowhite subclinical lesions.[6] We have treated 160 patients with vaginal and external anogenital condylomata acuminata electrosurgically[4], and the recurrence rates were similar irrespective of the presence or absence of coexistent diffuse acetowhite areas that were untreated.

Hard data on the biologic behavior of acetowhite, subclinical, HPV infections (flat condylomata) of the vagina and external anogenital skin are not available. However, the relative rarity of squamous cell carcinoma in these anatomical regions suggests that the potential of these lesions for progressing to invasive cancer is negligible.[7]

The mechanism(s), risks and rates of re-infection of previously treated patients by their monogamous sex partners with untreated HPV infections have not specifically been investigated. The available clinical data, although indirect, supports the hypothesis that partners in a stable sexual union are unlikely to "re-infect" each other. For example, recurrence rates in patients treated successfully for CIN by cryotherapy[8] or laser vaporization[9] but who failed to practice protected intercourse were not higher (4 and 6 per 1,000 women, respectively) than was the incidence rate of CIN in the general population. In another study, recurrence rates of approximately 35% have been noted after laser vaporization for external anogenital condylomata irrespective of whether the patients engaged in protected or unprotected intercourse.[4,10] Finally, in a large series of patients treated for CIN and vulvar warts with CO_2 laser vaporization, recurrence rates were essentially the same, 15% and 50% respectively, regardless of whether the partners were treated (Campion M., personal communication, 1991). Therefore, failures or recurrences after cytodestructive therapies such as cryo-, laser, or electrosurgery may be due to the subsequent activation of latent HPV DNA carried in the histologically normal genital skin adjacent to treated areas as opposed to reinfection.[10]

Equipment Required for Electrosurgery of External Genital Lesions

Electrosurgery for vaginal and anogenital tract disease requires much of the same basic equipment as required for electrosurgery of the cervix (see Chapter 4). Table 10.2 lists the equipment required for non-cervical applications. Most of the procedures are performed in the office, with maximum power outputs of approximately 30 watts cutting and 50 watts coagulation, respectively.

The major difference between the electrodes used for cervical lesions and those for the vagina and external anogenital skin is that the latter have shorter shafts. For vaginal lesions, the electrodes have a 9 - 10 cm long shaft (Figure 10.1), whereas for external anogenital lesions the shaft usually measures 5.5 cm in length (Figure 10.2). These short-shafted electrodes enable the physician's hand to reach close to the area to be treated providing good support to the hand during excision and fulguration procedures (Figure 10.3).

A steady hand is the major prerequisite for controlling the depth of excision with both the loop and microneedle electrodes. Deep cuts into the subepithelial tissues may lead to severe bleeding which may require suturing.

ELECTROSURGERY FOR HPV-RELATED DISEASES

Table 10.2

Basic Equipment and Instruments

Electrosurgical generator (ESU)
Fume evacuator
Loop/microneedle electrodes
Ball/macroneedle electrodes
Dental syringe and xylocaine solution
Insulated speculum, forceps and skin hooks

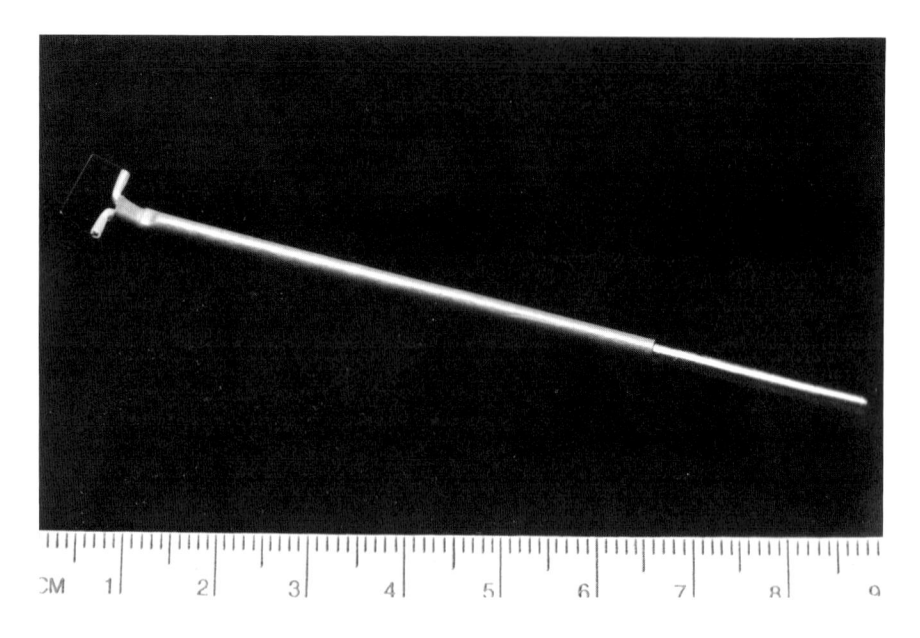

Figure 10.1. Loop electrode for vaginal lesion. The electrode has a 9 cm long insulated shaft and a 1.0 x 0.4 cm square-shaped loop bent at a 10° angle. This configuration helps to reach lesional tissues on the lateral vaginal walls.

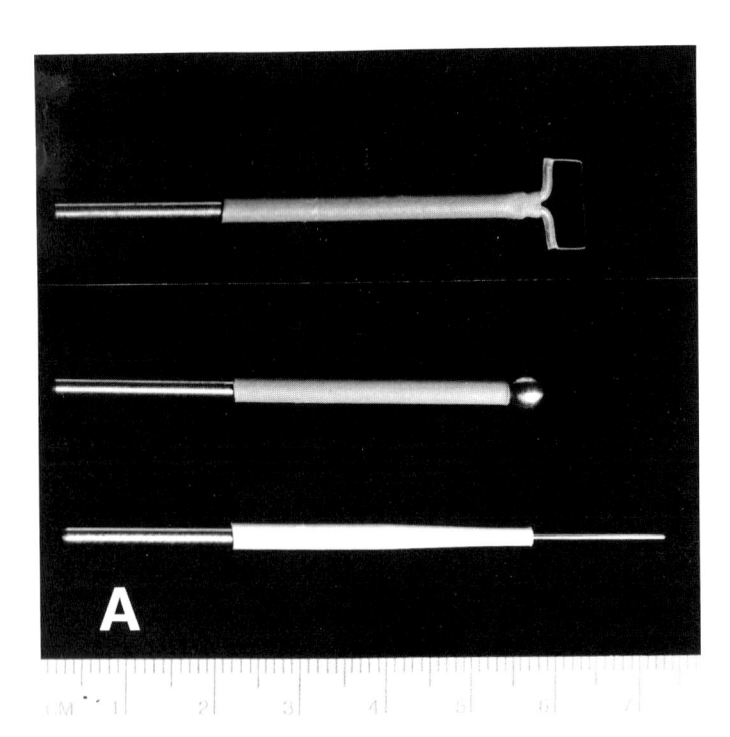

Figure 10.2. Loop, ball and needle electrodes. A) For excising small-sized condylomata and vulvar intraepithelial neoplasia the 1.0 cm x 0.4 cm loop electrode (upper) is used, whereas for fulguration the 5 mm ball and 1 mm macro-needle electrode are employed. The 5.5 cm shaft of these electrodes is insulated as is the crossbar of the loop. B) Ball electrode with a 12 cm long shaft used for fulgurating condylomata/intraepithelial neoplasia located on the lateral walls of the vagina.

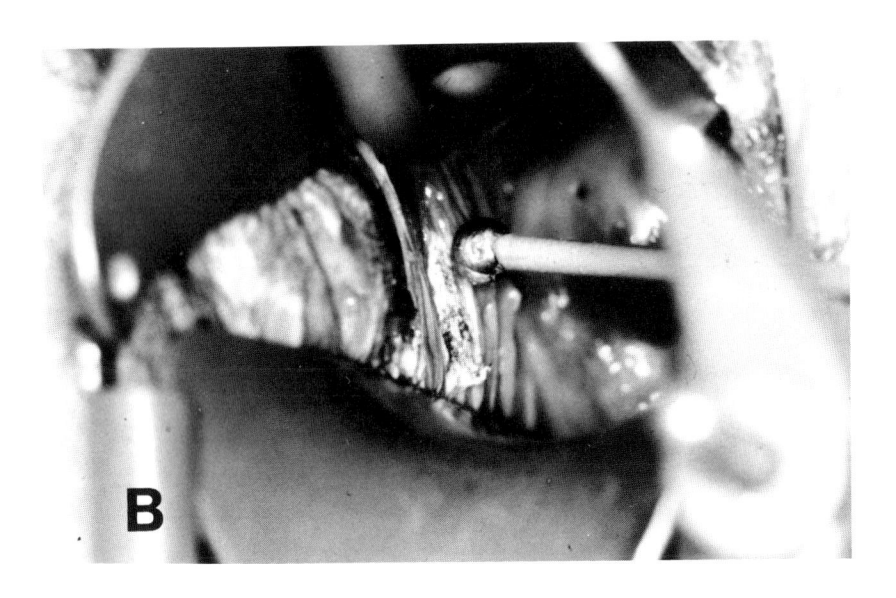

ELECTROSURGERY FOR HPV-RELATED DISEASES

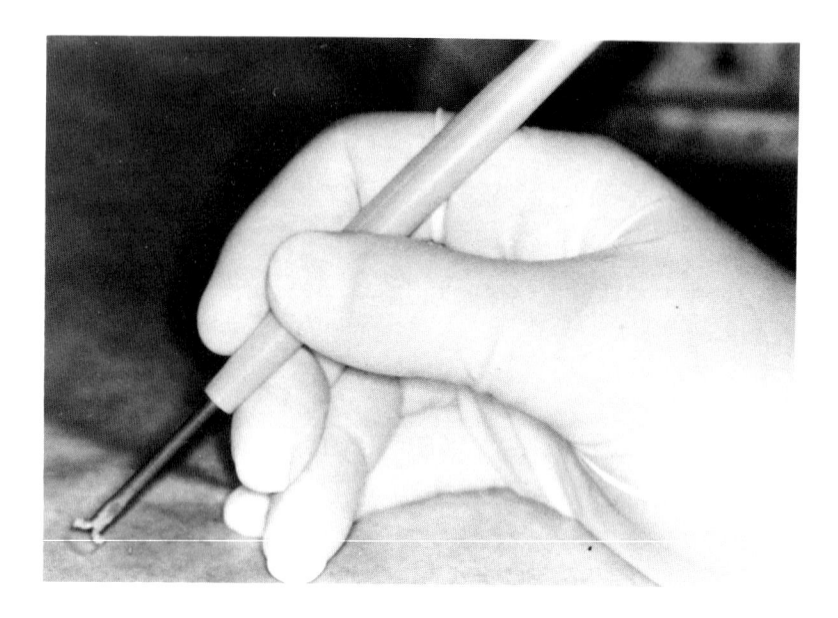

Figure 10.3. Depth control. The short shaft of the electrode permits positioning the operator's hand close to the lesional tissue. This provides good hand support and control of the depth of excision.

As required when excising cervical lesions, specially designed wire loop electrodes that have appropriate configurations and sizes should be used when excising vaginal and external anogenital disease. For condylomata acuminata and intraepithelial neoplasia of the external anogenital skin 1.0 cm x 0.4 cm loop electrodes are used (Figure 10.2). For vaginal condylomata, the 1 cm x 0.4 cm loop with a 10° angle (Figure 10.2) facilitates access to lesional tissues located on the vault and the lateral walls. The microneedle electrode is preferred for dissecting away lesions in which different tissue planes are to be penetrated during the procedure (Figure 10.4). Microneedle electrodes are particularly useful in cases of VIN in which areas with early invasion are suspected and for tumors of the vulva or the vagina with possible deep extension into the subjacent connective tissue where gradual, step by step dissection along the tissue planes is desirable rather than excising the entire lesion in one stroke with the loop electrodes. Smaller lesions and bleeding vessels can be fulgurated with either a 3 mm or a 5 mm ball electrode or a 1 mm macroneedle electrode (Figure 10.2A).

Electrosurgery of vaginal and external anogenital lesions requires some form of anesthesia. In patients in whom the anal canal, one half or more of the vagina, or two thirds of the vulva are involved, either a general, spinal or epidural anesthetic is required. In all other cases loop excision and fulguration

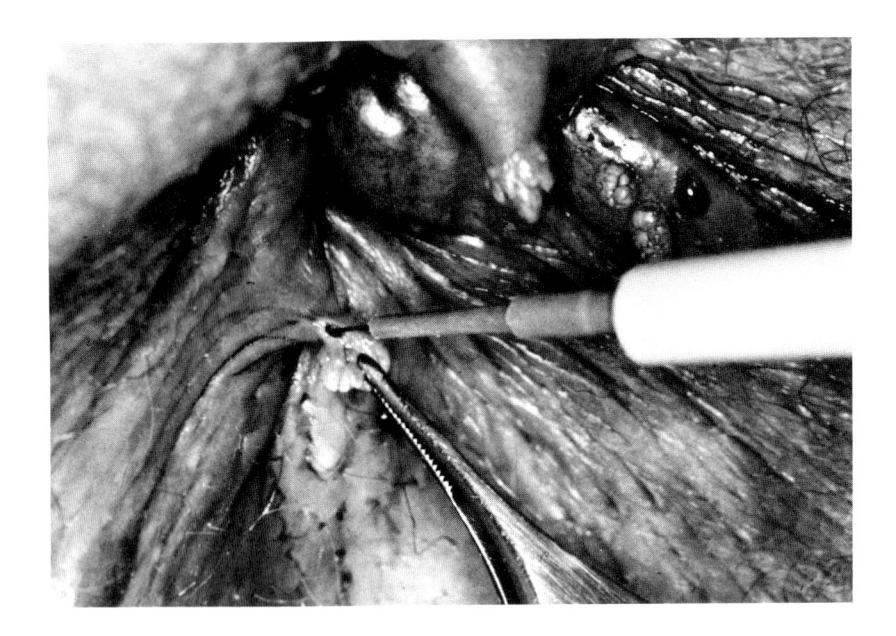

Figure 10.4. Microneedle electrode. The 5 mm x 0.5 mm tungsten wire needle is useful for excising or dissecting acuminate condylomata and intraepithelial neoplasia.

are performed under local anesthesia using 2% xylocaine with epinephrine in a concentration of 1:100,000 (except for the penis). To inject the anesthetic we use a dental-style syringe, cartridges containing 1.8 ml of 2% xylocaine solution, and 27 gauge needles (see Chapter 4). For anesthetizing the upper one-third of the vagina including the vaginal vault, a reinforced 27 gauge needle similar to that used for the cervix is helpful (see Chapter 4). A fume evacuation system is also needed to evacuate the plume of smoke generated by electrosurgery. The amount of smoke is negligible during excision, however, it is relatively abundant during periods of fulguration.

Electrosurgical excision of extra-cervical lesions requires good technical skills. During the first phase of the learning curve, excisions are easier to perform without magnification. However, the depth of excision is better controlled, and the treatment results are superior, when the loop electrodes are used under colposcopic guidance with a magnification of 4-7.5x. This requires that the operator has expertise in manipulating the electrodes under magnification.

ELECTROSURGERY FOR HPV-RELATED DISEASES

Accessories for Electrosurgery

Accessories for electrosurgery are summarized in Table 10.3 and illustrated in Figure 10.5.

Table 10.3

Accessories Needed for Electrosurgery of External Lesions

- 5% acetic acid (vinegar)
- Forceps, lens paper
- Fixative (10% formalin)
- Cotton-tipped applicators
- 2" x 2" and 4" x 4" gauzes
- Small biopsy punch
- Strong aqueous Lugol's solution
- Silver sulfadiazine cream

Five percent (5%) acetic acid solution is used to clean lesional tissue surfaces and identify acetowhite lesions. Ring- and fine-toothed forceps are needed to grasp lesions to be excised or dissected, and to place the excised specimens onto lens paper and then in neutral buffered formalin fixative solution. Acetic acid-soaked, cotton-tipped applicators are needed to wipe away the hard eschar produced by fulguration. Acetic acid-soaked 2" x 2" sponges are used to clean secretions from the vagina and to identify lesional tissues in the vaginal epithelium. When introduced into the anal canal, sponges soaked in saline prevent rectal gases from being ignited by the electrosurgical current.

A small biopsy punch is used to obtain histologic specimens from areas in which loop excision is not desired, such as the vaginal vault, periclitoral area, and the glans and frenulum of the penis. At the end of the procedure either silver sulfadiazine cream or silver sulfadiazine cream containing 5% benzocaine (Silcaine™) can be placed over the excised area.

ELECTROSURGERY FOR VAGINAL AND EXTERNAL ANOGENITAL LESIONS

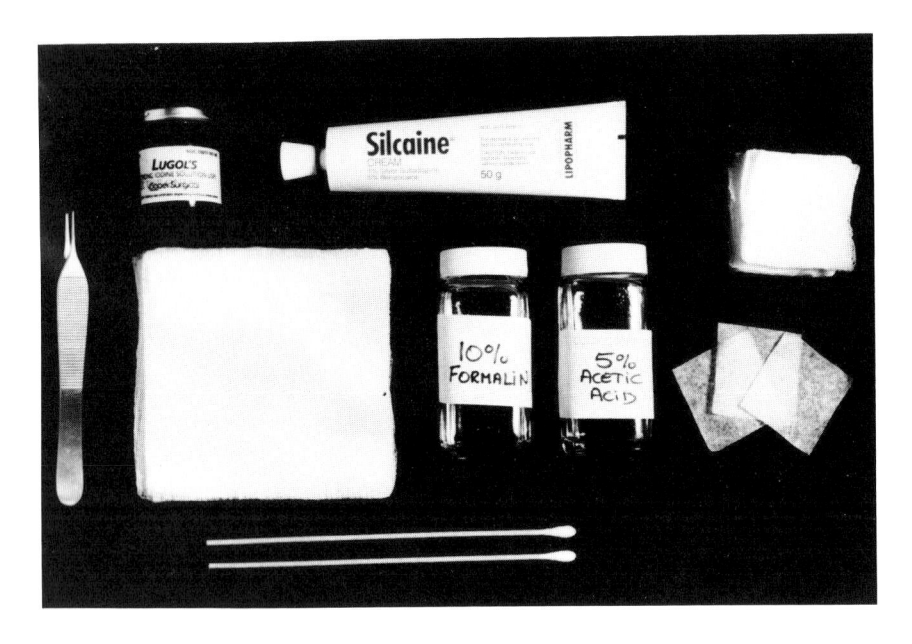

Figure 10.5. Accessories for electrosurgery. Strong aqueous Lugol's solution is needed for outlining vaginal lesions; Silcaine™ cream (Lipopharm, Montreal, CooperSurgical, Inc.) is used to treat the external anogenital skin after therapy; fine-toothed forceps are used for traction of lesions to be excised and for placing specimens on lens paper (right) and then in 10% neutral buffered formalin fixative; 4" x 4" and 2" x 2" sponges help to retain Silcaine™ cream on denuded areas and to apply 5% acetic acid solution to the vagina and external anogenital skin, respectively. The eschar after fulguration is wiped off with cotton-tipped applicators.

Technique of Electrosurgery

This is presented in detail in Chapter 11 (Electrosurgery of the Vagina and External Anogenital Tract: A Step-by-Step Guide). When the patient is managed under local anesthesia, the anesthetic solution is delivered superficially into the connective tissue layer under the lesion (Figure 10.6). Discomfort that may occur secondary to heat radiating from the wire electrode is prevented by extending the infiltration of the anesthetic solution to about a centimeter from the lesion, circumferentially. Infiltration will also elevate the lesion to be excised and, at the same time, provide a tissue space with low resistance to alternating current (Figures 10.7, 10.8). This provides protection from inadvertently excising too deeply. Since the water-rich tissue has little resistance to the high-frequency alternating current, this limits the thermocoagulation artifacts to a zone of less than 100 microns. In patients treated under general anesthesia, saline, rather than xylocaine, can be used to elevate the tissues.

ELECTROSURGERY FOR HPV-RELATED DISEASES

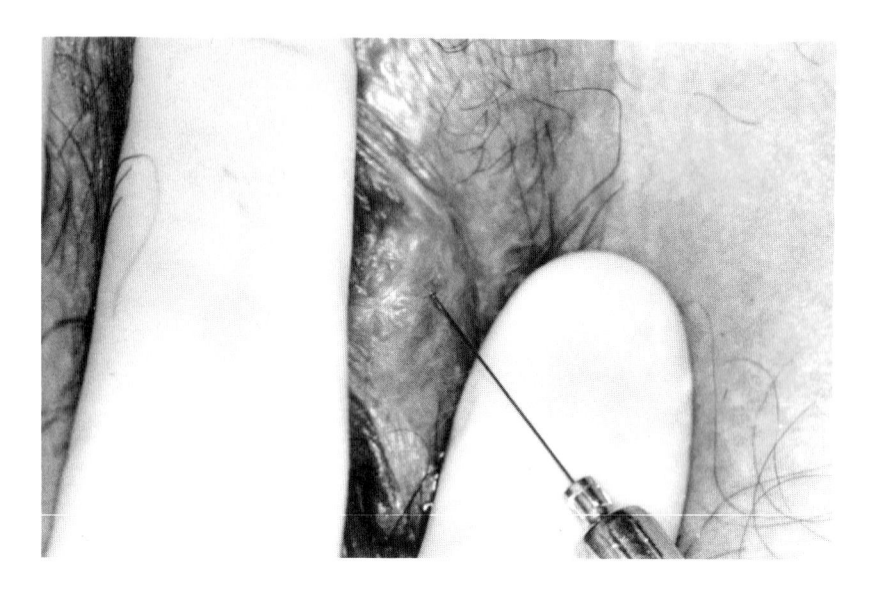

Figure 10.6. Injection of anesthesia. The lesion to be excised is elevated by infiltrating the anesthetic solution just beneath the lesional tissue. This "separates" the lesion from the underlying, supportive connective tissue providing for shallow penetration of the loop electrode.

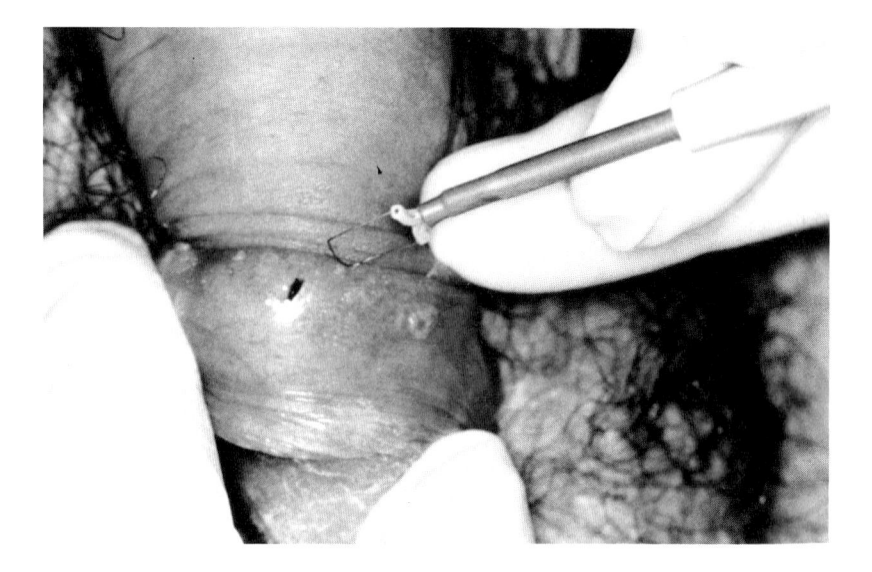

Figure 10.7. Local anesthesia. Elevating the lesional tissue from the adjacent papillary dermis with 2% xylocaine solution is particularly important in the non-hairy genital skin including the distal foreskin.

ELECTROSURGERY FOR VAGINAL AND EXTERNAL ANOGENITAL LESIONS

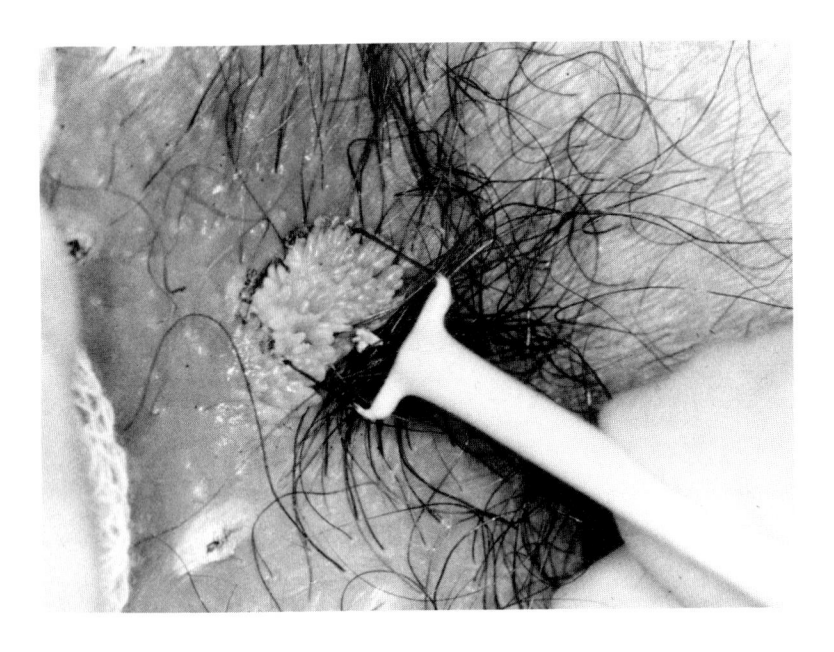

Figure 10.8 Loop excision. A condyloma acuminatum is excised with a square-shaped loop electrode.

As mentioned earlier, to control the depth of excision with the loop electrodes, the operator's hands must rest solidly near the excision site. Placing the fifth finger of the hand that holds the electrode on the index finger of the opposite hand, which is used to spread the skin at the site of excision, provides hand stability and good control of the depth of excision (Figure 10.9). This is particularly important when papular, or only slightly elevated lesions (VIN, VAIN, PAIN), are excised.

When the microneedle electrode is used, the lesional tissue is dissected along the desired tissue planes as when using a scalpel (Figure 10.4). The depth of excision is easier to control with the microneedle than with the loop electrode, for excision is carried out step by step with the microneedle rather than in a continuous stroke as with the loop electrode. Excisional procedures are carried out with a blended cutting current. The power output is set according to the size of the electrode being used.

ELECTROSURGERY FOR HPV-RELATED DISEASES

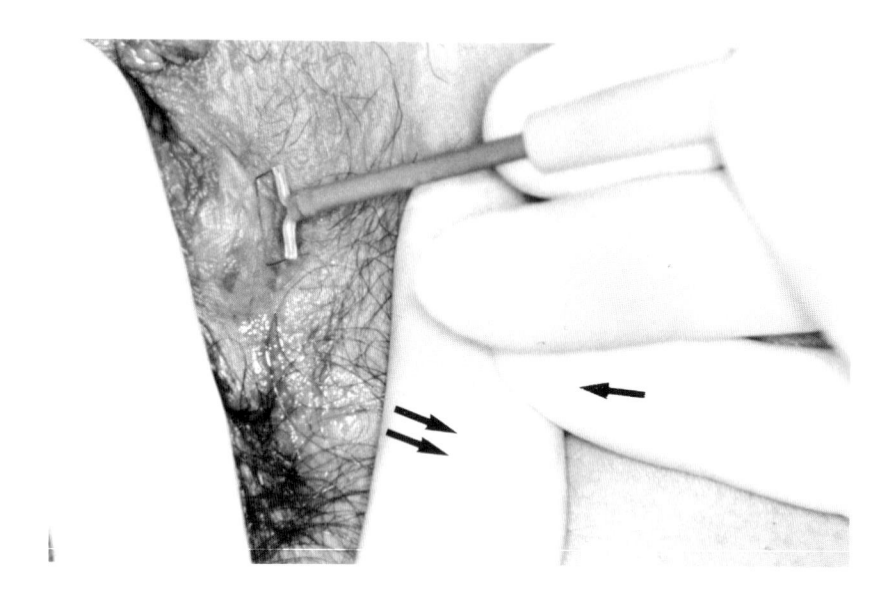

Figure 10.9. Depth control. This is achieved when the fifth finger (arrow) of the hand that is holding the loop electrode is placed on the index finger (double arrow) of the opposite hand which is used to expose the lesional tissue, in this case, a VIN.

Under some conditions, excision may be followed by significant bleeding (Table 10.4). For example, decidual polyps during pregnancy, polypoid granulation tissue at episiotomy sites or in the vaginal walls after hysterectomy, and voluminous perianal condylomata may bleed profusely if they are excised with a blended cutting current. In such situations the use of pure coagulation current rather than cutting current is suggested. Pure coagulation current can also be used to excise the pedicle of lesions to which traction is applied (Figure 10.10). If histological interpretation is required when using pure coagulation, the excision line should be chosen to be at a distance from the area to be diagnosed.

Table 10.4

Excisions That Can Result in Significant Bleeding

Decidual polyps during pregnancy

Polypoid granulation tissue at episiotomy sites or in vagina after hysterectomy

Voluminous perianal condylomata

Hemostasis at excision sites is obtained by fulgurating the bleeding vessels with either a ball or macroneedle electrode. Fulguration is also useful for destroying smaller acuminate or papular lesions, particularly in the vagina, labia, and perianal and intra-anal epithelium as well as for "brushing" the normal epithelium adjacent to treatment fields (Figure 10.11). As suggested previously, the epithelium adjacent to HPV-related lesions often contains HPV DNA in a nonexpressed (latent) form which can be activated by mechanical or humoral factors during, or soon after, therapy. Once the lesions become productive, clinically visible, seemingly "recurrent" disease can develop (Figure 10.12). Selectively removing the normal epithelium adjacent to surgical margins in patients with "recurrent" disease may reduce their recurrence rates.[11,12] Under ideal conditions, electrosurgical fulguration results in very superficial thermocoagulation of the treated tissue (Figure 10.13).

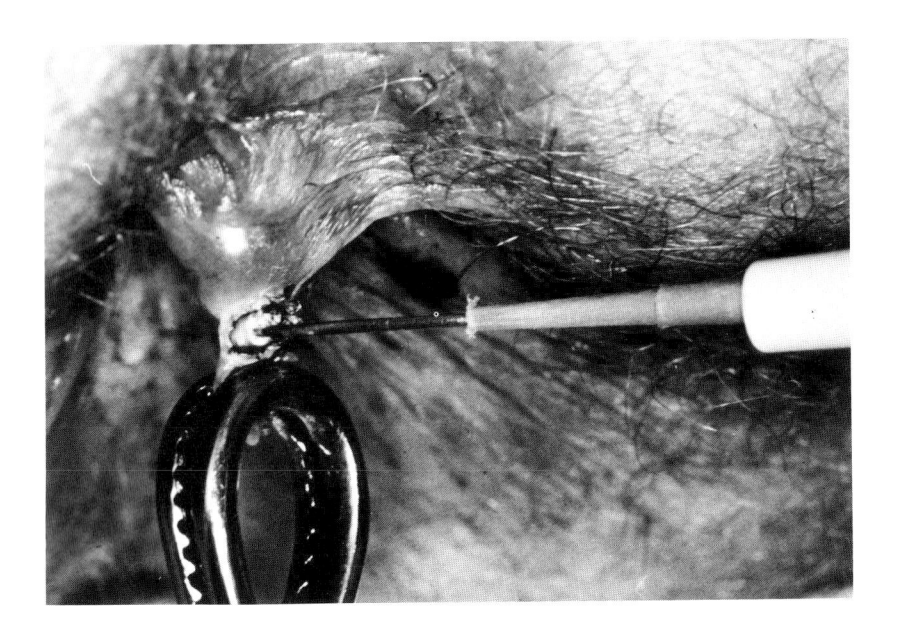

Figure 10.10. Macroneedle electrode. This 1.0 mm thick needle, when used in a coagulation power output mode, provides for the virtually bloodless excision of lesional tissues that are prone to bleed. Excisions with this electrode are best performed when traction is applied to tissues being excised.

ELECTROSURGERY FOR HPV-RELATED DISEASES

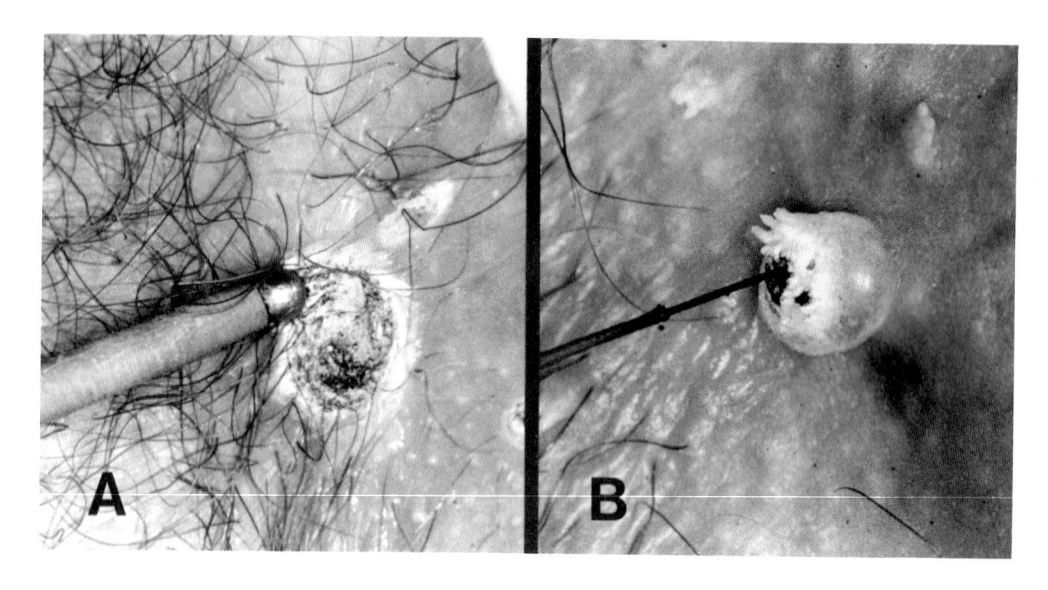

Figure 10.11. Fulguration. A) A ball-shaped electrode is used to fulgurate small, acuminate, papular or flat lesions. The procedure provides also for excellent hemostasis of bleeding vessels at excision sites. B) A macroneedle electrode is particularly appropriate for electrosurgically fulgurating small lesional tissues. The condylomatous tissue is destroyed and separated from the adjacent papillary dermis by steaming (bubbling) and superficial thermocoagulation.

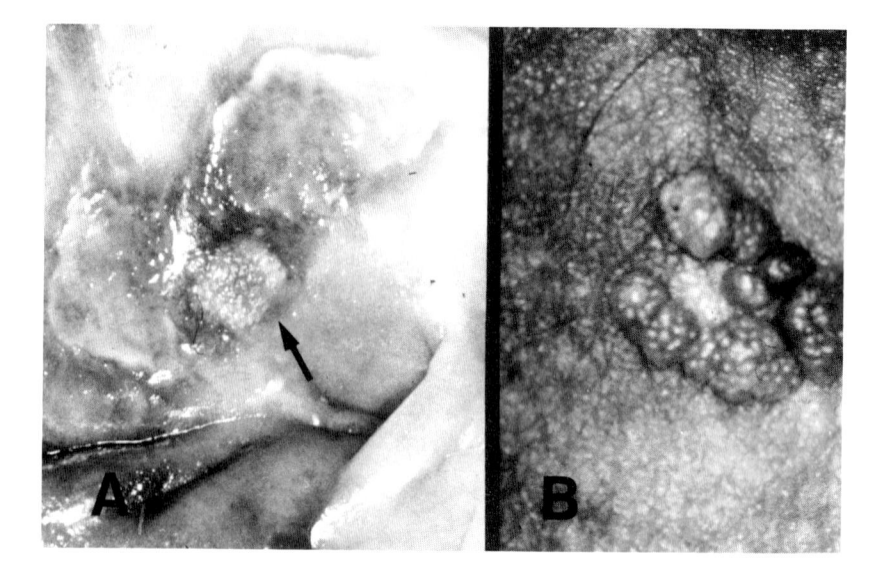

Figure 10.12. Recurrent condylomata A) Three weeks after laser vaporization for vulvar condylomata, a new lesion has appeared at the laser margin (arrow) despite the patient being sexually abstinent. B) Multiple condylomata surrounding previously treated lesion, producing the so-called "ring" recurrence pattern. *(Used with permission from reference 4.)*

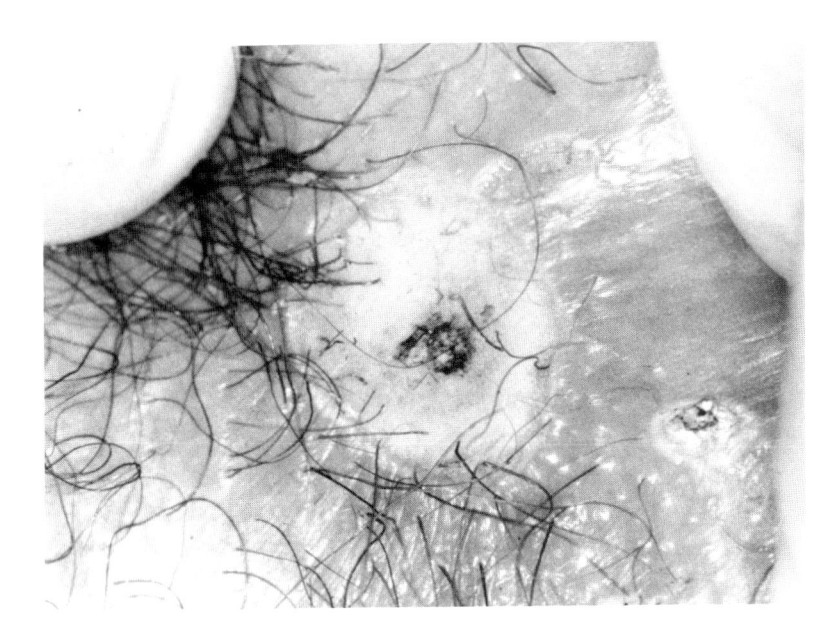

Figure 10.13. Electrosurgically excised/fulgurated genital skin. The central area corresponds to an excised acuminate condyloma with deep rete pegs. The pericentral area has a finely granular surface and a yellowish, chamois leather-type clinical appearance corresponding to the second surgical plane. The peripheral area next to the intact skin is whitish, granular and corresponds to the "electrobrushed" normal epithelium adjacent to the lesional tissue.

Superficial thermocoagulation is obtained when arcing occurs between the tissue and the electrode, which is rapidly swept over the surface. When the electrode is placed in direct contact with the tissue, desiccation, rather than fulguration, occurs and desiccation produces deep thermal damage. This should be avoided.

The eschar produced by fulguration is relatively hard and must be removed by saline-soaked, cotton-tipped applicators. Once the eschar is cleaned away from the fulgurated tissues, the base can be colposcoped to determine if lesional tissue is still present. If lesional tissue remains, another tissue layer is fulgurated. The procedure may be repeated until the desired depth has been obtained. Condylomata acuminata have rete pegs that extend only superficially (about 0.5 mm) into the subepithelial connective tissue. Intraepithelial neoplasia of the hairy skin of the external anogenital tract, on the other hand, may extend deeper into the subjacent hair follicles and sebaceous glands of the non-hairy skin[13] (Figure 10.14).

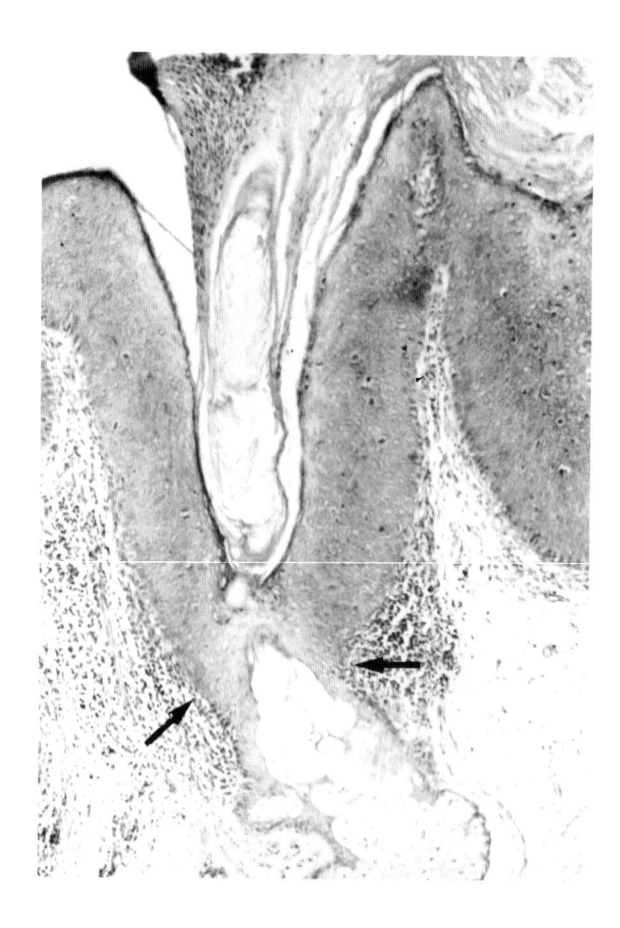

Figure 10.14. Vulvar intraepithelial neoplasia (VIN) with extension into pilosebaceous units of vulvar skin. In most instances, the disease does not extend further than the first sebaceous gland unit (arrows).

In a series of 62 cases of vulvar intraepithelial neoplasia (VIN), hair follicle and sebaceous gland involvement was observed in 31% and 21% of the surgically excised specimens, respectively, and in 99.5% of the cases, the depth of involvement did not exceed 2 mm in the hair follicles and 1 mm in the sebaceous glands.[13] These depths correspond to the second and first surgical tissue planes, respectively (Figure 10.13). The former has a whitish, fibrillar appearance, whereas the latter appears as yellowish chamois leather.[14] These studies indicate that it is appropriate to limit the depth of tissue penetration to the first surgical plane when the disease involves the vagina and the non-hairy areas of the external anogenital skin and to the second surgical plane when intraepithelial neoplasia is located on the hairy genital skin.

Fortunately, the vast majority of intraepithelial neoplasms involve the non-hairy skin of the external anogenital region. In cases in which the adjacent normal-appearing epithelium is fulgurated ("brushed"), the denuded lamina propria (in the vagina) and the papillary dermis (external anogenital skin) has a whitish, finely granular appearance (Figure 10.13). This corresponds to the denuded stromal papillae of the first tissue plane (Figure 10.15).

After electrosurgery, the cleaned, denuded areas are covered by a 1% silver sulfadiazine cream with 5% benzocaine (Silcaine™) (Figure 10.6) or, if not available, silver sulfadiazine alone. The advantage of Silcaine™ over silver sulfadiazine alone is its superior pain relieving properties. In a double-blind, prospective study of 40 patients randomized for silver sulfadiazine and Silcaine™ after electrosurgery and laser ablation of the external anogenital skin, pain was more often relieved by Silcaine™ cream than Silvadene™ cream ($p<0.01$).[15]

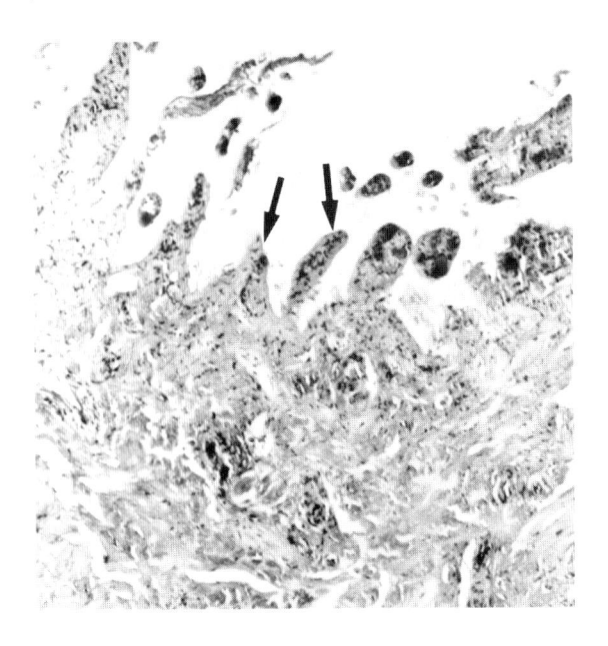

Figure 10.15. Histology of "electrobrushed" epithelium. The epithelium has been "brushed" off from the supportive papillary dermis. The granular colposcopic appearance of this area corresponds histologically to denuded, varying sized papillae (arrows).

Post-Operative Management

The details of post-operative management of patients with external anogenital tract electrosurgery are detailed in Chapter 11. Depending upon which anatomic area being treated, the patients are give written instructions for self care. In patients in whom one third or more of the vagina has been denuded, intravaginal application of Sultrin™ cream prevents coaptation of the epithelium and stenosis of the vagina.

We have observed no greater incidence of side effects or complications in patients who were sexually abstinent than in those who were not after therapy for HPV-related vaginal and external anogenital skin disease. Therefore, sexual abstinence is not required.

The patients who have been treated for extensive vulvar lesions benefit from Sitz baths. The discomfort associated with tissue destruction is generally relieved by topical Silcaine™ or silver sulfadiazine cream mixed with either 5% lidocaine gel or 20% benzocaine ointment.

The patients who are treated for peri/intra-anal condylomata and/or intraepithelial neoplasia are given stool softeners in addition to topical creams to minimize the discomfort associated with bowel movements during the first 10 to 14 postoperative days. The patients are asked to return at one week after treatment to insure that no infection has developed and at six to eight weeks to assess the progress of healing and to look for recurrent disease. The majority of recurrences are observed six weeks after treatment; they are relatively uncommon after a six-month, disease-free period in patients with condylomata but are frequent in patients with intraepithelial neoplasia.

At six to eight weeks post-treatment, recurrent lesions are generally uncommon and are easily removed by punch biopsy or fulguration. If, clinically and colposcopically, the patients are found to be disease-free at six to eight weeks after treatment, they are reexamined at three to four months and 12 months postoperatively and, if found to be normal, are followed annually thereafter.

Results of Electrosurgery for Treating External Anogenital Lesions

In a series of 220 patients with lower genital tract condylomata and intraepithelial neoplasia, one half of the lesional area was treated with electrosurgical excision/fulguration and the other half with CO_2 laser excision/vaporization (Figure 10.16A-E).

The healing time (mean of 14 days) and the rate and duration of postoperative discomfort were similar in the areas treated by electrosurgery or CO_2 laser.[4,5] These results were expected as the depth of tissue penetration was similar in areas treated by electrosurgery and CO_2 laser vaporization (Figure 10.16 D).

For condylomata acuminata and intraepithelial neoplasia involving the non-hairy skin, the tissue removal did not exceed the first surgical plane (papillary dermis), whereas for intraepithelial neoplasia involving the hairy skin, the depth of penetration was limited to the superficial aspect of the second surgical plane (superficial reticular dermis)[4,14] (Figure 10.17A-D).

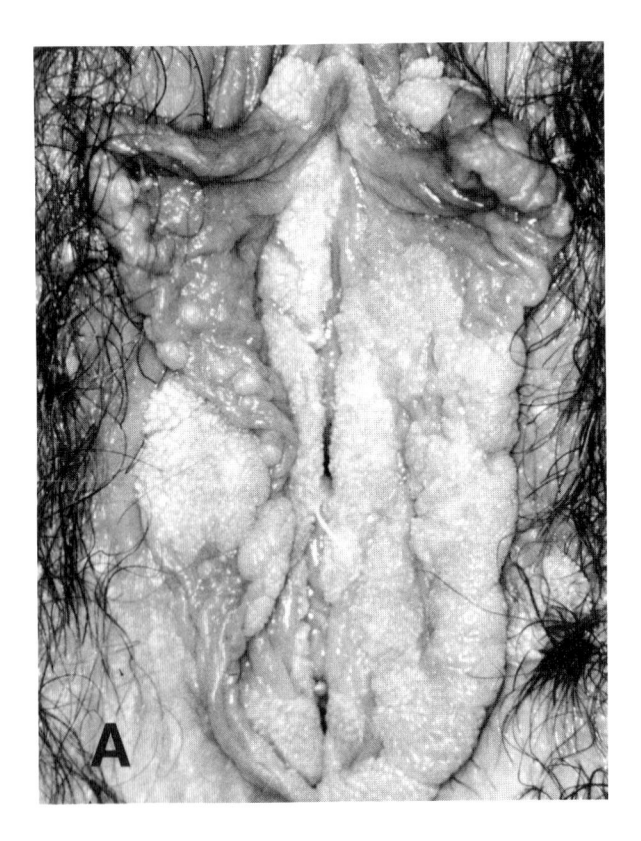

Figure 10.16. Vulvar condylomata. A) Extensive vulvar condylomatosis prior to treatment. B) CO_2 laser vaporization of condylomata of the right labia.

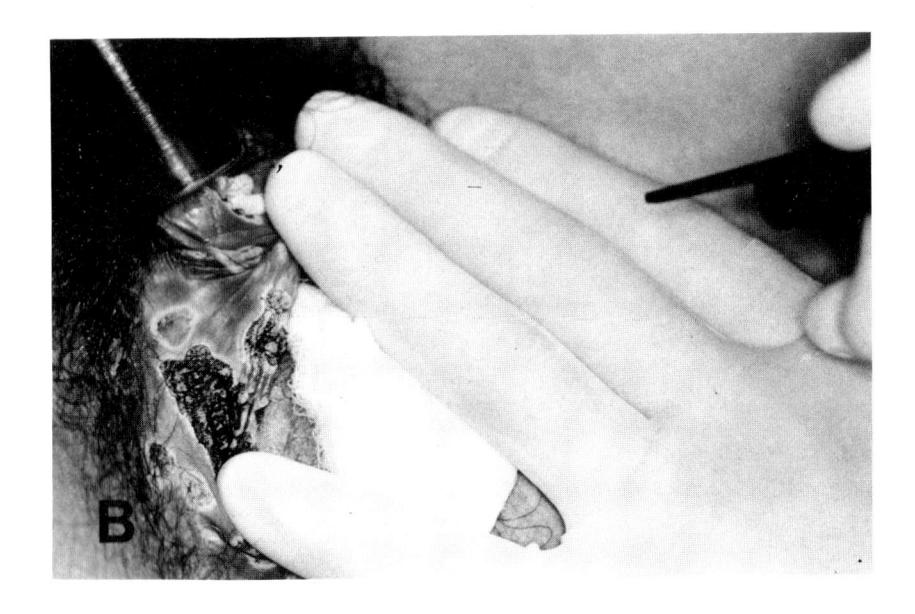

ELECTROSURGERY FOR HPV-RELATED DISEASES

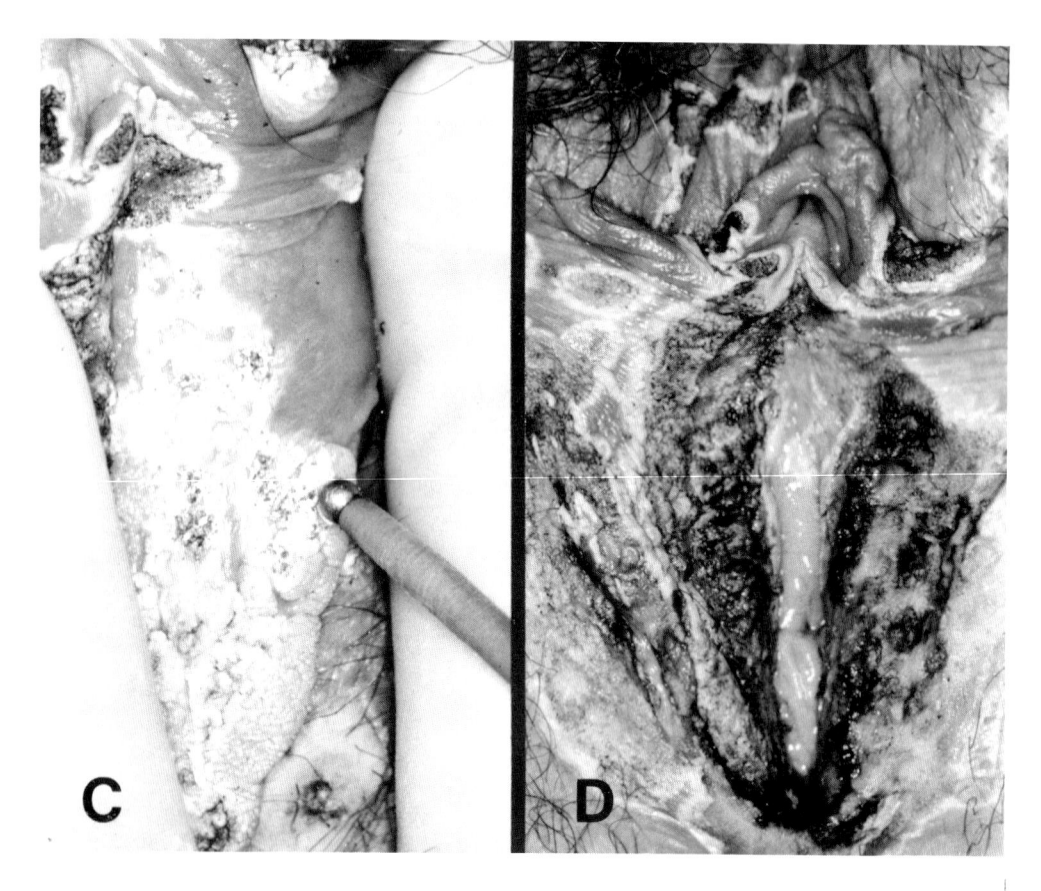

C) Fulguration of condylomata of the left labia with the ball electrode. D) Vulvar skin after CO_2 laser vaporization and electrosurgery. Note that depth of tissue destruction is limited to the first surgical plane.

The recurrence rate in the 160 patients that were treated for vaginal and external anogenital condylomata by electrosurgery and laser treatment (for whom follow-up is available) was 53% (Table 10.5). After multiple treatments (mean of 2.5), the complete response rates were increased to 76%. There was no difference in the recurrence rates between electrosurgically and laser treated areas (Table 10.6).

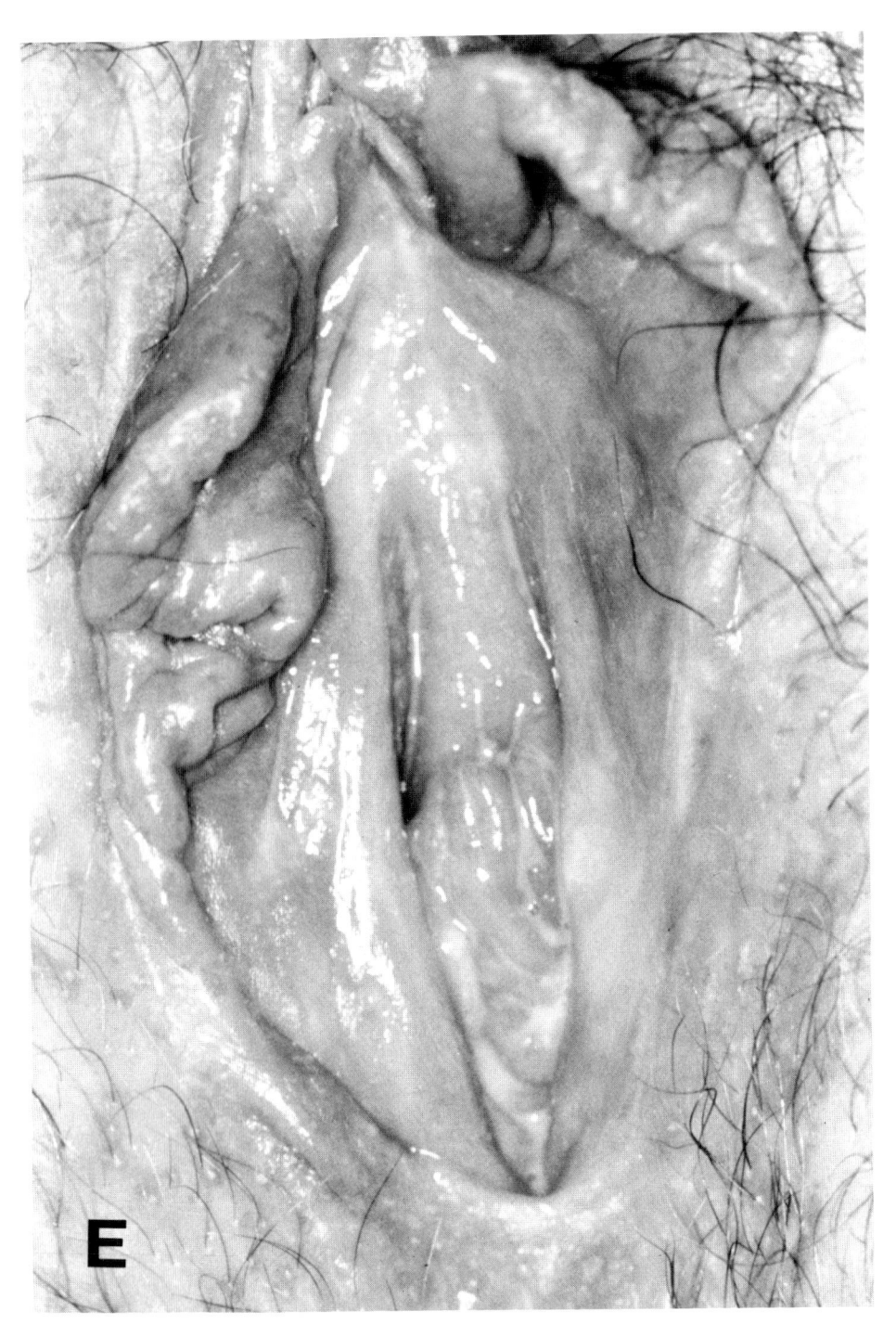

E) Same vulva at 6 weeks post-laser/electrosurgery. Healing has been completed, the new vulvar skin is devoid of lesions and it is both physiologically functional and cosmetically adequate. *(Used with permission from 4.)*

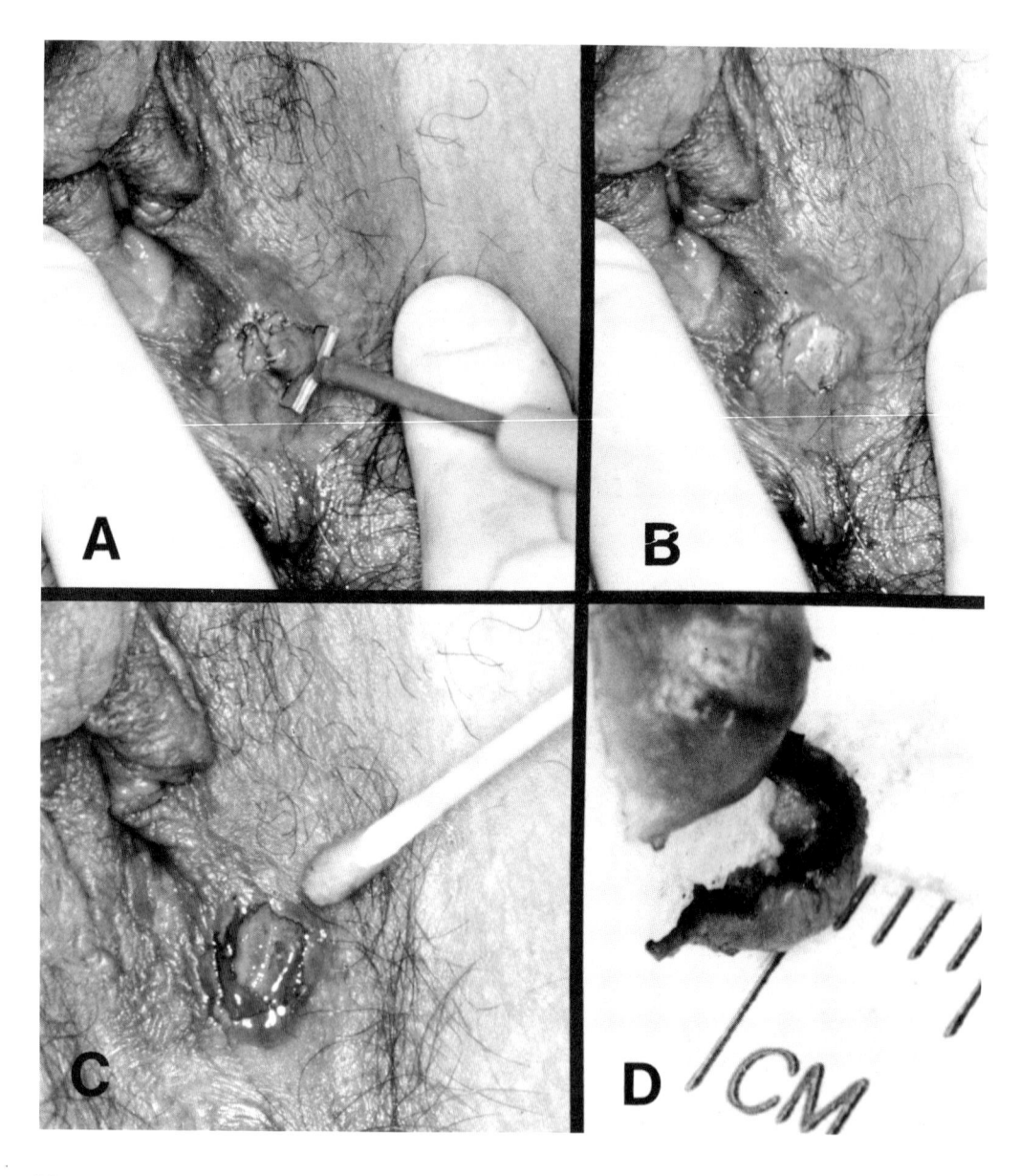

Figure 10.17. Electrosurgical excision of vulvar intraepithelial neoplasia (VIN). A) Loop electrode excising previously anesthetized VIN. Note the close proximity of the hand holding and moving the electrode to the lesion. This position provides excellent support for the operator's hand and facilitates control of the depth of excision. B) Excised lesion prior to its removal from the tissue bed. C) The crater measures approximately 1 mm in depth. D) The 1 mm depth is verified in the excised tissue specimen.

Table 10.5

Treatment Results Using Electrosurgery for Vaginal and External Anogenital Condylomata

Treatments	Complete Response* No. (total)	%
Single Treatment	85/160	53
Multiple Treatments	37/71	52
All Treatments	122/160	76

* Follow-up from 6 - 18 mos.; mean is 8 mos.

Table 10.6

Recurrence Rates of Condylomata in Areas Treated by Electrosurgery vs. Laser

Method of Therapy	Recurrence Rates* No.	%
Electrosurgery and laser	59	83
Electrosurgery only	5	7
Laser surgery	7	10
Total	71	100

* After a single treatment.

In another series of 60 patients treated with electrosurgery for intraepithelial neoplasia, the complete remission rate after multiple treatment sessions was 53% (Table 10.7).

Table 10.7

Treatment Results Using Electrosurgery for Intraepithelial Neoplasia*

Lesion	Complete Response* No. (total)	%
VAIN	3/7	43
VIN	22/40	55
PAIN**	7/13	54
Total	32/60	53

*all received more than one treatment, maximum 6 treatments, mean 3; **all but one also had VIN

Unlike the experience of some, we found no negative influence of age, sex, cigarette smoking, coexistence of subclinical, acetowhite lesions, or CIN grade on treatment results. On the other hand, response to therapy was less favorable in patients (particularly homosexual men) with intra-anal warts ($p < 0.01$), with lesions larger than 3 cm^2 (p 0.05), and with lesions of less than one year's duration ($p < 0.02$) than it was in patients with none of these characteristics.[4]

SIDE EFFECTS AND COMPLICATIONS

The side effects and complications after electrosurgery for external anogenital skin lesions are similar to those reported after CO_2 laser vaporization[11,12] (Table 10.8).

Provided tissue destruction of the external anogenital skin is limited to the second surgical tissue plane and the postoperative instructions are carried out, abscesses, fistulas, labial coaptation and scarring are uncommon.

A list of complications in patients treated electrosurgically for vaginal lesions is given in Table 10.9. Some patients develop a brownish vaginal discharge which occasionally becomes malodorous. The odor is caused by anaerobic organisms with or without Trichomonas vaginalis infection. Active bleeding at one to seven days after electrosurgery is relatively rare and is controlled by fulgurating the bleeding vessels with the macroneedle electrode in the office.

Table 10.8

Complications of Electrosurgery in Patients with External Anogenital Lesions*

Complication	No.	%
Pain (Mod. to Severe)	66	30**
Vitiligo	8	4
Hypertrophic Scars	4	2
Total	78/220	36

*Includes 160 patients with condylomata and 60 with intraepithelial neoplasia. ** Mostly in patients with extensive peri/intra-anal disease.

Table 10.9

Complications of Electrosurgery in Patients with Vaginal Lesions*

Complication	No.	%
Vaginal discharge	4	22
Infection	1**	4
Post-op Bleeding	1	4
Total	6/23	26

*Includes 16 patients with condylomata and 7 with intraepithelial neoplasia. ** Also had discharge.

REFERENCES

1. Simmons, P.D., Langlet, F. and Thin, R.N.T. Cryotherapy versus electrocautery in the treatment of genital warts. *Br. J. Vener. Dis.* 53:49-53, 1981.
2. Stone, K.M., Becker, T.M., Hadgu, A. and Kraus, S.J. Treatment of external genital warts: A randomized, clinical trial comparing podophyllin, cryotherapy, and electrodesiccation. *Genitourin. Med.* 66:16-19, 1990.
3. Billingham, R.P. and Lewis, F.G. Laser vs. electrical cautery in the treatment of condylomata acuminata of the anus. *Surg. Gynaecol. Obstet.* 155:865-867, 1982.
4. Ferenczy, A., Behelak, Y., Haber, G., Wright, T.C. and Richart, R.M. Treating vaginal and external anogenital condylomata with loop electrosurgical excision/fulguration procedure (LEEP) vs. laser ablation. Submitted, 1991.
5. Ferenczy, A. Comparison of CO_2 laser ablation and loop electrosurgical excision procedure (LEEP) for the treatment of vulvar intraepithelial neoplasia (VIN), Abstract. The Society of Gynecologic Oncologists Annual Meeting, March 15-18, 1992.
6. Condylomata International Collaborative Study Group. Recurrent condylomata acuminata treated with recombinant interferon alpha-2a. A multicenter double-blind placebo-controlled clinical trial. *J.A.M.A.* 265:2684-2687, 1991.
7. Ferenczy, A. Intraepithelial neoplasia of the vulva. In *Gynecological Oncology, Fundamental Principles and Clinical Practice.* 1, 3rd ed. M. Coppleson, ed. Churchill Livingstone, London, 1992.
8. Richart, R.M., Townsend, D.E., Crisp, W., *et al.* An analysis of "long-term" follow-up results in patients with cervical intraepithelial neoplasia treated by cryotherapy. *Am. J. Obstet. Gynecol.* 137:823-826, 1980.
9. Valverde, M.A. and Ferenczy, A. Laser ablation of cervical intraepithelial neoplasia: A preliminary study of recurrence rates. *J. Gynecol. Surg.* 5:295-299, 1989.
10. Ferenczy, A., Mitao, M., Nagai, N., *et al.* Latent papillomavirus and recurring genital warts. *N. Eng. J. Med.* 313:784-788, 1985.
11. Ferenczy, A. Laser treatment of patients with condylomata and squamous carcinoma precursors of the lower female genital tract. *Ca-A Cancer J. for Clinic.* 37:334-347, 1987.
12. Ferenczy, A. Laser treatment of genital human papillomavirus infections in the male patient. In *Lasers in Gynecology.* J. Dorsey, ed. *Obstet. Gynecol. Clin. North Amer.* 18:525-535, 1991.
13. Shatz, P., Bergeron, C., Wilkinson, E.J., *et al.* Vulvar intraepithelial neoplasia and skin appendage involvement. *Obstet. Gynecol.* 74:769-774, 1989.
14. Reid, F., Elfont, E.A., Zirkin, R.M. and Fuller, T.A. Superficial laser vulvectomy: II. The anatomic and biophysical principles permitting accurate control over the depth of dermal destruction with carbon dioxide laser. *Amer. J. Obstet. Gynecol.* 152:261-271, 1985.
15. Ferenczy, A., Arseneau, J. and Franco, E. Pain-relieving effectiveness of silver sulfadiazine with 5% benzocaine (Silcaine™) and without benzocaine (Silvadene) after CO_2 laser vaporization and low-voltage diathermy for anogenital condylomata; a double-blind, prospective study on 40 patients. In preparation.

CHAPTER 11

ELECTROSURGERY OF THE VAGINA AND EXTERNAL ANOGENITAL TRACT: A STEP-BY-STEP GUIDE

ELECTROSURGERY OF VAGINAL LESIONS

Treatment Procedure

Patients are always treated under colposcopic guidance at 4 to 7.5x magnification.

Step 1 Place patient in the lithotomy position and attach a return electrode pad to the thigh.

Step 2 Insert insulated speculum and connect suction smoke evacuator tube to the suction system.

Step 3 Apply strong aqueous iodine solution to identify the margins of the lesional tissues.

Step 4 Elevate lesional tissues to a height of 0.5 to 1.0 cm above the adjacent normal epithelium by infiltrating the subepithelial connective tissue stroma with the anesthetic solution. Best results are obtained when the point of the needle is placed just beneath the epithelium (Figure 11.1). If the patient is treated in the office, inject 2% xylocaine with 1:100,000 epinephrine to anesthetize all treatment fields. For the upper 1/3 of the vagina an extended needle or a specially designed "cervical syringe" (Figure 4.17) may be required. If electrosurgery is performed under general or epidural/spinal anesthesia instead of local anesthesia, the lesional tissue can be elevated by injecting saline into the subepithelial connective tissue. Wait three minutes to obtain the desired anesthesia effect.

Step 5 Select appropriate electrode for the electrosurgery. Large exophytic lesions, or flat intraepithelial neoplasms of the vagina in which histologic diagnosis is desired are best excised using shallow rectangular electrodes such as those measuring 1.0 cm wide by 0.4 cm deep. Angling the electrode approximately 10 degrees off center makes the electrode easier to use in the vagina.

ELECTROSURGERY FOR HPV-RELATED DISEASES

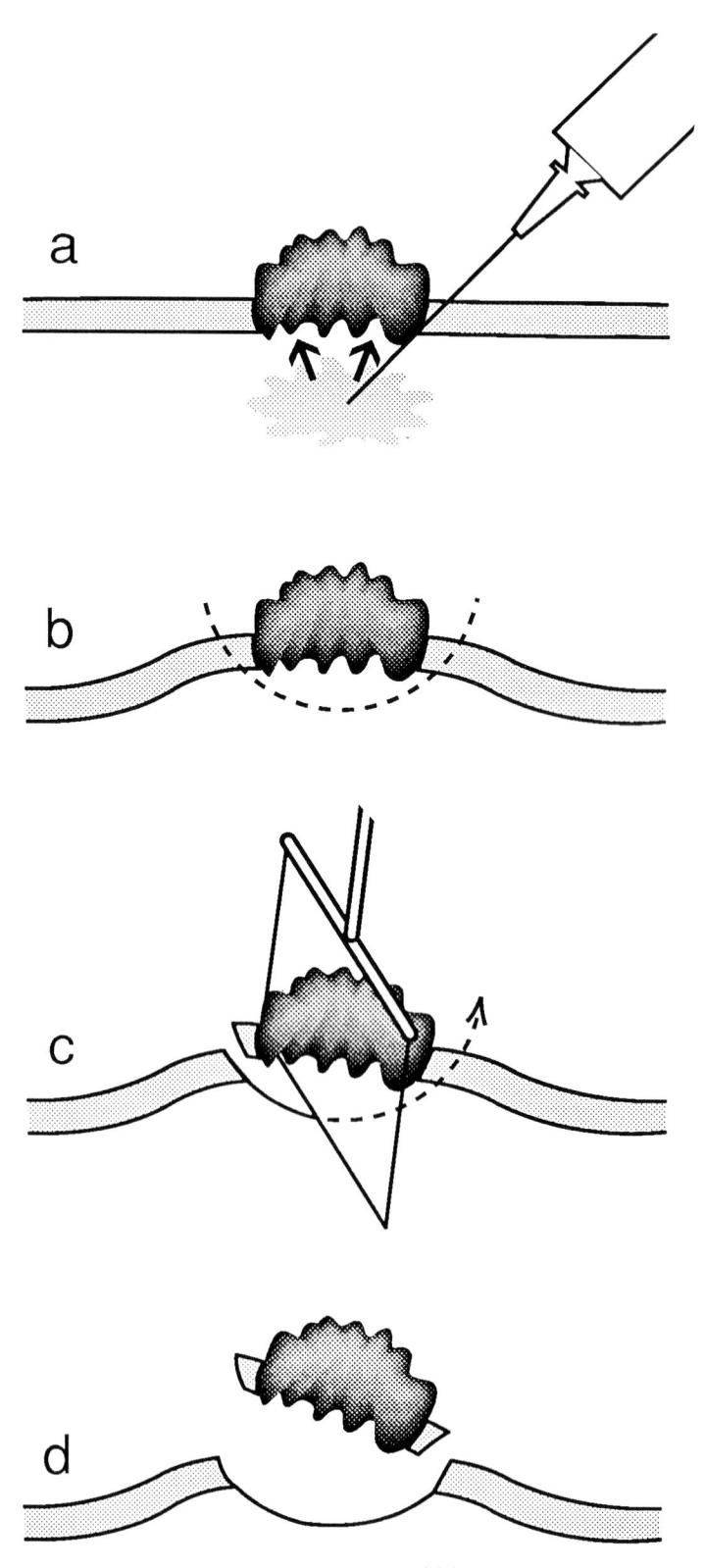

Figure 11.1. Schematic illustration of local anesthesia and depth of excision. A) The subepithelial connective tissue is infiltrated with local anesthetic solution by placing the needle just beneath the lesional tissue. B) The lesion is elevated from the underlying supportive connective tissue. C) The lesion is excised through the infiltrated subepithelial connective tissue. D) The crater's depth is at the level of the adjacent normal epithelium-connective tissue junction.

ELECTROSURGERY OF THE VAGINA AND EXTERNAL ANOGENITAL TRACT

Step 6 Select the appropriate power settings. Always make certain that the ESU is maintained in "Standby Mode" until the actual procedure is begun. The power settings that will be used for a particular application will depend on the size and design of the electrode, whether fulguration or cutting is desired, as well as the electrosurgical generator which is used. Table 11.1 lists the appropriate settings for one of the generators.

Step 7 Turn vacuum suction "on".

Step 8 Activate ESU and begin electrosurgery.

Hints for Electrosurgical Excision with Loop or Needle Electrodes

When excising lesional tissue, it is important to have a stable hand; this can be secured by placing the shaft of the loop electrode on the posterior blade of the speculum (Figure 11.2). This position will give excellent support to the operator's hand and help control the depth of excision. Do not open the speculum too widely because an over-stretched vagina enhances deep tissue penetration. The speculum should be opened only until the vaginal folds are "flattened out".

Table 11.1

Power Settings for Electrodes Used for Vaginal and External Genital Lesions*

Electrodes	Power Setting
Loop Style 1.0 x 04 cm.	Blend 26 watts
Ball Style 3 mm.	Coagulation 30 watts
5 mm.	50 watts
Macroneedle	Coagulation 30 watts
Microneedle	Blend 16 watts

* recommended values for the CooperSurgical LEEP™ System 6000.

The lesion should be excised with a continuous motion without stopping, if at all possible. Stopping the excision or stalling the electrode may produce excessive thermal damage and prevent accurate interpretation by the pathologist. After lesions are excised they are placed onto lens paper and put in the fixative solution.

Hints for Fulguration

The best approach to VAIN lesions located in the vaginal vault is to sample the lesions histologically using a small biopsy punch and then to fulgurate the lesion with the ball electrode. Prior to fulguration, moisten the area to be treated with saline-soaked vaginal swabs to enhance the transfer of electric sparks to the tissue.

For fulguration, the ball or macroneedle electrode is placed very close to, but not in actual contact with, the lesional tissue. The foot switch is activated and electric sparks are generated (Figure 11.3). The electrode is then swept across the area relatively rapidly, always keeping the electrode close to, but not in contact with, the lesional epithelium.

For lesions in the vaginal vault, particularly in post-hysterectomy patients, the tunnels ("dog ears") at 3 and 9 o'clock and in the upper 1/3 of the vagina, may be exposed for electrosurgery by applying traction with a skin hook (Figure 11.3).

Once fulguration has been completed, the hard eschar is wiped off with saline-soaked, cotton-tipped applicators or large vaginal swabs.

The colposcopic appearance of the denuded areas should be whitish-yellowish. This corresponds to the subepithelial connective tissue stroma at a depth of 0.5 mm to 1 mm from the adjacent normal epithelium.

Step 9 At the completion of therapy the denuded areas are treated with 4 gms of intravaginal Sultrin cream and the patient is discharged with an external pad and an instruction sheet.

Problems That Can Develop Postoperatively

Postoperative Bleeding

The bleeding area(s) is/are identified, cleaned with acetic acid, and anesthetized with 2% xylocaine with epinephrine (1:1,000,000). Hemostasis is achieved by fulgurating the area using either the 5 mm ball or the 1 mm macroneedle electrode and "coag" power outputs.

ELECTROSURGERY OF THE VAGINA AND EXTERNAL ANOGENITAL TRACT

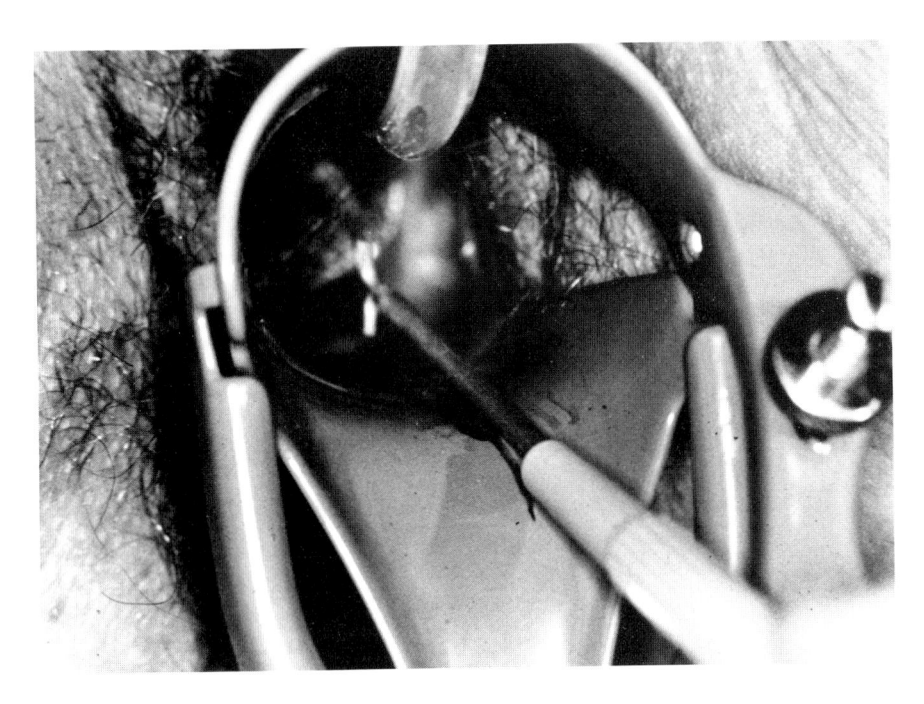

Figure 11.2. Loop excision of vaginal lesions. To help support the hand and obtain a uniform motion when excising vaginal lesions, the shaft of the loop electrode is rested on the posterior blade of the insulated speculum.

Postoperative Infection

Clean the vagina with 5% acetic acid. Prescribe a single 2 gm dose of Metronidazole and have the patient begin vaginal douches with a peroxide solution (1 tbsp. in 3 cups of warm water), once a day for 7 days. If discharge is associated with abdominal pain and fever, prescribe antibiotics.

ELECTROSURGERY OF EXTERNAL ANOGENITAL LESIONS

Treatment Procedure

Step 1   Clean areas to be treated with 5% acetic acid solution. Never use alcohol solution to prepare a patient for electrosurgery as it is flammable and may ignite when surgery is begun.

Step 2.   Place saline-soaked 2" x 2" gauze sponge into anal canal to prevent igniting rectal methane gases.

ELECTROSURGERY FOR HPV-RELATED DISEASES

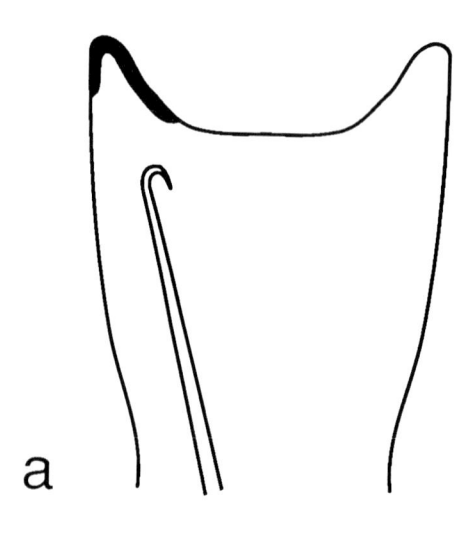

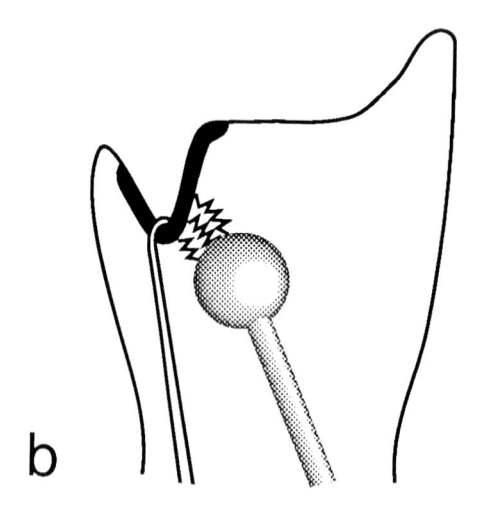

Figure 11.3. Schematic illustration of fulguration of vaginal vault lesion. A) The lesional tissue (in black) in the tunnels ("dog ears") is exposed by pulling out the apex of the tunnel with an insulated Iris (skin) hook. B) The everted tunnel lesion is then fulgurated using long sparks. These are obtained when the ball electrode is close to, but not in contact with, the lesional tissue.

ELECTROSURGERY OF THE VAGINA AND EXTERNAL ANOGENITAL TRACT

Postoperative Instructions

Table 11.2

Postoperative Instructions after Electrosurgery of Vaginal Lesions

You may develop vaginal spotting for up to 6 days. This is normal. **If spotting persists longer than 6 days or profuse bleeding develops, please call the office.**

You may also develop a brown-black vaginal discharge which may last for a few days to 2 weeks. This is normal. **If discharge becomes malodorous and/or is associated with pelvic pain, please call the office.**

Apply 4 gms of Sultrin cream with an applicator 3 times a week for 2 weeks.*

Refrain from intercourse for 4 weeks.

Avoid vigorous exercise and lifting heavy weights over the head for 2 weeks.

Please return to the office in 3 months.

only for patients with extensive treatment (the doctor will tell you if this applies to you)

Step 3 Apply strong aqueous iodine solution to identify the margins of the lesional tissues.

Step 4 Elevate lesional tissues to a height of 0.5 to 1.0 cm above the adjacent normal epithelium by infiltrating the subepithelial connective tissue stroma with the anesthetic solution. This is rapidly achieved with a 27 gauge dental needle which is introduced just underneath the lesional tissue. The solution is delivered to the papillary dermis (Figure 11.1A). If the patient is treated in the office, inject 2% xylocaine with 1:100,000 epinephrine to anesthetize all treatment fields. If electrosurgery is performed under general or epidural/spinal anesthesia instead of local anesthesia, the lesional tissue can be elevated by injecting saline into the subepithelial connective tissue. Wait three minutes to obtain the desired anesthesia effect.

ELECTROSURGERY FOR HPV-RELATED DISEASES

Step 5   Select appropriate electrode for electrosurgery. Large, exophytic, acuminate condylomata and extensive intraepithelial neoplasia of the external anogenital area are "debulked" by excision using a 1.0 cm x 0.4 cm condyloma loop or the microneedle electrode. Short-shafted electrodes are best for external lesions. Flat lesions or bleeding excision sites are fulgurated with the short-shafted 5 mm ball and/or the macroneedle electrode.

Step 6   Select the appropriate power settings. Always make certain that the ESU is maintained in "Standby Mode" until the actual procedure is begun. The power settings that will be used for a particular application will depend on the size and design of the electrode, whether fulguration or cutting is desired, as well as the electrosurgical generator which is used. Table 11.1 lists the appropriate settings for one of the generators.

Step 7   Turn vacuum suction "on".

Step 8   Activate ESU and begin electrosurgery.

Hints for Electrosurgical Excision

In addition to using loop electrodes, electrosurgical excision may also be performed using the microneedle tungsten electrode. Acuminate condylomata are grasped with an insulated ring forceps and VIN may be grasped with surgical forceps (Figure 11.4). The warts are then dissected along the first surgical plane (non-hairy skin) or along the second surgical plane (hairy skin) of the external anogenital skin.

Hints for Fulguration

For fulguration, the lesional tissue is first moistened with saline or 5% acetic acid solution and the ball electrode or macroneedle electrode is placed close to, but not on, the area to be fulgurated. The area is then lightly fulgurated. It is important to make certain that the electrode is not placed in direct contact with the skin because this will result in desiccation rather than fulguration and cause too much tissue damage.

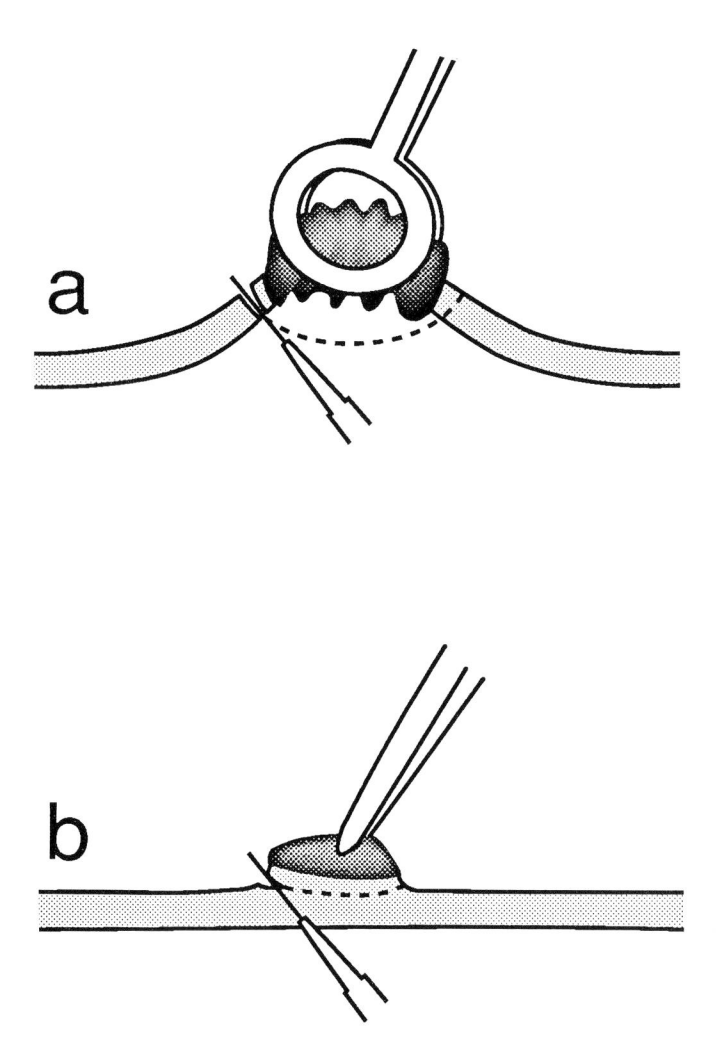

Figure 11.4. Schematic illustration of electrosurgical excision of A) condyloma and B) VIN with the microneedle electrode; mechanical traction is applied to the lesion for faster and better control of the excision.

To determine the depth of destruction and to obtain good healing it is important that all the eschar be wiped off the fulgurated area using a cotton-tipped applicator dipped in saline. Because the eschar produced by fulguration is hard and solidly attached to the underlying tissue, it is necessary to hold the cotton-tipped applicator close to the cotton tip; otherwise the wooden handle may break. A rough-surfaced cleaning pad for removing the eschar from large treatment fields can also be used.

Once the fulgurated areas are free of eschar, inspect them with the colposcope and, if residual disease is noted, repeat fulguration by rapidly sweeping the electrode over the incompletely denuded treatment fields. Wipe the areas and inspect them again for possible residual disease. The appropriately treated and cleaned areas should have a whitish to yellowish hue, chamois-like appearance corresponding to the papillary dermis (first surgical plane) and to the reticular dermis (second surgical plane), respectively (Figure 11.5). For VIN lesions on the hairy skin ablate to the second surgical plane.

After fulguration of the lesional tissue, 5 mm of adjacent normal-appearing skin may be treated by lightly "brushing" it with either the ball or macroneedle electrode. This is achieved by rapidly sweeping the electrode over the epithelium.

Step 9 At completion of electrosurgery, the treatment fields are covered with a thick layer of 1% silver sulphadiazine and 5% benzocaine (can be mixed by the patient or purchased as Silcaine™) or, if not available, silver sulphadiazine alone. The layer of cream is retained by 4" x 4" dressing gauzes.

Postoperative Instructions

Complete postoperative instructions are given to the patients (Tables 11.3, 11.4).

Problems That Can Develop Postoperatively

Postoperative Discomfort

If prescribed medications are insufficient to relieve/control pain (rather uncommon), a mixture of 1% silver sulphadiazine cream with 5% benzocaine, or Silcaine™, may be applied every 1 to 2 hours a day for 5 to 7 days. If an infection develops, the patient should be treated with appropriate antibiotics.

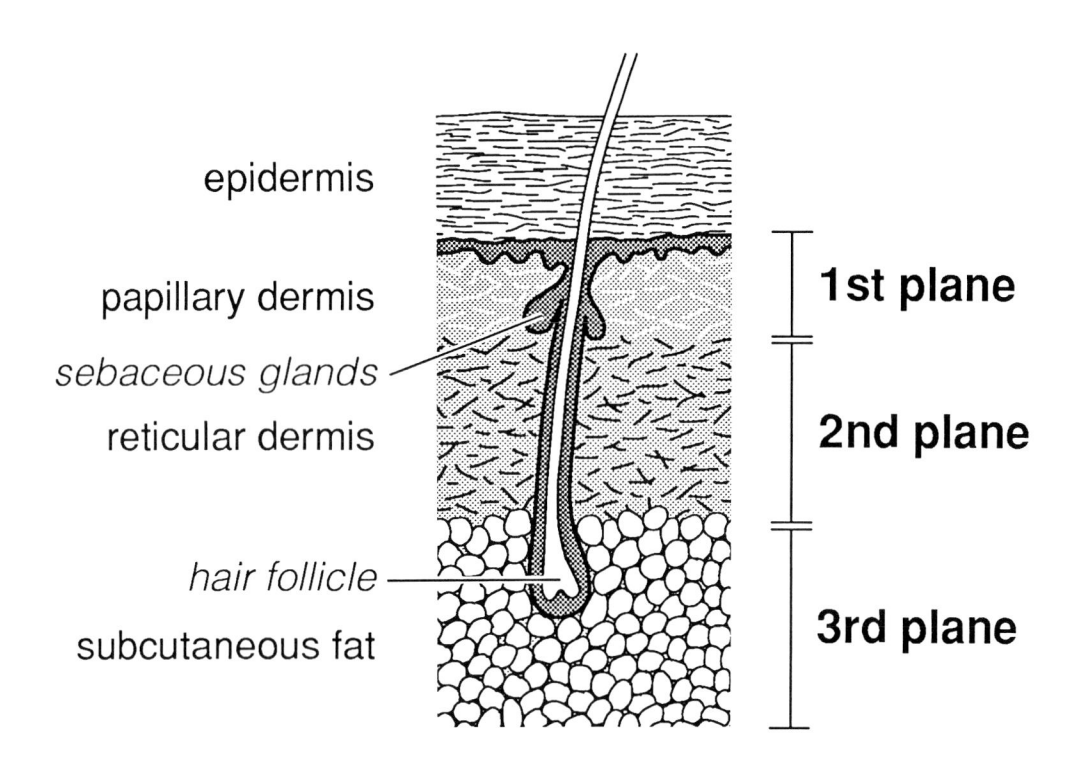

Figure 11.5. Schematic illustration of tissue planes. The first surgical tissue plane extends from the basal layer of the epithelium to the papillary-reticular dermis junction. The second plane consists of the reticular dermis, and the third surgical plane includes the subcutis. Note the presence of hair follicles at that level; fulguration of the third tissue plane often leads to scarring and alopecia of the hairy genital skin.

Recurrent Disease

If there are only a few lesions, they can be excised with a biopsy punch using local anesthetic with 2% xylocaine. Monsel's paste or gel can be applied to the excision sites to control minimal bleeding. Once hemostasis has been obtained the excess Monsel's is wiped away. The wounds are then covered with silver sulphadiazine cream or Silcaine™ and dressing gauzes.

If recurrent lesions are relatively extensive, electrosurgery is repeated as described above.

Table 11.3

Postoperative Instructions for Patients Treated Electrosurgically for Vulvar Lesions

Within 4-12 hours after surgery, you may experience mild to moderate discomfort that can be controlled by a prescription pain reliever (will have been prescribed by your physician if expected to be needed). If a transient increase in pain occurs, this can be relieved by applying an ice pack to the area. **If severe or throbbing pain persists, please call the office.**

Soak your vulva by sitting in a bath of sea water for 20 minutes twice a day until healing is completed (about 2-3 weeks). (Make sea water by adding 1/4 cup of natural sea salt or "Instant Ocean Salt" to 1/4 gallon of warm water. These can be bought at a health food or tropical fish store.)

At each bath, separate the inner and outer vulvar lips from each other, using either a Q-tip or your clean finger. This is done by putting either the Q-tip or your finger at the entrance to the vagina, and then moving it upwards until it touches the clitoris. (This is necessary to prevent the vulvar lips from "gluing" together during healing.)

After your bath, gently dry the area with a clean towel or hair dryer set on low heat and then apply a thick layer of 1% silver sulphadiazine or Silcaine™ cream to the wounds and between the lips. (This will reduce the pain and help prevent the vulvar lips from sticking together.)

Table 11.4

Postoperative Instructions for Patients Treated Electrosurgically for Penile Lesions

Irrigate treated areas with warm sea water twice daily until healing is completed (about 2-3 weeks). (Make sea water by adding 1/4 cup of natural sea salt or "Instant Ocean Salt" to 1/4 gallon of warm water. These can be bought at a health food or tropical fish store.)

After irrigating the treated areas, gently dry them with a clean towel or hair dryer set on low heat and then apply a thick layer of 1% silver sulphadiazine or Silcaine™ cream (this will help to reduce the pain).

Apply a gauze dressing over the treated areas to prevent rubbing against underwear.

Return to the office 6 weeks from today **or earlier should the area become red, hot, swollen or painful. If new warts develop, return at once.**

ELECTROSURGERY FOR INTRA-ANAL LESIONS

Treatment Procedure

A Fleet enema is always prescribed 12 hours prior to electrosurgery. It is best to carry out electrosurgery under colposcopic guidance.

Step 1   Treatment is performed under general/epidural or spinal anesthesia.

Step 2   Insert an insulated anal speculum equipped with a fume evacuation tube and connect the tube to the smoke evacuation system.

Step 3   Insert 2" x 2" saline-soaked sponges into the rectum 5 cm above the treatment fields to prevent igniting methane gases.

Step 4   Select the appropriate electrode. Fulguration is preferred over excision since the latter may produce bleeding which obscures the treatment field. A 5 mm ball electrode or a macroneedle electrode is preferred for intra-anal fulguration. If histologic diagnosis is

ELECTROSURGERY FOR HPV-RELATED DISEASES

desired, specimens may be obtained with a punch biopsy before fulguration is begun.

Step 5 Select the appropriate power settings. Fifty watts in the coagulation mode is used with the 5 mm ball electrode and 30 watts in the coagulation mode with the macroneedle electrode.

Step 6 Turn vacuum suction "on".

Step 7 Begin fulguration.

Step 8 Remove sponge from rectum.

Step 9 Apply 1% silver sulphadiazine or Silcaine™ cream in the intra-anal and perianal treatment fields and place a dressing gauze on the perineum to retain the cream.

Step 10 Discharge patient with instruction sheet.

Hints for Fulguration of Intra-anal Lesions

Open the anal speculum blades just until the epithelial folds are "stretched out". The speculum should be held throughout the procedure and the anus should not be overdilated. Overdilation can lead to rupture of the epithelium, deep penetration into the supporting connective tissue, and profuse bleeding.

Start from the perianal skin and proceed gradually into the anal canal. If bleeding develops, apply pressure on the bleeding site with a rectal swab and coagulate it with the macroneedle electrode.

Large, pedunculated, bleeding-prone, acuminate warts are best treated by grasping them with a ring forceps and excising them. Use the macroneedle electrode at 30 watts of coagulation power output. By using this technique, bleeding is usually minimal.

Once fulguration/excision is completed, as much eschar as possible is wiped off with cotton-tipped applicators or a cleaning pad. Eschar-free treatment fields appear to heal faster and with less discomfort.

Postoperative Instructions After Electrosurgery for Intra-Anal Lesions

Complete printed postoperative instructions are given to the patient (Table 11.5).

Problems That Can Develop Postoperatively

Postoperative Infection

If a postoperative infection develops prescribe appropriate antibiotics for 14 days. If an abscess occurs, drain it.

Recurrent Disease

If a few lesions develop, excise them under local anesthesia with a biopsy punch. If multiple lesions recur, repeat electrosurgery as described above.

Table 11.5

Postoperative Instructions for Patients Treated Electrosurgically for Intra-anal Lesions

Rectal bleeding, particularly after bowel movements, may occur for several days to 3 weeks. This is normal. **If bleeding persists for longer than 3 weeks or is excessive, return to office.**

Return to office should the treated areas become red, swollen and painful. If new warts develop, return to office at once.

Take Sitz baths in sea water twice a day, each for 10 to 15 minutes until healing is completed (about 2-3 weeks). If discomfort is not relieved, take Sitz baths in tea. (Make sea water by adding 1/4 cup of natural sea salt or "Instant Ocean Salt" to 1/4 gallon of warm water. These can be bought at a health food or tropical fish store. Make tea with 4 tea bags for 1/2 gallon of water.)

After Sitz baths, gently dry the treated areas with a clean towel or hair dryer set on low heat and then apply a thick layer of silver sulphadiazine or Silcaine™ cream (this will help to reduce the pain).

Apply a gauze dressing over the treated areas to prevent rubbing against underwear.

Take 2 capsules of Colace™ (10 mg each) and a glass of Metamucil™ at bedtime for 10 days.

If excessive discomfort develops, place an ice bag on anus and apply 1% silver sulphadiazine with 5% benzocaine or Silcaine™ every 1 to 2 hours a day for 5 to 7 days.

Return to the office in 6 weeks.

CHAPTER 12

THE PATHOLOGY OF SPECIMENS PRODUCED USING LOOP ELECTRODES

A common concern for clinicians who are contemplating electrosurgical loop excision procedures is that the loop electrode will produce so much thermal damage in the excised specimen that it will be uninterpretable histologically. In our experience, the amount of thermal damage in the specimen is directly related to the type of procedure which is performed, the adequacy of the equipment used to perform it, the power which is applied, and the degree to which sound electrosurgical principles are followed. Provided the proper equipment and technique are used, the excised specimen should be of sufficient quality to allow the pathologist to rule in or rule out invasive cancer. The histologic interpretation of adequately excised lesional tissues, including intraepithelial neoplasia, is not a problem.

THERMAL INJURY IN TISSUES EXCISED ELECTROSURGICALLY

A number of studies have documented the effects of the CO_2 laser on cervical tissues and have chronicled the reparative process after laser surgery. The type of thermal injury that is produced when using electrosurgery is similar to that produced using the CO_2 laser.[1,2] When a CO_2 laser is used to produce a "crater" in the cervix, the crater is covered by a thin layer of ash. Beneath the carbon ash there is a zone of necrotic tissue that can measure up to 500 microns (1/2 mm) in depth.[3] Histologically, in both electrosurgically-excised and CO_2 laser-excised tissues there are two different zones of injury.[2] The most peripheral zone is the most severely distorted histologically and is characterized by a narrow band of charring and carbonization with cells which are vacuolated and highly distorted. This zone is thought to arise secondary to the direct absorption of either the infrared energy of the laser or the electrical energy of electric sparks and occurs as cells in this zone are partially vaporized.[3] This most peripheral zone of injury seldom measures more than 100 microns in thickness and, in the vast majority of specimens, it is less than 50 microns in greatest thickness (Figure 12.1A). Zones of injury this narrow do not destroy a sufficient amount of tissue to create a diagnostic problem for the pathologist. The second zone of thermal injury is internal to the peripheral zone and is almost always substantially thicker than the more peripheral zone. It is identifiable in tissue sections principally by changes in its staining characteristics, i.e., increased eosinophilia, and by the smudging of the cell outlines and nuclei. This zone is produced as heat dissipates into the tissue and is secondary to propagated heat coagulating the cellular and extracellular proteins rather than direct absorption of infrared or electrical energy. This eosinophilic zone of secondary injury is highly variable and can range from 100 microns to more than 800 microns in thickness.

Although only a few studies have characterized how different electrosurgical variables affect these two zones of injury, several studies have investigated the influence of various parameters on these two zones when the injury is produced by the CO_2 laser. The peripheral zone of injury and carbonization produced by the CO_2 laser is relatively invariable in thickness.[3] Changing neither the power density nor the speed at which the laser is moved has an effect on the thickness of this zone. In contrast, the second zone of tissue coagulation is much more variable and increases in thickness as the time that the tissue is lasered increases but is not affected by increases in the power density.[3]

The healing of the cervical epithelium after laser ablation has also been analyzed.[4] At 5 to 8 days after laser ablation, the lasered area is covered by a dense slough of necrotic tissue. Under this slough there is histological evidence of tissue necrosis to a depth of up to 600 microns. Adjacent to the necrotic area there is a dense, acute, inflammatory infiltrate. By 8 days, a thin layer of squamous epithelium begins to migrate over the edges of the necrotic areas. This layer of epithelium is only a few cells in thickness and the cells composing it are flattened. They are best observed histologically and are often inapparent colposcopically. By 12 days, the epithelial ingrowth has extended further over the necrotic area and, colposcopically, a thin rim of translucent white epithelium can be seen at the edges of the lasered area. Fifteen days after laser therapy, patches of epithelium begin to appear in the center of the lasered area that are not contiguous with the sheets of epithelium advancing from the edges of the defect. These central patches appear to migrate out from columnar epithelium that lines the bases of residual crypts that were not destroyed during laser therapy. Over the next 2 weeks, a progressive re-epithelialization of the defect develops and, by 4 weeks, the entire defect is almost always covered by squamous epithelium.

DIRECT COMPARISON OF THERMAL EFFECTS PRODUCED USING ELECTROSURGERY AND CO_2 LASER

Several studies have compared the extent of thermal injury induced in various tissues with the CO_2 laser and electrosurgically. In one study published by Montgomery et al.[1], CO_2 laser and electrosurgery were compared for making incisions in dog's skin. The laser incision took longer to make than the electrosurgical incision but the extent of blood loss was similar with the two procedures. Histologically, the areas of excision using either the laser or electrosurgery had a similar extent of thermal injury 2 weeks after the operation. Recently, we completed two studies that have directly compared the extent of thermal damage in specimens excised using electrosurgery with that in tissue excised using the CO_2 laser.[2,5]

In the first study we analyzed 40 cervical loop excision specimens and 11 laser excisional cervical conization specimens (Table 12.1).[2] In this study the extent of thermal damage was directly measured on multiple histological sections of the excised tissue using a micrometer. In both types of specimens

Table 12.1

Thermal Damage in Cervical Specimens Removed With CO_2 Laser and Loop Electrosurgical Procedure

Method	Extent of Thermal Damage (microns)		
	Mean	Minimum	Maximum
Laser (n = 11)	411	130	750
Electrosurgery (n = 40)	396	150	830

the total width of thermal injury was similar. The total zone of histologically observable thermal damage in specimens obtained using the electrosurgical loop measured from 150 to 830 microns in thickness, with a mean thickness of 396 microns. In specimens excised with the CO_2 laser this zone ranged from 130 to 750 microns in thickness and had a mean thickness of 411 microns. There was no significant difference between the extent of thermal injury produced electrosurgically and that produced with the CO_2 laser (Figure 12.1A and B).

Although the types and total thickness of thermal injury produced by the CO_2 laser are remarkably similar to that produced by electrosurgery, the CO_2 laser consistently was found to produce a higher degree of carbonization than did the electrosurgical procedure and consistently produced more distortion of the epithelium at the edge of the specimens than did the electrosurgical procedure (Figure 12.2A and B).

In our series of excised cervical specimens, we found that the area of thermal coagulation produced electrosurgically, although, obvious at the light

ELECTROSURGERY FOR HPV-RELATED LESIONS

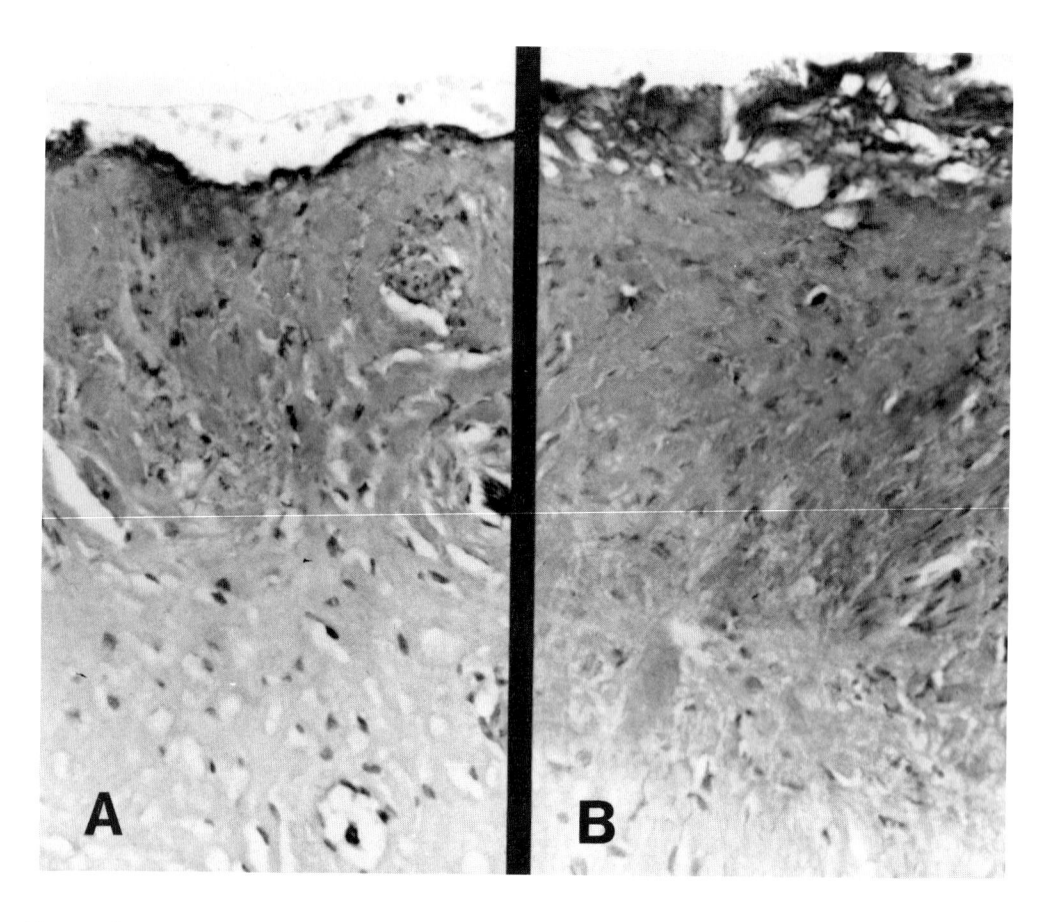

Figure 12.1. Extent of thermal injury in electrosurgically excised and CO_2 laser excised tissues. A) Electrosurgically excised cervical tissue. The most peripheral zone of injury measures approximately 50 microns in thickness and is characterized by extensive carbonization, vacuolation of cells and charring. The inner zone of thermal injury measures approximately 350 microns in thickness and is characterized by a change in the staining pattern. B) CO_2 laser excised cervical tissue.

microscopy level, did not produce sufficient tissue or cytological distortion to create diagnostic problems. This is because the pathologist can "read through" the thermally coagulated areas and can easily distinguish between normal epithelium and CIN and between CIN and invasion. In contrast, the extensive carbonization and distortion produced using the CO_2 laser made many of the laser-excised specimens more difficult to analyze. It may also have precluded the colposcopist's being able to evaluate the base of the excised area. This is generally easy to evaluate when the tissue has been excised electrosurgically. When considering this data, it is important to note that the CO_2 laser excisional

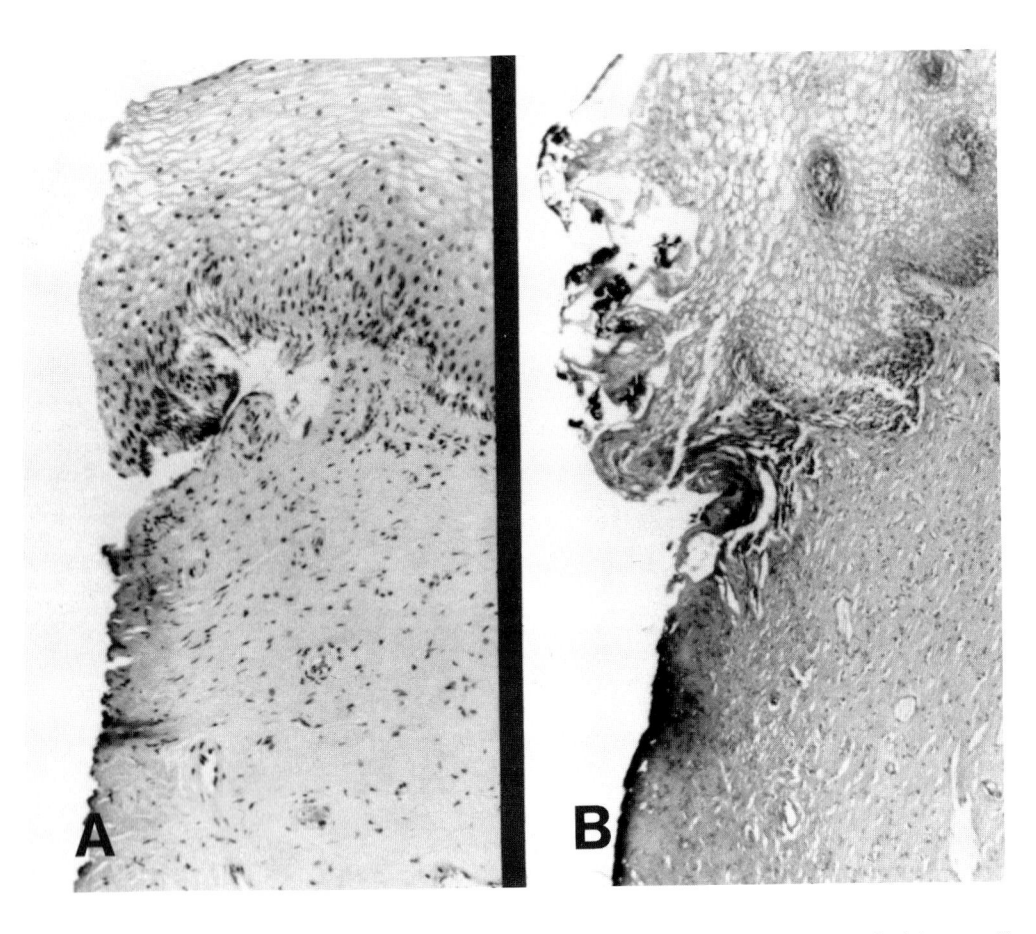

PATHOLOGY OF SPECIMENS PRODUCED USING LOOP ELECTRODES

Figure 12.2. Edges and margins of electrosurgically excised and CO_2 laser excised cervical tissues. A) Electrosurgically excised cervical tissue. The margin of the excised tissue has some charring and artifact but the pathologist can tell that invasive cancer is not present. B) CO_2 laser excised cervical tissue. The margin of the CO_2 laser excised tissue has much more damage, with epithelial denudation and vacuolization of cells.

conizations in this study were obtained by a clinician (Alex Ferenczy) who is highly skilled in this technique and who was performing more than 100 laser conizations each year. In our consultation practices, we have found that significantly more thermal damage is frequently present in laser excisional conization specimens excised by clinicians with less experience. It is these effects that have led some institutions to prohibit their clinicians from performing CO_2 laser excisional conizations (see Chapter 13).

ELECTROSURGERY FOR HPV-RELATED LESIONS

We have also completed a study comparing thermal damage produced using either CO_2 laser or electrosurgery at lower genital sites other than the cervix in 20 patients (Table 12.2).[5] The results obtained in this second series of 20 patients with vaginal and external anogenital condylomata were remarkably similar to those obtained in the cervical study. Electrosurgically excised lesional tissue contained thermocoagulation to a varying extent along the excision lines. The mean thickness of thermocoagulation was essentially identical for electrosurgical and laser excision, 0.35 and 0.31 mm respectively. The most significant thermal effects in these non-cervical specimens were fragmentation and coagulation of the lesional epithelium, particularly at the edges of the excision (Figure 12.3). Despite the extensive damage that was occasionally present in the excised tissues, diagnosing disease histopathologically was not a problem. When electrosurgical excision was performed through a xylocaine or saline infiltrated subepithelial connective tissue layer, the thermocoagulation zone often measured less than 50 microns in thickness (Figure 12.4).

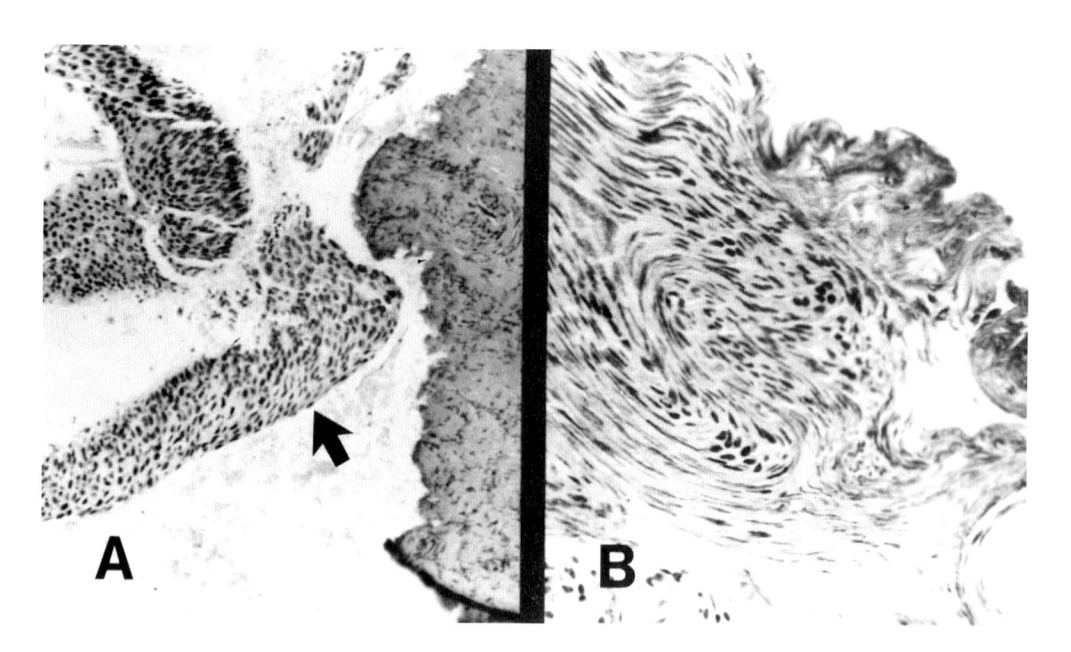

Figure 12.3. Tissue effects of electrosurgery at external genital sites. A) Neoplastic epithelium (arrow) at edge of excised specimen is fragmented and separated from papillary dermis. B) Epithelium with severe coagulation artifacts.

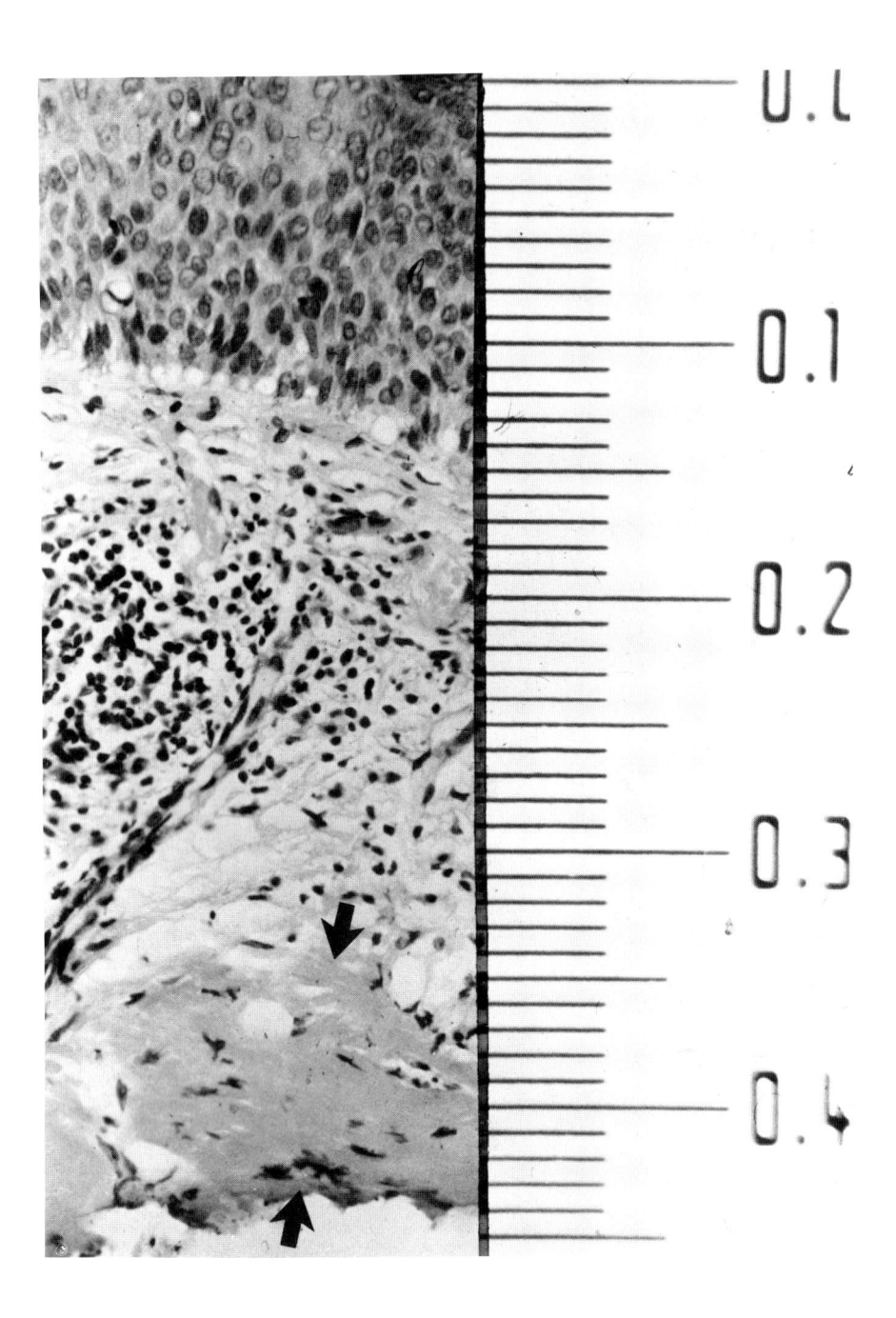

Figure 12.4. Tissue effect of electrosurgical excision of external anogenital sites. A steady, relatively slow motion with the loop electrode, appropriately set cutting current and subepithelial infiltration of anesthetic solution are associated with thermal injury limited to a 100 micron zone (arrows).

Table 12.2

Extent of Thermal Defect in Specimens Excised by Electrosurgery and CO_2 Laser

Method	Extent of Thermal Damage (microns)		
	Mean	Minimum	Maximum
Electrosurgical Excision	335	90	757
Laser excision	310	100	638
Fulguration	650	250	1120
Laser vaporization	628	215	1355

FACTORS THAT CAN INFLUENCE THERMAL DAMAGE TO SPECIMENS

It is critical to think out what is to be done before doing it when using electrosurgical equipment. When an excision procedure is to be performed, it is important to be certain that the electrosurgical unit's power setting is on cut or blend. A common error is to set the controls on coagulation rather than blend, or to forget to change the setting from coagulation to blend. This error should be obvious when the clinician begins to cut and finds that the procedure is not going well. However, particularly when the surgeon is not experienced with this technique, the tendency is to continue the procedure and assume there is something wrong with the tissue, rather than there is something wrong with the equipment settings. The surgeon should learn very quickly what is to be expected in different organs using the standard array of loop, needle, and ball electrodes and should immediately stop the procedure if it is not proceeding in the expected fashion. When the expected events are not occurring, the operator should reevaluate the settings, the equipment, and all the points at which an error could occur before starting the procedure again. It is also important to match the power setting with the electrosurgical tip which is being used. Each manufacturer should supply the operator with the recommended power settings for the standard loop, needle and ball electrodes that can be used with their electrosurgical unit. In general, the power settings which are recommended by the manufacturers should be used, but they may have to be varied to some degree depending on the skill of the operator, the speed with which the procedure is performed, the type of tissue and the particular electrode being used (Table 12.3). With experience, an evaluation of all these becomes second nature and there is seldom a problem matching the proper power setting to the site and conditions of the procedure being performed.

Table 12.3

> **Factors Affecting Correct Power Settings.**
>
> Skill of operator.
> Speed at which procedure is performed.
> Type of tissue being excised.
> Water content of tissue.
> Particular electrode being used.

If too much power (wattage) is used for a given loop size, or if the loop is pressed against the tissue to produce electrodesiccation, the thermal damage will be increased. Similarly, if the loop wire is too thick or if a loop that has previously been used and allowed to develop a carbonized layer is used without scouring off the carbonization, excessive thermal damage will occur (Table 12.4). All these points should be examined before the procedure is begun.

Table 12.4

> **Factors Increasing Thermal Damage**
>
> Too much power for a given loop size.
> Moving the loop too slowly.
> Stopping and starting the procedure.
> Pressing loop too firmly against the tissue.
> Too thick an electrode wire.
> Previously used, carbonized electrode.

It is important that the operator always keep in mind the difference between desiccation, fulguration and electrosurgical cutting. For most of the nonexcisional procedures which will be performed in the male and female lower anogenital tract epithelium, fulguration rather than desiccation should be used.

Much more extensive tissue damage is produced when the electrode is put in direct contact with the tissue and desiccation occurs, than when a spark is generated between the electrode and the tissue resulting in fulguration. The operator should be certain to use desiccation only when that is the indicated procedure.

The most commonly performed gynecological procedure using electrosurgical loops is removal of tissue from the cervix in a patient with an abnormal Pap smear and a CIN lesion which has been identified colposcopically. Although thermal damage will always be produced at the margins of the tissue in direct contact with the electrosurgical loop or needle, the area of greatest thermal damage will be at the point at which the loop is completely embedded in the cervix and there is full contact between the electrode and the cervical tissue. If the procedure is halted before the full sweep through the tissue is complete and then restarted with the electrode embedded in the tissue, substantially greater thermal damage will occur than if the tissue is excised with one continuous, flowing sweep. In the event that a loop excision must be stopped midway through a procedure (i.e., if a stall occurs), the operator should remove the loop, move to the other side of the lesion and start again, meeting the original line of excision.

PROCESSING OF EXCISED TISSUES

When preparing tissues for pathological examination the pathologist must orient the tissue in order to process it appropriately, make sections which are taken in the proper plane, and have the tissue embedded appropriately by the laboratory technician (Table 12.5). When tissues are placed in fixatives they

Table 12.5

Requirements for
Complete Pathological Examination

Correct orientation of specimens.
Sections taken perpendicularly to the surface.
Histopathologic analysis of the entire specimen.

PATHOLOGY OF SPECIMENS PRODUCED USING LOOP ELECTRODES

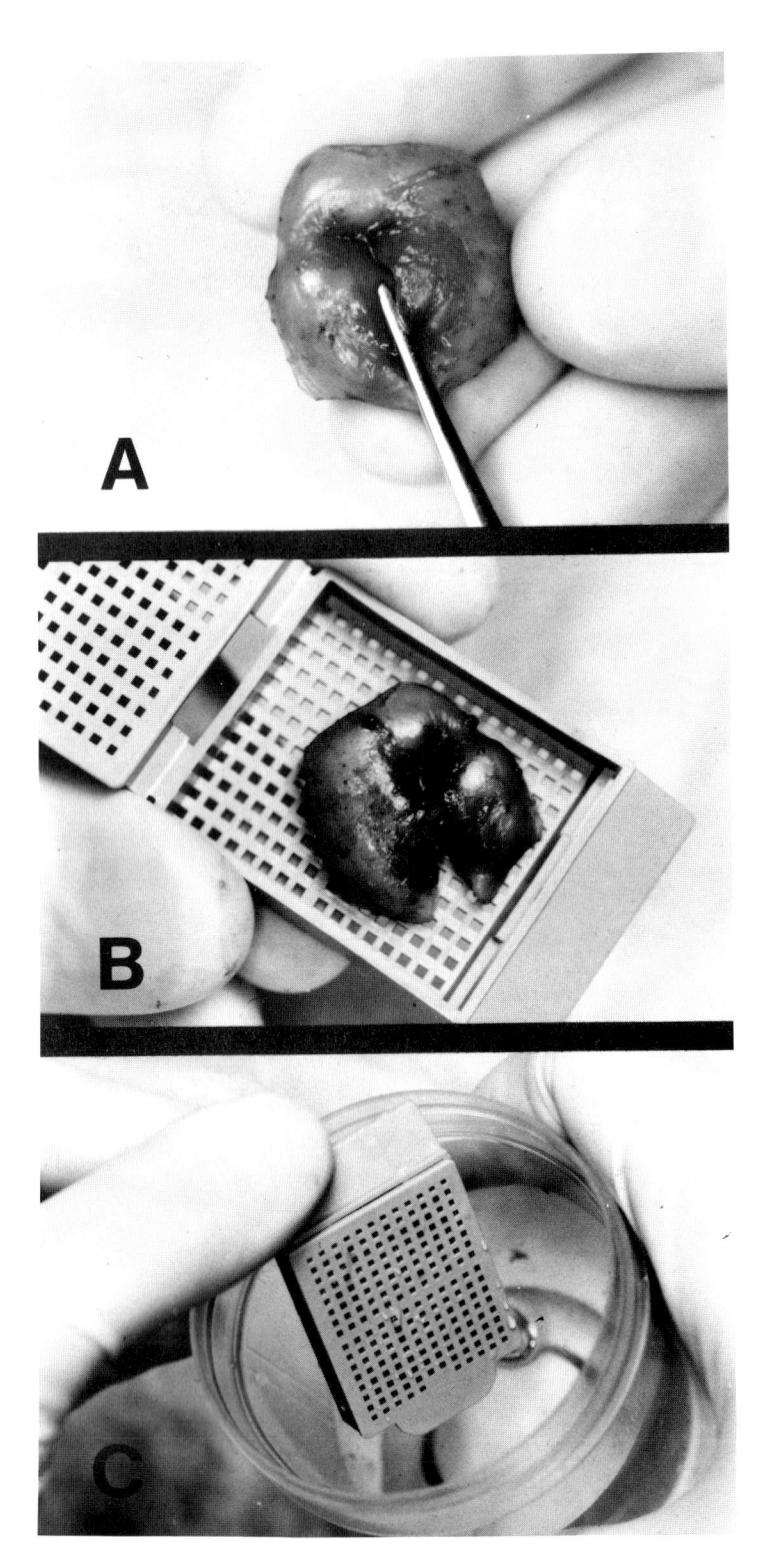

Figure 12.5. Procedure for processing cervical excisional specimens for pathology. A) Excised specimen is opened with a scissors. B) Specimen is placed in a plastic histopathology "cassette". C) The entire cassette is placed in a container of formalin.

contract and lose 15-20% of their volume. This is commonly accompanied by twisting and turning if the tissue is placed directly into a container of fixative. Such twisting makes it extremely difficult for the pathologist to orient the specimen correctly. For specimens excised with loop electrodes, one way to avoid twisting and turning of the tissue is for the operator to place the tissue in a plastic cassette of the type which is commonly used in pathology laboratories to process tissues for histology. These cassettes can readily be obtained from the pathology laboratory. To use them, the cervix should be opened with a pair of scissors after which the now linearized donut can be placed stroma-side down in the cassette, the top snapped in place, and the entire cassette dropped in the fixative (Figure 12.5). When multiple strips are made, one or more strips can be placed in cassettes in a similar fashion. An alternative to using cassettes is to pin the tissue out on a piece of cork or a piece of paraffin. This is slightly more cumbersome to perform and requires a larger container of fixative than is generally available in the physician's private office. This may be, however, the procedure of choice if the operation is performed in a surgicenter or other in-hospital type facility.

INFORMING THE PATHOLOGY LABORATORY THAT THEY WILL BE GETTING A NEW TYPE OF SPECIMEN AND LACK OF IMPORTANCE OF MARGINS

There is one final caveat with regard to thermal damage in excised tissues. As some pathologists have not had experience with electrosurgically-excised tissues, it is highly recommended that the surgeon discuss the procedures with his pathologist(s) before submitting the tissues and make the pathologist(s) aware that, although thermal coagulation will be seen, it should not create problems in diagnosis. One point that should be covered in this discussion is whether surgical margins need to be assessed in the specimens. In the idealized loop excision specimen, the entire CIN lesion or atypical transformation zone is excised in a single pass with the electrode. In such a specimen, the surgical margins are relatively easy to assess histopathologically.

However, in our opinion, there is no clinical benefit from knowing the status of the excisional margins. This has been well documented by multiple studies of patients who have had positive margins on cone biopsies.[6,7] In over 70% of these patients, no residual disease was detected in either subsequent hysterectomy specimens or in clinical follow-up (several months later). The reason why residual disease regresses in the majority of patients is unknown but may be related to reparative processes and the stimulation of an immune response. Regardless of the mechanism, the clinical importance is that no further treatment is needed in those patients with positive cone biopsy margins who have no residual disease at follow-up examination. Similar arguments can be made for loop excision specimens and no clinical action need be taken purely on the basis of a positive margin in squamous lesions.

An additional argument against assessing the clinical margins is that many loop excisional procedures require multiple passes of the electrode making it difficult for the pathologist to know what a "true" surgical margin is. In addition, in many cases, residual CIN is fulgurated and, therefore, a "true" margin is not submitted for histopathologic assessment.

REFERENCES

1. Montgomery, T.C., Sharp, J.B., Bellina, J.H. and Ross, L.F. Comparative gross and histological study of the effects of scalpel, electric knife, and carbon dioxide laser on skin and uterine incisions in dogs. *Lasers in Surgery and Medicine* 3:9-22, 1983.
2. Wright, T.C., Richart, R.M., A. Ferenczy, A. and Koulos, J. Comparison of specimens removed by CO_2 laser conization and loop electrosurgical excision procedures. *Obstet. & Gynecol.* 79:147-153, 1991.
3. Stafl, A., Wilkinson, E.J. and Mattingly, R.F. Laser treatment of cervical and vaginal neoplasia. *Am. J. Obstet. Gynecol.* 128:128-136, 1977.
4. MacLean, A.B. Healing of cervical epithelium after laser treatment of cervical intraepithelial neoplasia. *Br. J. Obstet. Gynecol.* 91:697-706, 1984.
5. Ferenczy, A., Behelak, Y., Haber, G., Wright, T.C. and Richart, R.M. Treating vaginal and external anogenital condylomata with loop electrosurgical excision/fulguration procedure (LEEP) vs. laser ablation. *Am. J. Obstet. Gynecol.,* submitted, 1992.
6. Andersen, E.S., Nielsen, K. and Larsen, G. Laser conization: Follow-up in patients with cervical intraepithelial neoplasia in the cone margin. *Gynecol. Oncol.* 39:328-331, 1990.
7. Schulman, H. and Cavanagh, D. Intraepithelial carcinoma of the cervix: The predictability of residual carcinoma of the uterus from microscopic study of the margins of the cone biopsy speciman. *Cancer* 14:796-800, 1961.

CHAPTER 13

CLINICAL IMPLICATIONS OF ELECTROSURGICAL EXCISION PROCEDURES

EARLY THERAPIES FOR CERVICAL CANCER PRECURSORS

Although it took many years for the medical community to recognize that cancer precursor lesions of the cervix existed, once that concept was accepted, investigators and clinicians searched for simple and effective methods for managing patients with these preinvasive cervical lesions. Initially, when little was known about the natural history of cervical cancer precursors, radical therapeutic modalities were the rule and patients were commonly treated by methods that differed only in degree from those that were being used to treat

Table 13.1

Early Therapeutic Modalities For Treating Cervical Cancer Precursors

Histologic Diagnosis	Therapeutic Modality
"Dysplasia"	Large cone biopsy
Carcinoma-*in situ*	Radiation therapy or hysterectomy

invasive cancer. Some patients with carcinoma-*in situ* of the cervix, for example, were treated with radiation therapy and others, even if young, were treated with hysterectomy. Women with "lesser degrees" of cervical intraepithelial abnormalities than carcinoma *in situ* which were often referred to as "dysplasias" were customarily treated with large, radical cervical conizations. This approach to treating cervical cancer precursors had a number of obvious drawbacks. The most important drawback was that the radical therapies being used were associated with significant morbidity and side effects. Most cervical cancer precursors are diagnosed in women of the reproductive ages, many of whom have not yet completed childbearing. The use of radiation therapy or hysterectomy to treat lesions that only have a potential for being malignant is certainly less than desirable in women wishing to maintain fertility if other, less

LOOP EXCISIONAL PROCEDURES

"radical", therapeutic modalities are available. Similarly, the conizations used to treat cervical "dysplasia" were less than an optimal therapeutic modality since large cone biopsies are frequently associated with significant morbidity. In a recent review by Luesley, *et al.* of the complications associated with 915 cone biopsies, it was reported that 14% of the procedures were associated with significant bleeding, 17% were associated with cervical stenosis, and 5% were associated with subsequent infertility or complications in the ensuing pregnancies (Table 13.2).[1] Similar complication rates have been reported in

Table 13.2

Complications of Cone Biopsies

Complication	%
Significant Bleeding	
Operative	6%
Postoperative	8%
Cervical stenosis	17%
Infertility	4%
Pregnancy complications	1%

other large series of cone biopsies.[2-4] In addition to their high rates of complications, cold knife cones have a number of other disadvantages. These include the fact that they require good surgical skills, limiting their use to trained surgeons, and that they require general anesthesia and are, therefore, usually performed in operating rooms or surgicenters, which adds significant expense to the procedure.

Despite the fact that these therapeutic modalities were less than optimal, many physicians continued to use them throughout the 1970s and early 1980s. "Extended hysterectomy" and, in some centers, pelvic lymph node dissection, only disappeared from the recommended treatment procedures for carcinoma-*in situ* 10 to 15 years ago.

Table 13.3

> **Disadvantages of Cold Knife Cones**
>
> High level of complications
> Moderate surgical skill required
> General anesthesia required
> Performed in operating room/surgicenter

CONSERVATIVE THERAPIES FOR MANAGING CERVICAL INTRAEPITHELIAL NEOPLASIA

During the 1960s and 1970s, the natural history of cervical cancer precursors was well characterized.[5-9] On the basis of these studies, it became widely recognized that cancer precursors, prior to the subsequent development of invasive cancer, did not have the potential for metastasizing. Moreover, during this same time period, other studies demonstrated that complete removal of precursor lesions (including carcinoma-*in situ*) by less "radical" methods could result in a "cure", provided the lesion was totally eradicated.[10-12] On the basis of these and other advances, the concept of cervical intraepithelial neoplasia (CIN) was introduced in the early 1970s to refer to all forms of precursors to squamous cell carcinoma of the cervix, and outpatient treatment protocols began to be commonly used for treating CIN lesions.[13-15] Triage

Table 13.4

> **Conservative Modalities for Treating CIN**
>
> Electrosurgical Fulguration
> Electrocautery ("Hot cautery")
> Cryotherapy
> CO_2 laser ablation
> CO_2 laser cone
> Wire loop excision

protocols for conservatively managing CIN that were based on colposcopic assessment were formulated in the 1970s. The protocols were commonly referred to as "conservative" treatment options since they were less "radical" than radiation therapy, hysterectomy, or cone biopsies. These triage rules required that the clinician have good colposcopy skills, that accurate biopsies be taken on all patients and that an endocervical curettage be performed, if the patient was not pregnant.[16] The original outpatient protocols for treating CIN

Table 13.5

Colposcopic Triage Requires

Good colposcopy skills
Accurate biopsies
Endocervical curettage (non-pregnant)

used electrosurgical fulguration that was applied to the lesional tissue using a large ball electrode and a spark gap-type electrosurgical generator.[17,18] Both fulguration and electrocautery ("hot cautery") produced cure rates of about 90% (Chapter 5). Despite the high success rate, they suffered from being difficult to control, producing substantial tissue damage, being associated with severe uterine contractions due to galvanic stimulation of the uterine corpus, and being irritating to the physician as well as the patient, because of the large amount of smoke produced. After the introduction of cryotherapy in the 1970s, spark gap electrosurgical fulguration was almost totally abandoned and cryotherapy became the treatment of choice for patients with CIN lesions in whom invasion had been ruled out.[19-21]

Cryotherapy was a remarkably safe procedure, which was easy to teach and learn, and served gynecology well for over 20 years. Its principal side effects included a profuse watery discharge in a high proportion of the treated patients that often lasted two to three weeks and was often malodorous, a rate of cervical stenosis and cervical narrowing that approached 5% in some series, and vasomotor reactions with flushing and discomfort in many patients.[21] Another significant drawback to cryotherapy was that it was not very effective for larger lesions that could not easily be covered with a single application of the cryoprobe.[22,23]

CLINICAL IMPLICATIONS OF ELECTROSURGICAL EXCISION PROCEDURES

Table 13.6

Problems with Cryotherapy

Profuse watery discharge
Slow to heal (4 months)
Ablative procedure
Cervical narrowing/stenosis
Flushing and discomfort common
Not effective for large lesions

However, cryotherapy had a number of advantages that led to its wide acceptance. These included the fact that it was easy to teach, learn and use, and was inexpensive and highly effective.[24,25]

Table 13.7

Advantages of Cryotherapy

Easy to teach and learn
Easy to use
Mature engineering
Inexpensive
Highly effective

In the late 1970s, CO_2 laser ablation was introduced as an alternative to cryotherapy and excisional methods for treating CIN and HPV-related lesions of the anogenital tract.[26,27] Initially, the indications for CO_2 laser ablation of CIN were identical to those for cryotherapy—it was used for cervical lesions in which colposcopy was satisfactory and in which cervical biopsies had ruled-out the presence of invasive cancer. However, as experience with the CO_2 laser for treating CIN increased, the technique of CO_2 laser excisional conization was introduced.[28-30] Laser excisional conizations are used in patients with unsatisfactory colposcopy in whom a further diagnostic test is required. CO_2 laser excisional conizations make the laser both a diagnostic and a therapeutic modality. After CO_2 laser began to be used for treating CIN lesions, laser ablation of HPV-related cancer precursors of the vagina, vulva, perineal, perianal, and penile epithelium was also introduced.[31] As with the cervix, CO_2 laser ablation of external lesions was generally preceded by multiple, colposcopically-directed, punch biopsies to rule out invasive cancer. Other

Table 13.8

CO_2 Laser for Treating HPV-Related Disease	
Laser ablation	Therapeutic modality for CIN, VIN, VAIN, PIN, PAIN
Laser excisional conization	Combined diagnostic and therapeutic modality in patients with CIN.

advantages of laser over cryosurgery included the fact that laser produced much less discharge than did cryosurgery and that healing was very rapid after laser ablations. Cervical healing is generally complete within one month.[32,33]

Table 13.9

Advantages of CO_2 Laser Ablation

Office/surgicenter procedure
Can be performed rapidly
Little discharge
Rapid healing

However, CO_2 laser ablation also had some disadvantages compared to cryotherapy. First, the equipment is very expensive and is difficult to maintain. Moreover, the technique is technically quite demanding and is difficult to teach and learn. Because of its technical difficulty, the surgeon also needs to perform a large number of cases to become skilled and needs to have a high case load to maintain expertise.

Table 13.10

Difficulties of CO_2 Laser Ablation

Equipment is expensive

Technique is demanding and difficult to learn and teach

Requires high case load to maintain expertise

The debate as to whether CO_2 laser therapy or cryotherapy was the preferred treatment modality for the treatment of CIN (prior to the development of loop excisional protocols), revolved around side effects, complications, efficacy and the cost of treatment.[25] It was generally agreed that CO_2 laser ablation provided a higher cure rate on the initial treatment of CIN than did cryotherapy but that, if those patients who were failures on the initial treatment were re-evaluated and re-treated, the results were virtually identical. The one group of CIN lesions for which CO_2 laser was consistently found to be superior to cryotherapy were large (3 quadrant or larger) lesions, especially those which extended onto the vagina.[23] These lesions do not respond well to cryotherapy, but are often adequately treated with a single CO_2 laser treatment.

Despite the fact that the end results using CO_2 laser and cryotherapy were the same and the cost of CO_2 laser ablation was substantially greater than cryotherapy, the two techniques both became widely used and were thought to be complimentary to one another. CO_2 laser ablation was commonly used for the larger lesions and cryotherapy for the smaller lesions. For the treatment of external HPV-related lesions, CO_2 laser therapy gradually became ascendent and, for the past decade, was viewed by most clinicians as the treatment of choice for VIN, VAIN, PIN, and PAIN lesions.

DEVELOPMENT OF INVASIVE CANCER AFTER CONSERVATIVE THERAPY

As experience with various forms of conservative management increased, it became well documented that squamous cell carcinomas of the cervix occasionally developed in patients with CIN who have been treated with either cryosurgery or laser ablation (Table 13.11). The first report of invasive cancer developing after cryosurgery was by Sevin, who reported on 8 patients who were seen in referral.[34] On the basis of this initial report, Townsend and Richart established a registry among members of the Society for Gynecological

Oncology (SGO) in which all members were requested to report cases of invasive cervical cancer developing after cryosurgery. Analysis of the SGO registry cases revealed a number of important facts.[35,36] One was that, in the majority of patients who developed invasive cancer, the triage rules for evaluation of an abnormal Pap smear had been violated. In many of these

Table 13.11

Development of Invasive Cancer After Conservative Therapy

Authors	# cases reported	# or source of patients
Sevin (1979)	8	Referrals
Townsend (1981)	110	Registry
Webb (1985)	11	Referrals
Pearson (1989)	9	3,738

patients an endocervical curettage had not been obtained, or a cervix, in which biopsy-proven CIN was not detected despite an abnormal Pap smear, was frozen. Since these cases were either referrals or registry cases, the incidence of invasive cancer after conservative therapy is not known. It is very difficult to arrive at precise figures for how often invasive cancers are missed during triage. Based on a variety of different lines of evidence, Ferenczy has estimated that approximately 0.1 - 0.2% of patients evaluated colposcopically for an abnormal smear will have an invasive lesion that is missed during triage even when the Pap smear is performed and read by qualified personnel, an endocervical curettage is well taken and read, and multiple cervical biopsies are taken (Table 13.12).[37]

One of the largest series trying to measure directly the incidence of missed invasive cancers is that of Pearson and co-workers.[38] They reported that nine patients out of 3,738, who were treated with laser ablation at a colposcopy clinic in an eight and a half year period between 1979 and 1988, subsequently developed microinvasive or invasive squamous cell carcinoma of the cervix.

Table 13.12

> ### Colposcopically Missed Cancers
>
> **Occurs in approximately 0.1-0.2% of patients with abnormal smears evaluated with:**
>
> Colposcopy
> High quality cytology
> Well-taken and read endocervical curettage
> Multiple punch biopsies

With the publication of over 150 cases of invasive cancer of the cervix developing after cryotherapy or laser, and with the anecdotal reports of patients with invasive cancer of the vulva who had been treated inappropriately by CO_2 laser ablation, it is clear that, although conservative treatment modalities for CIN are largely effective and associated with minimal complications and side effects, the triage of patients presenting with an HPV-related lesion can occasionally result in errors of classification. The principal triage goal of colposcopic evaluation is to distinguish those patients who have no lesion from those who have a precursor which can be treated on an outpatient basis, and those who have invasive cancer who must be treated appropriately. This triage largely rests upon the ability of the colposcopist to identify those lesions most likely to harbor invasive cancer and to obtain appropriate biopsies (and in the case of the cervix, an endocervical curettage) to rule in or out the presence of invasion. It is clear that the vast majority of patients are appropriately triaged and receive appropriate care. It is also clear, however, that a very small, but important, number of patients who are thought to have a cancer precursor have invasion, and that an ablative, outpatient approach to the management of these lesions will be inappropriate and will result in substantial morbidity and, sometimes, even in death.

There are a number of possible reasons for the failure to detect invasive cancers in some patients (Table 13.13). It is evident from recent studies that some patients with invasive cancer, particularly microinvasion, will have lesions in which the characteristic "atypical vessels" fail to reach the surface and cannot be detected even by the most highly skilled colposcopist. It is probably also true that some colposcopists fail to recognize the atypical vessels associated with invasive cancer at the time of colposcopy.[39] In a recent study of 196 large

Table 13.13

Reasons for Missing Invasive Cancers

Atypical vessels don't reach surface
Disease in canal and not detected
Colposcopist fails to recognize diagnostic changes
Biopsy taken at incorrect site
Endocervical curettage not performed

excisional conization specimens obtained from patients who had CIN lesions that were considered to fulfill the criteria for conservative management, McIndoe et al. detected two microinvasive carcinomas and one adenocarcinoma-in situ lesion that had been missed during triage.[30] Another worrisome finding in this study was that 16 patients had a 2 to 3 grade more severe intraepithelial lesion diagnosed on the excisional biopsy specimen than on the colposcopically-directed biopsy (Table 13.14).[30]

Table 13.14

Accuracy of Colposcopically-Directed Biopsies

Change in diagnosis	%
To microinvasion	1%
To adenocarcinoma-*in situ*	0.5%
To a 2 to 3 grade more severe lesion	8%

For most private practitioners, seeing an invasive cancer is a rare event. Only about 13,000 invasive squamous cell carcinomas of the cervix were diagnosed in the U.S. in 1990 and the average gynecologist will see less than one cancer each year.[40] This means that most colposcopists don't have much experience in recognizing invasive cancers and, in at least one large series, the majority of invasive cancers missed colposcopically were missed by clinicians with less than 3 years of experience performing colposcopy. Although missing invasive cancer during the triage procedure of colposcopy, biopsy, and endocervical curettage is generally considered a "diagnostic error", it is likely that, in some cases, the biology of the lesion is more responsible for the inaccurate diagnosis than is a lapse in procedure. Nonetheless, the end result is the same—a patient may be treated as having a cancer precursor when she, in fact, has cancer.

FAILURE TO DIAGNOSE ADENOCARCINOMAS OF THE CERVIX

Another area of concern with regards to our ability to diagnose cancers colposcopically is adenocarcinomas of the endocervix. This lesion, which was relatively uncommon at the time colposcopic triage rules were first formulated, is now being seen more frequently. The reasons for this apparent increase in adenocarcinomas are complex and probably include an increased recognition of the lesion on the part of pathologists and the fact that squamous cell cancer precursors are easily detected cytologically, but glandular precursors are more difficult. Therefore, cytologic screening programs designed to detect cervical cancer precursors may have had a proportionally greater effect in reducing the incidence of squamous compared to glandular carcinomas. Whatever the cause, this apparent increase is problematic, since it is clear from a number of published case reports and anecdotal stories that adenocarcinoma-*in situ* and early endocervical adenocarcinoma looks like normal endocervix colposcopically. In addition, these lesions can occasionally be found deep in the canal at sites that may not be observable with the colposcope and they often coexist with CIN lesions.

Table 13.15

Endocervical Glandular Neoplasia

Difficult to detect cytologically

Adenocarcinoma-*in situ* looks like normal endocervix colposcopically

May be found deep in canal

May coexist with CIN

LOOP EXCISIONAL PROCEDURES

SHALLOW LASER EXCISIONAL CONIZATIONS

Because of the increasing recognition that triage errors may occur and that adenocarcinomas-*in situ*, or early endocervical adenocarcinomas may not be detectable by colposcopy, a growing number of investigators have recommended that precursor lesions not be treated by ablative methods, but by excisional methods instead. This has lead some advocates of CO_2 laser treatment protocols to recommend the routine use of shallow laser conization rather than laser ablation for treating all CIN lesions.[28-30] The proponents of the routine use of shallow laser cones argue that the results will be the same as with laser ablations, but that invasive cancers should not be missed because all the tissue will be available for pathological diagnosis.

When properly executed, shallow laser excisional conizations provide an adequate pathological specimen and have a complication rate that is not significantly greater than that of laser ablations. The problem with the general recommendation that laser cones be used for the management of CIN rather than laser ablation is that it is technically much more difficult to perform a laser cone than an ablation. Therefore, in actual practice, the tissue specimens produced for pathologic analysis using shallow laser excisional cones are often of such poor quality that they are not useful. In a histopathologic review of 77 laser conization specimens, Howell *et al.* found that laser excisional conization specimens frequently had extensive thermal coagulation artifact, epithelial denudation and so much charring and distortion that the pathologist could not interpret the margins (Table 13.16).[41] In our experience, the laser cone is more difficult to perform than cryosurgery or laser ablasion, and requires a

Table 13.16

Histology of Laser Cones

Laser Artifact	% of Cases
Negative for CIN	39%
Extensive epithelial denudation	36%
Extensive coagulation artifact	13%
Unreadable margins	14%

continuing case load in order to gain the requisite skills and to maintain them (Table 13.17).

A major drawback to the CO_2 laser is its high cost. Not only is the initial purchase price high, but maintenance costs are also high and this frequently limits its use to laser suites or surgicenters (Table 13.18).

The CO_2 laser continues to play a role in treating HPV-related lesions of the lower genital tract, but its role is limited principally to the treatment of some of the flat white lesions of the external genitalia which are better managed by ablation than excision. Under these circumstances, however, it is of critical importance that the lesions be biopsied adequately to rule out invasive cancer before laser ablation is undertaken.

Table 13.17

Problems with CO_2 Laser Conization

Difficult to teach and learn

Requires large experience to become and stay skilled

Good manual skills required

Excisional tissues may be so damaged that ablation occurs when intent is to excise.

Table 13.18

Cost Considerations of Therapies for CIN

	Cryotherapy	CO_2 Laser	Loop Excision
Equipment	$1,200	$35,000 up	$4,000
Maintenance	Low	High	Low
Disposables	Low	High	High
Venue	Office	Laser suite	Office
Skill level	Low	High	Low

Despite the excellent results that can be achieved with this technique by some practitioners, many clinicians in private practice do not have a sufficient number of patients with abnormal smears flowing through their practices to be able to generate the case load that is required to become a highly skilled laser surgeon. In addition, many practices cannot afford the relatively expensive laser instrumentation and rely instead on cryotherapy as the principal, office-based treatment modality for CIN. This has lead to a dichotomy between the recommendations made by the clinicians based in tertiary care centers who publish in medical journals and teach colposcopy courses, and the practicality of applying those recommendations in private practices.

ADVANTAGES OF LOOP ELECTROSURGICAL EXCISION TECHNIQUES FOR TREATING CIN

The application of electrosurgical principles and techniques to the diagnosis and treatment of HPV-related lesions in the male and female lower anogenital tract eliminates most of the problems associated with CO_2 laser conization, CO_2 laser ablation, and cryotherapeutic ablation (Table 13.19). Particularly for the cervix, loop excision of CIN can readily be taught, can readily be learned, and can readily be applied by the practicing gynecologist even when he or she sees only a relatively small number of patients with abnormal smears. The principal advantage of electrosurgical loop or needle excision procedures is that they provide a pathologic back-up to the

Table 13.19

Comparison of Therapies for CIN

	Cryotherapy	CO_2 Laser	Loop Excision
Discharge	Large	Mild	Mild
Tissue Specimen	No	If conization	Yes
Recessed SCJ	Frequent	Uncommon	Uncommon
Large Lesions	No	Yes	Yes
Skill Level	Low	High	Low

colposcopist's diagnostic impressions. Although good training in colposcopy and the acquisition of diagnostic colposcopy skills remain a prerequisite for managing patients with CIN electrosurgically, should a colposcopist fail to make the distinction between the atypical vessels seen in invasive cancer and the atypical transformation zone associated with CIN, it is still unlikely that invasive cancer will be missed, because the entire abnormal transformation zone or, in the case of flat lesions of the external genitalia, the entire area of abnormal epithelium, will be removed and available for histological examination. This simple fact is sufficient to recommend these procedures as the principal diagnostic and therapeutic modality for all HPV-related cervical lesions and for a significant proportion of HPV-related lesions of the vagina and external genitalia as well.

ARGUMENTS AGAINST THE ROUTINE USE OF THE LOOP EXCISION PROCEDURE

The major argument that has been raised against the routine use of the loop procedure for treating all cases of CIN is that it removes larger amounts of tissue than do alternative procedures and that significant morbidity and long term sequelae might, therefore, occur. For the cervix, we strongly recommend using as the "standard loop" a fine tungsten loop electrode which measures 1.5 to 2 cms across the base and no more than 8 mm in depth. This type of loop makes it difficult to remove inadvertently too much tissue from the cervix and to produce significant damage. This style loop electrode can be used to treat more than 90% of the lesions which are seen in clinical practice, and will generally allow removal of the lesions with a single pass. If additional tissue needs to be

Table 13.20

Arguments Against Loop Excisions
Removes too much tissue
Will encourage over-treatment

removed because of residual glands, or to complete the excision of the entire transformation zone after the initial pass has been made, the tissue can be removed by additional judicious passes with the electrode without compromising the integrity of the cervix. When very large loops, such as the 2.5 x 2.5 cm loops (which have been illustrated in the original articles on loop excision) are used, it is possible to remove so much cervical tissue that the cervix virtually disappears. We strongly recommend that such large loops not be used except in exceptional circumstances.

Provided proper loop selection is used, the amount of tissue which is removed during the loop procedure is no greater than that which is destroyed during either cryotherapy or CO_2 laser ablation, or removed during shallow CO_2 laser conization. The fact that the amount of tissue removed and the way that it is removed using either the loop electrode or a CO_2 laser is virtually identical should allow extrapolation of long-term clinical outcomes obtained using the CO_2 laser to cervical loop procedures. A recent brief report by

Table 13.21

Pregnancy After Cervical Loop Excision

Outcome	No.
1st trimester miscarriage	3
2nd trimester miscarriage	2
Delivery 28-36 weeks	2
Delivery >36 weeks	37
Total # of pregnancies	**44**

Bigrigg *et al* on the effects of cervical loop excision procedures on pregnancy outcome suggests that this is indeed the case since no adverse effects on number of miscarriages, birth weight, or length of labour were detected (Table 13.21).[42] Similarly, for the electrosurgical treatment of external lesions, the data from CO_2 laser ablation should be directly relevant and the results of loop treatment should be similar to those published for CO_2 laser ablation.

Another argument that has been raised against the loop procedure is that it is so easy to perform that it will encourage the over-treatment of patients with low-grade CIN lesions whose lesions may regress spontaneously and who may not need further treatment. In assessing whether low-grade CIN lesions should be treated, it is important to note that 30% of such lesions contain "high oncogenic risk" HPV types, i.e., HPV types 16, 18, 33, 45, 56.[43,44] Although the majority of the types which produce low-grade CIN lesions are of "low oncogenic risk" or "novel types" (i.e., types that have not yet been characterized) those which contain "high oncogenic risk" types are cytologically and histologically indistinguishable from the others.[45] It is also important to note that up to 20% of patients with a low-grade CIN lesion are found to harbor more than one viral type when sensitive detection methods are used to evaluate the lesions.[44]

Since it is virtually impossible to distinguish histopathologically between the low-grade CIN lesions that contain "high oncogenic risk" HPV types from those containing other HPV types, in our opinion, all low-grade CIN lesions should be treated. It must be emphasized, however, that our therapeutic approach requires that the pathologist or cytopathologist utilize strict criteria for diagnosing low-grade CIN (or low-grade SIL) and not indiscriminately diagnose reparative or atypical metaplastic processes as being CIN (or SIL).

One argument against treating all low-grade precursors is that it is fruitless to attempt to treat HPV-related lesions because it may be difficult to eradicate the virus. It is now clear that this argument has little clinical validity. In latently infected cells (as discussed in Chapter 6), no clinical or histopathological effects are noted. Unless a change in the relationship between the virus and the host occurs, there is no evidence that these latent infections have deleterious effects, since a productive infection must intervene between latency and the development of neoplasia. As all productive infections will be accompanied by a cytopathogenic effect which will generally be accompanied by colposcopically-visible lesions, a patient who is colposcopically and cytologically negative over repeated examinations may, for practical purposes, be considered not to be infected, not to be infectious, and not be at proximate risk for developing neoplasia. The important point to remember is that we treat lesions and not viruses. We treat only lesions, we do not treat HPV infections.

If the colposcopic lesions are eradicated and no cytopathogenic effect persists, the patient can be regarded as a cure. This has been substantiated by the results of a long term, multicenter follow-up study of more than 2,800 women who had been treated with cryosurgery (Table 13.22) involving more than 40,000 patient years of follow-up.[46] Once colposcopic lesions have been eradicated, women who had CIN are at no greater risk of developing CIN than the general population.[46]

Table 13.22

Long-term Follow-up of Women After Cryosurgery

2,839 patients treated with cryosurgery and followed for at least 1 year after 3 consecutive negative smears.

Risk of developing a new CIN was 1 in 200 over a 14 year period.

Risk of redeveloping CIN is that of the general population.

LOOP EXCISIONAL PROCEDURES

"SEE AND TREAT"

One of the advantages of an excisional rather than an ablative approach that has been stressed throughout this book is that it allows selected patients to undergo both diagnosis and treatment in a single sitting. This approach, which has been labeled "See and Treat" by Luesley and co-workers in the United Kingdom, has a number of potential advantages over the conventional triage procedure for patients with abnormal Pap smears.[47]

Conventional triage protocols require that patients with an abnormal smear be evaluated colposcopically at their first visit, at which time cervical biopsies and an endocervical curettage are obtained. The patient is then sent home and the biopsy samples are sent to the pathology laboratory. After a delay of approximately 1 week, the pathology results become available. Provided the entire lesion was colposcopically visible, there was a reasonable agreement between the cytology, biopsy and colposcopic results and invasion was not identified or suspected, the patient is scheduled for another visit at which time conservative treatment would be performed.

Although this approach has been highly successful in reducing cervical cancer, there are several disadvantages to it that are overcome with the "See and Treat" protocol (Table 13.22). The first is that the delay between taking the cervical biopsy and informing the patient of her actual diagnosis can be a period of considerable anxiety for many patients. Not only was the patient initially told that she had an abnormal Pap smear and then had to wait several days to weeks to have colposcopy, but at the colposcopy visit she was told that an abnormal area was present on her cervix and that a biopsy was required "to absolutely rule out the presence of cancer". Understandably, patients often find this to be an emotionally upsetting experience.

Another consideration both to the community and to the patient is that the patient has a sexually transmitted disease and should consider herself to be potentially infectious to her sexual partners until definitive treatment is performed. This provides a potential risk to the community as a whole and may also be a source of concern to the patient.

A third problem with the conventional triage approach is that the patient and the clinician must schedule two office visits for the triage and treatment to be completed. As more women enter the work force and must leave work in order to attend the gynecologist's office and with increasing pressure on the clinician to reduce the costs of health care, this has also become an important consideration.

In the United Kingdom "See and Treat" has been used at some colposcopy centers for several years and the results reported from these centers

CLINICAL IMPLICATIONS OF ELECTROSURGICAL EXCISION PROCEDURES

Table 13.23

Advantages of "See and Treat"

Reduces patient anxiety by eliminating wait between biopsy and treatment.

Eliminates an office visit.

Reduces potential for transmission of sexually transmitted disease.

---

have been encouraging. In the recent report of Luesley *et al.* 65% of the patients with CIN attending their clinic were managed with this approach at a single visit[48] and in a study by Bigrigg *et al.*[49] 90% of 1,000 women with abnormal smears were diagnosed and treated at their first visit. In the United Kingdom, where there is an emphasis on reducing the costs of health care and where considerable delays can occur in obtaining a colposcopy appointment, "See and Treat" has been considered a success.

However, careful analysis of the results obtained in the United Kingdom with "See and Treat" suggest that modifications may be required before this protocol will be widely accepted in the United States. "HPV effects", or atypia with koilocytosis, are terms often used indiscriminately by pathologists to refer to minor histopathologic changes such as perinuclear halos in the absence of nuclear atypia (see Chapter 6). These changes are not considered sufficient to warrant treatment in some centers in the United States. In the Luesley series, 22% of patients treated with "See and Treat" had this diagnosis (Table 13.24).[47] Therefore, up to 25% of the women treated in the United Kingdom using "See and Treat" protocols probably would not have received treatment in some centers in the United States using conventional triage protocols. It is unlikely that this apparent over-treatment would actually cause harm to patients. In fact, it may be beneficial since elimination of the transformation zone should place the patient at very low risk for subsequently developing cervical cancer. However, in the United States, it seems unlikely that a 25% over-treatment rate will be considered acceptable by most clinicians. The key is to be certain that the cytologist/pathologist uses the appropriate criteria to ensure that only "real" HPV-related lesions are diagnosed as abnormal.

Table 13.24

Histologic Diagnosis of "See and Treat" Specimens

Histological Diagnosis	% of cases
No lesion identified	5%
Atypical with koilocytosis	22%
CIN	71%
Squamous cell carcinoma	0.7%
Adenocarcinoma *in situ*	1%

A key difference between "See and Treat" and biopsy-based triage protocols is that with "See and Treat" the Pap smear becomes a test which relegates the patient to a treatment path rather than playing its traditional role as a screening test. Cervical cytology is well accepted to be effective for detecting patients at high risk for developing cervical cancer but is not very useful as a diagnostic test. There are two reasons for this. One is that some patients' lesions are underclassified by cytology. In underclassifications, patients with low grade SIL or with atypical cells suggestive but not diagnostic of SIL on cytology, have high grade CIN, or even invasive cancer, detected on colposcopy and cervical biopsy. Cases that are underclassified by cytology do not present a problem for "See and Treat" since the cervix contains disease. It is the converse misclassification which causes problems for patients managed with "See and Treat". These are women who are diagnosed as having cervical disease on cytology, but in whom a cervical lesion is not detected on colposcopy and cervical biopsy. Such patients are a problem with "See and Treat" protocols since, after loop excision, no CIN will be detected in the excised specimen. As originally practiced in the 1960s and 1970s, cervical cytology was a highly specific test, (i.e., when a smear was diagnosed as being abnormal there was a high probability that the patient had disease). Unfortunately, over the last 5 years cytologists are increasingly diagnosing smears with even very minor degrees of atypia as being abnormal. This problem appears to have been aggravated by the recent introduction of the Bethesda System for classifying Pap smears, since Bethesda specifically allows smears with "HPV-related changes" to be diagnosed as having low-grade SIL.[50] Despite the fact that the grouping of CIN 1 with HPV-related changes is based on well established virologic data, in practice, this grouping appears to be causing a marked increase in the number of patients cytologically diagnosed as having SIL since many cytologists over-diagnose HPV-related changes. Although this is a problem of educating the cytologist rather than an inherent problem of the Bethesda System terminology, the implications for "See and Treat" are enormous since many people who lack histopathologic/colposcopic cervical disease are being given the diagnosis of low-grade SIL.

Because of the above considerations, if "See and Treat" is to work in the United States, it is mandatory that the colposcopists be skilled enough to determine which patients with abnormal smears actually have a clinically significant lesion and which do not.

For those patients with abnormal smears (low-grade or high-grade SIL) with easily recognizable CIN at colposcopy "See and Treat" is an acceptable and useful approach. However, in patients with a low-grade SIL on cytology who lack a clear-cut CIN lesion, the best approach, in our opinion, is to biopsy possible lesions and await the results of the biopsy before proceeding with loop excisional treatment. Using this balanced approach, the clinician and patients will gain the advantages of "See and Treat" while avoiding the pitfalls of over-treatment.

We strongly recommend that only clear-cut CIN lesions be treated using the "See and Treat" approach. In women with an abnormal smear and colposcopically equivocal lesions, we recommend initial triage with a directed cervical biopsy prior to electrosurgery.

IMPLICATIONS OF THE LOOP EXCISION PROCEDURE FOR DEVELOPING COUNTRIES

There is one final important clinical implication of the loop excision procedure. Although the electrosurgical excision procedures have been used principally in Western Europe and North America, they have the potential for making a much greater impact in the less-developed countries where treatment modalities for cervical precursors have generally been unavailable. In Western countries, cytology screening is widely available and there has been a dramatic reduction in the incidence of invasive cancer of the cervix and deaths from cervical cancer over the past 25 years. The decrease in the cervical cancer death rate has largely been due to the ability of cytology to detect precursor lesions, the ability of the colposcopist to identify them, and the ability of the clinician to eradicate the precursor lesions and prevent the subsequent development of cervical cancer. In contrast, in most of the developing world, cytology is generally unavailable, clinicians are frequently not trained in colposcopy and diagnostic and therapeutic procedures for eradicating the cancer precursors are not available to the vast majority of the population. As a consequence, in much of the developing world cervical cancer is the leading or second leading cause of death from cancer among women. In some countries, as many as 5% of adult female deaths are attributable to cancer of the cervix. Although screening for anogenital tract neoplasia remains a technical problem for the less-developed countries, electrosurgical excisional and treatment procedures should substantially increase the ability of clinicians to diagnose and inexpensively treat the patients once high-grade precursor lesions have been identified. Because the equipment is relatively inexpensive, because the procedure is easy to learn, and because it is associated with such a low rate of side effects and complications, it is ideally suited for the settings found in so many less-developed countries and for the general lack of medical skills found in many of their health care systems. These procedures deserve to be evaluated in such settings and to become a part of the armamentarium of care which is desperately needed.

REFERENCES

1. Luesley, D.M., McCrum, A., Terry, P.B., et al. Complications of cone biopsy related to the dimensions of the cone and the influence of prior colposcopic assessment. *Br. J. Obstet. Gynecol.* 92:158-164, 1985.
2. Bushnell, L.F. Prevention of complications in cervical conization. *Am. J. Obstet. Gynecol.* 22:190-198, 1963.
3. Holdt, D.G., Jacobs, A.J., Scott, J.C. and Adam, G.M. Diagnostic significance and sequelae of cone biopsy. *Am. J. Obstet. Gynecol.* 143:312-315, 1982.
4. Larsson, G., Gullberg, B. and Grundsell, H. A comparison of complications of laser and cold knife conization. *Obstet. Gynecol.* 62:213-217, 1983.
5. Nasiell, K., Roger, V. and Nasiell, M. Behavior of mild cervical dysplasia during long-term follow-up. *Obstet. Gynecol.* 67:665-669, 1986.
6. Richart, R.M. and Barron, B.A. A follow-up study of patients with cervical dysplasia. *Am. J. Obstet. Gynecol.* 105:386-393, 1969.
7. Koss, L.G., Stewart, F.W., Foote, F.W., et al. Some histological aspects of behavior of epidermoid carcinoma in situ and related lesions of the uterine cervix. *Cancer* 16:1160-1211, 1963.
8. Hall, J.E. and Walton, L. Dysplasia of the cervix: a prospective study of 206 cases. *Am. J. Obstet. Gynecol.* 100:662-671, 1968.
9. Kottmeier, H.L. Evolution et traitement des epitheliomas. *Revue Francaise de Gynecol et d'Obstetrique* 56:821-826, 1961.
10. Kolstad, P. and Klem, V. Long-term follow-up of 1121 cases of carcinoma-*in situ*. *Obstet. Gynecol.* 48:125-129, 1975.
11. Burghardt, E. and Holzer, E. Treatment of carcinoma-*in situ*: Evaluation of 1609 cases. *Obstet. Gynecol.* 55:539-545, 1980.
12. Creasman, W.T. and Rutledge, F. Carcinoma-*in situ* of the cervix. *Obstet. Gynecol.* 39:373-380, 1972.
13. Richart, R.M. Natural history of cervical intraepithelial neoplasia. *Clin. Obstet. Gynecol.* 10:748-784, 1967.

14. Richart, R.M. Cervical intraepithelial neoplaia: A review. *Pathology Annual.* Somers, ed. Appleton-Century-Crofts, East Norwalk, CT, pp. 301, 1973.
15. Richart, R.M. and Townsend, D.E. Outpatient therapy of cervical intraepithelial neoplasia with cryotherapy or CO_2 laser. In H.J. Osofsky, ed. *Advances in Clincial Obstetrics and Gynecology.* Williams and Wilkins, Baltimore. pp. 235-246, 1982.
16. Richart, R.M., Crum, C.P. and Townsend, D.E. Workup of the patient with an abnormal Papanicolaou smear. *Gynecol Oncol.* 12:S265-S276, 1981.
17. Younge, P.A., Hertig, A.T. and Armstrong, D. A study of 135 cases of carcinoma-*in situ* of the cervix at the Free Hospital for women. *Am. J. Obstet. Gynecol.* 58:867-895, 1949.
18. Richart, R.M. and Sciarra, J.J. Treatment of cervical dysplasia by outpatient electrocauterization. *Am. J. Obstet. Gynecol.* 101:200-205, 1968.
19. Crisp, W.E., Asadourian, L. and Romberger, W. Application of cryosurgery to gynecolgic malignancy. *Obstet Gynecol.* 30:668-673, 1967.
20. Ostergard, D.R. Cryosurgical treatment of cervical intraepithelial neoplasia. *Obstet. Gynecol.* 56:231-233, 1980.
21. Townsend, D.E. Cryosurgery for CIN. *Obstet. Gynecol. Surv.* 34:828, 1979.
22. Ferenczy, A. Comparison of cryo- and carbon dioxide laser therapy for cervical intraepithelial neoplasia. *Obstet. Gynecol.* 66:793-798, 1985.
23. Townsend, D.E. and Richart, R.M. Cryotherapy and carbon dioxide laser management of cervical intraepithelial neoplasia: A controlled comparison. *Obstet. Gynecol.* 61:75-78, 1983.
24. Creasman, W.T., Hinshaw, W.M. and Clarke-Pearson, D.L. Cryosurgery in the managment of cervical intraepithelial neoplasia. *Obstet. Gynecol.* 63:145-149, 1984.
25. Wetchler, S.J. Treatment of cervical intraepithelial neoplasia with the CO_2 laser: Laser versus cryotherapy. A review of effectiveness and cost. *Obstet. Gynecol. Surv.* 39(8):469-473, 1984.
26. Stafl, A., Wilkinson, E.J. and Mattingly, R.F. Laser treatment of cervical and vaginal neoplasia. *Am. J. Obstet. Gynecol.* 128:128-136, 1977.
27. Bellina, J.H. and Seto, Y.J. Pathological and physical investigations into CO_2 laser-tissue interactions with specific emphasis on cervical intraepithelial neoplasia. *Lasers in Surgery and Medicine* 1:47-69, 1980.
28. Partington, C.K., Turner, M.J., Soutter, W.P., *et al.* Laser vaporization versus laser excision conization in the treatment of cervical intraepithelial neoplasia. *Obstet. Gynecol.* 73:775-778, 1989.
29. Baggish, M.S. A comparison between laser excisional conization and laser vaporization for the treatment of cervical intraepithelial neoplasia. *Am. J. Obstet. Gynecol.* 155:39-44, 1986.
30. McIndoe, G.-A., Robson, M.S., Tidy, J.A., *et al.* Laser excision rather than vaporization: The treatment of choice for cervical intraepithelial neoplasia. *Obstet. Gynecol.* 74:165-168, 1989.
31. Baggish, M.S. The ghosts of lasers past, present, future: A synopsis of the CO_2 laser in gynecology. *Lasers in Surgery and Medicine* 4:135-138, 1984.
32. Fahmy, K., Sammour, M.B., Lamki, H., *et al.* Healing of the cervix after laser treatment. *Colposcopy & Gynecologic Laser Surgery.* 4(1):29-35, 1988.
33. MacLean, A.B. Healing of cervical epithelium after laser treatment of cervical intraepithelial neoplasia. *Br. J. Obstet. Gynecol.* 91:697-706, 1984.
34. Sevin, B.-U., Ford, J.H., Girtanner, R.D., *et al.* Invasive cancer of the cervix after cryosurgery. Pitfalls of conservative management. *Obstet. Gynecol.* 53:465-471, 1979.
35. Townsend, D.E., Richart, R.M., Marks, E. and Nielsen, J. Invasive cancer following outpatient evaluation and therapy for cervical disease. *Obstet. Gynecol.* 57:145-149, 1981.

36. Townsend, D.E. and Richart, R.M. Diagnostic errors in colposcopy. *Gynecol. Oncol.* 12:S259-S264, 1981.
37. Ferenczy, A. Management of the patient with an abnormal Pap smear. In *Gynecologic Oncology. Controversies in Cancer Treatment.* S.C. Ballon, ed. GK. Hall Medical Publishers, Boston, 1982
38. Pearson, S.E., Whittaker, J., Ireland, D. and Monaghan, J.M. Invasive cancer of the cervix after laser treatment. *Br. J. Obstet. Gynecol.* 96:486-488, 1989.
39. Benedet, J.L., Anderson, G.H. and Boyes, D.A. Colposcopic accuracy in the diagnosis of microinvasive and occult invasive carcinoma of the cervix. *Obstet. Gynecol.* 65:557-562, 1985.
40. American Cancer Society. *Cancer Facts and Figures-1990.* American Cancer Society, 1990
41. Howell, R., Hammond, R. and Pryse-Davies, J. The histologic reliability of laser cone biopsy of the cervix. *Obstet. Gynecol.* 77:905-911, 1991.
42. Bigrigg, M.A., Codling, B.W., Pearson, P., *et al.* Pregnancy after cervical loop diathermy. *Lancet.* 337:119, 1991.
43. Lorincz, A.T., Reid, R., Jenson, A.B., *et al.* Human papillomavirus infection of the cervix: Relative risk associations of 15 common anogenital types. *Am. J. Obstet. Gyn.,* in press, 1992.
44. Lungu, O., Sun, W.X., Felix, J., *et al.* Restriction of human papillomavirus types in high-grade cervical intraepithelial neoplasia: A polymerase chain reaction analysis. Submitted, 1991.
45. Willet, G.D., Kurman, R.J. and Reid, R. Correlation of the histological appearance of intraepithelial neoplasia of the cervix with human papillomavirus types. *Int. J. Gynecol. Pathol.* 8:18-25, 1989.
46. Richart, R.M., Townsend, D.E., Crisp, W., *et al.* An analysis of "long-term" follow-up results in patients with cervical intraepithelial neoplasia treated by cryotherapy. *Am. J. Obstet. Gynecol.* 137:823-826, 1980.
47. Luesley, D.M., Cullimore, J., Redman, C.W.E., *et al.* Loop diathermy excision of the cevical transformation zone in patients with abnormal cervical smears. *B.M.J.* 300:1690-1693, 1990.
48. Luesley, D.M., McCrum, A., Terry, P.B., *et al.* Complications of cone biopsy related to the dimensions of the cone and the influence of prior colposcopic assessment. *Br. J. Obstet. Gynecol.* 92:158-164, 1985.
49. Bigrigg, M.A., Codling, B.W., Pearson, P., *et al.* Colposcopic diagnosis and treatment of cervical dysplasia at a single clinic visit: Experience of low-voltage diathermy loop in 1000 patients. *Lancet* 336:229-231, 1990.
50. National Cancer Institute Workshop. The 1988 Bethesda system for reporting cervical/vaginal cytologic diagnoses. *J.A.M.A.* 262:931-934, 1989.